Hypothalamus- Pituitary
Ovaries
Testicles

Endocrinology 360
A trilogy for the study of Endocrinology

Volume III.

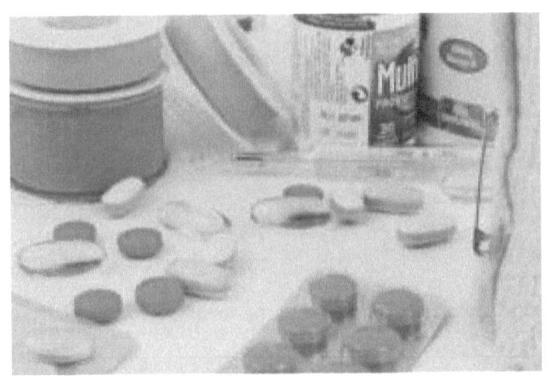

Dr. Mario Vega Carbó
Endocrinologist

Edition 2021

To my parents, Lucia and Nicolás, my brothers Angela, Nicolás and Manuel, my children Luiba, Fidel, Mario and Rocío, my grandchildren Richard and Andy.

To my two great friends from the "Vladimir I. Lenin" Pre-University Institute of Exact Sciences in Havana, they influenced as much as my parents, in my ethical and humanist training: José Raúl Lorenzo Sánchez, today a great philatelist, teacher and cyberneticist, and Benito Andrés Saínz González eminent professor and cardiologist.

To doctors José Fernández Sotolongo, gastroenterologist, and Carlos Valmañto Sánchez, a microbiologist, both excellent specialists and researchers, with whom I shared all the medical training at the "Salvador Allende" Hospital in Havana.

To my formal tutor Silvia Marín, an expert pediatrician in nutrition, and my informal tutor Maite Cabrera, an endocrinologist and an expert in reproductive biology, who gave me all of their experiences during my stay at the Endocrinology institute .

My greatest gratitude, to each professional who feels served with this text

Content

Presentation 1394
Introduction 1398
Part VII. Hypothalamus- Pituitary... 1401
   Chapter 252. Pineal Gland, Hypothalamus, and Pituitary . 1402
   Chapter 253. Neuroendocrinology 1410
   Chapter 254. Oxytocin 1413
   Chapter 255. Melatonin, Serotonin, Dopamine 1416
   Chapter 256. Pineal Tumors.. 1421
   Chapter 257. Endocrine - Hypothalamic Syndromes......... 1425
   Chapter 258. Pictures of the Sellar Region 1428
   Chapter 259. Pituitary Incidentaloma 1433
   Chapter 260. Hypothalamic Pituitary Dysfunction............ 1437
   Chapter 261. Polydipsic Polyuric Syndrome 1440
   Chapter 262. Central Diabetes Insipidus............................ 1445
   Chapter 263. Nephrogenic Diabetes Insipidus................... 1451
   Chapter 264. Primary Polydipsia 1455
   Chapter 265. Syndrome of Inappropriate ADH Secretion . 1458
   Chapter 266. Short Stature 1463
   Chapter 267. GH Deficiency in the Child.......................... 1469
   Chapter 268. GH Deficiency in the Adult.......................... 1474
   Chapter 269. Secondary Adrenal Insufficiency 1479
   Chapter 270. Secondary Hypothyroidism 1483

Chapter 271. Secondary Hypogonadism.................................. 1488

Chapter 272. Panhypopituitarism.. 1493

Chapter 273. Sheehan Syndrome 1499

Chapter 274. Craniopharyngioma 1503

Chapter 275. Non-functioning Pituitary Tumor................... 1507

Chapter 276. Galactorrheas.. 1511

Chapter 277. Hyperprolactinemia 1515

Chapter 278. Hyperprolactinemia and Pregnancy 1520

Chapter 279. Prolactinomas 1523

Chapter 280. Prolactinoma and Pregnancy 1528

Chapter 281. Thyrotropinomas 1531

Chapter 282. Gonadotropic Adenomas 1536

Chapter 283. Cushing's Disease 1539

Chapter 284. Nelson Syndrome 1543

Chapter 285. Acromegaly 1547

Chapter 286. Tall Stature 1552

Chapter 287. Pituitary Metastasis 1556

Chapter 288. Pediatric Pituitary Tumor 1559

Chapter 289. Pituitary Tumor and Pregnancy.................... 1563

Chapter 290. Cysts of Rathke's Bursa................................ 1567

Chapter 291. Pituitary Granulomas..................................... 1570

Chapter 292. Sellar Arachnoidocele 1574

Chapter 293. Pituitary Apoplexy 1578

Chapter 294. Hypophysitis.. 1583

Chapter 295. Surgery of the Pituitary 1587

Chapter 296. Radio and Pituitary Chemotherapy 1591

Part VIII. Gonadal Conditions.. 1594

Chapter 297. Endocrinologic Gynecology.......................... 1595

Chapter 298. The Ovaries 1598

Chapter 299. Disorder of Sex Development 1602

Chapter 300. Normal Puberty 1610

Chapter 301. Precocious Thelarchy 1614

Chapter 302. Precocious Adrenarche 1617

Chapter 303. Pubertal Gynecomastia 1621

Chapter 304. Precocious Puberty 1625

Chapter 305. Delayed Puberty 1632

Chapter 306. Turner Syndrome 1638

Chapter 307. Primary Amenorrhea 1644

Chapter 308. Oligomenorrhea and Secondary Amenorrhea
.... 1648

Chapter 309. Premenstrual Syndrome 1653

Chapter 310. Dysfunctional Uterine Bleeding 1658

Chapter 311. Polycystic Ovarian Syndrome 1664

Chapter 312. Adolescents with Polycystic Ovaries 1670

Chapter 313. Hydroxyprogesterone 1674

Chapter 314. Hyperandrogenism 1678

Chapter 315. Hyperhidrosis 1683

Chapter 316. Hirsutism 1688

Chapter 317. Acne 1692

Chapter 318. Androgenic Alopecia 1697

Chapter 319. Clitoromegaly 1701

Chapter 320. SHBG 1705

Chapter 321. Antiandrogens 1708

Chapter 322. Hormonal Contraception 1712

Chapter 323. Female Infertility 1718

Chapter 324. Ovarian and Antimullerian Reserve 1724

Chapter 325. Anovulation 1727
Chapter 326. Inducers of Ovulation 1732
Chapter 327. Endometriosis 1736
Chapter 328. Recurring Abortions 1741
Chapter 329. Artificial Insemination 1745
Chapter 330. In Vitro Fertilization...................................... 1749
Chapter 331. Pregnancy Hormonal Adjustments 1753
Chapter 332. Female Sexual Dysfunction........................... 1758
Chapter 333. Fibrocystic Condition of the Breast.............. 1764
Chapter 334. Functional Tumors of the Ovaries 1769
Chapter 335. Climacteric Syndrome 1775
Chapter 336. Premature Ovarian Failure 1778
Chapter 337. Female Hormone Replacement 1782
Chapter 338. Transgender Teen 1786
Chapter 339. Transgender Woman 1790
Chapter 340. Transgender Man... 1793
Chapter 341. Andrology... 1796
Chapter 342. The Testicles... 1799
Chapter 343. Anabolic Steroids 1804
Chapter 344. Ambiguous Genitalia..................................... 1809
Chapter 345. Prepubertal Male Hypogonadism 1813
Chapter 346. Micropenis... 1817
Chapter 347. Cryptorchidism.. 1821
Chapter 348. Kallmann Syndrome...................................... 1827
Chapter 349. Klinefelter Syndrome 1831
Chapter 350. Noonan Syndrome... 1835
Chapter 351. Functional Testicular Tumors....................... 1839
Chapter 352. Male Infertility 1845

Chapter 353. Spermatogram 1851
Chapter 354. Oligospermia 1855
Chapter 355. Erectile Dysfunction 1860
Chapter 356. Orchiectomy 1865
Chapter 357. Chemical Castration 1868
Chapter 358. Adult Gynecomastia 1871
Chapter 359. Andropause 1876
Chapter 360. Male Hormone Replacement 1880
Key Topics in Endocrinology 1885
   I. Suspicious clinical symptoms and signs of endocrine disease 1886
   II. Role of dynamic tests in the diagnosis of endocrinopathies 1895
   III. Interaction and referral of the endocrinologist with other specialists 1904
   IV. Epidemiology of endocrine diseases according to the stages of life 1913
   V. Endocrine: Specialist in nutrition, metabolism, hormones and reproduction 1920
   Final thoughts 1928
      General index 1931
   Epilogue 2045
   About the Author 2049

Endocrinology 360

A trilogy for the study of endocrinology

Presentation

Endocrinology is one of the medical areas that has experienced the most advances in recent years. Thanks to technological advances and scientific discoveries, we can recognize that the delicate balance that efficiently maintains functions in the body depends, in large part, on chemical communications between cells, which are produced by hormone / chemical interactions with receptors cell phones.

In this way, it is mandatory that doctors in any area, especially those of clinical subspecialties, know the basic notions of endocrine mechanisms and their alterations, since the consequences of these are related to various diseases, from cardiovascular diseases to neurological syndromes. Ideally, every health professional should be familiar with the principles of endocrinology to provide better patient care.

Below is a trilogy for the study of this medical subspecialty, Endocrinology 360, it is a collection of three texts that invite you to travel through the main subdivisions of endocrinology, starting from the physiological understanding of the organism's systems, in order to recognize their pathological alterations, endocrine diseases and their consequences, up to the therapeutic measures, considering both medications and lifestyle modifications and new innovative treatment options.

To study endocrinology, this specialty is divided into three large areas, which in turn group eight sections corresponding to the organs of the endocrine system, their functions, their alterations, and treatment options; in addition to presenting a new vision of medical practice, with chapters that talk about the importance of nutrition and dietetics to address different health conditions and enhance the benefits of treatment.

This academic journey begins by addressing Dietetics, Nutrition, Metabolism, and Diabetes mellitus. The first three are auxiliary sciences of endocrinology that help to understand how the processes that maintain the organism's homeostasis, cellular functions (respiration, ATP production and heat) work under physiological conditions, and how the regulatory systems that coordinate these processes are maintained.

This first volume highlights the importance of non-pharmacological measures for the success of therapy, mainly those that involve positive changes in life habits related to food, nutrition and dietetics. We will know the composition of the nutrients present in food, and how what we eat modifies the course of diseases; as well as the specific dietary recommendations for each pathology.

In the same way, the most recent evidence on diabetes mellitus, new nomenclatures and classifications, pathophysiological mechanisms, and reviews of traditional therapeutic options are presented, also presenting modern alternatives.

Next, the topics related to the metabolic axis and the water and electrolyte balance are discussed in the second volume: Thyroid, Parathyroid and Adrenal. The function of these glands is crucial to activate the biochemical reactions in all the cells of the body, and to maintain the balance of the internal environment with a stable composition of ions that act as cofactors in many cellular reactions and that maintain the membrane potentials in the cells through balanced and constant flow by ion pumps.

The pathologies that affect these glands, both due to deficiency and excess in the production of their respective hormones, are manifested with a set of systemic signs and symptoms that in turn compromise the function of other organs and systems of the body. These diseases constitute syndromes whose causes can be pathophysiological alterations of the glands, or others (poisoning, environmental factors, other diseases) that affect their function.

The last round of the endocrinology journey invites you to discover the Hypothalamic-Pituitary-Gonadal axis (ovaries and testes). It is a volume dedicated to the study of the endocrinology of the reproductive organs, their functions, starting from the beginning of the hormonal signals that lead to the appearance of female and male characters and somatic sexuality, to the conditions that modify and alter the regulation of these systems, triggering menstrual cycle disturbances and fertility problems, among others.

Endocrinology 360 is a comprehensive collection that groups the subareas of study of endocrinology according to their interactions and common functions, presenting a review of the concepts and definitions already known together with the new updates that have resulted from the latest research in this area to promote the practice of medicine based on the best evidence.

Now... let's begin the study of Endocrinology.

Introduction

Volume III. Hypothalamus-Pituitary, Ovaries, Testicles

The third part of this trilogy focuses on the study of the gland responsible for controlling and regulating the synthesis and secretion of practically all the other hormones, we are talking about the pituitary, as well as addressing the relationships that coordinate it through the releasing peptides of the hypothalamus, and the effects of their secretion in the different organs, especially in the gonads, which occupy the last part of this book.

The pituitary gland was one of the first glands described, with an embryological origin that led to the fusion of two lobes, a posterior one, closely related to the nervous system and with a storage function for hypothalamic hormones (oxytocin and ADH), and an anterior lobe (adenohypophysis) responsible for the production of seven main hormones that act as promoter and / or regulatory factors of the synthesis of the rest of the endocrine hormones, acting on the thyroid, growth, adrenal glands, and gonads.

In addition to knowing its anatomical constitution and its function, it is equally important to discuss the main pathologies that can compromise pituitary function. Such is the case of some congenital diseases, syndromes acquired from systemic conditions such as cardiovascular diseases or autoimmune processes, which secondarily affect pituitary function.

For its part, the discovery of the hypothalamus as a gland has been a relatively recent finding that has expanded the knowledge and advances in the field of neuroendocrinology. The hypothalamus is a diencephalic region located inferior to the subthalamic sulcus, composed of a series of nuclei formed by specialized neurons that secrete releasing and regulating factors of pituitary hormones, and in addition, they fulfill functions in the maintenance of internal homeostasis through the control temperature, the wake-sleep cycle, appetite, among other functions. We will also discuss the possible alterations of hypothalamic function from the point of view of endocrinology, where we will find that environmental factors, such as stress and lifestyle.

As the final section of this book and of the journey through the great areas of endocrinology, we present a section dedicated to the study of the gonads, ovaries and testes, considering their physiological endocrine function, their role in sexual development and differentiation, both from The physical as well as the psychic point of view, discussing not only the diseases that affect sexual development and fertility, but also issues that are currently a point of debate, such as gender dysphoria and other aspects of sexual identity.

In this way we present the *volume III of Endocrinology 360*, a trilogy of books that condenses the large areas of this medical subspecialty, presenting anatomical, physiological, pathological and therapeutic aspects, supported by current evidence, discussed with the author's professional experience.

And now… *Hypothalamus-Pituitary, Ovaries and Testicles.*

Dr. Mario Vega Carbó
Endocrinologist

Part VII. Hypothalamus- Pituitary

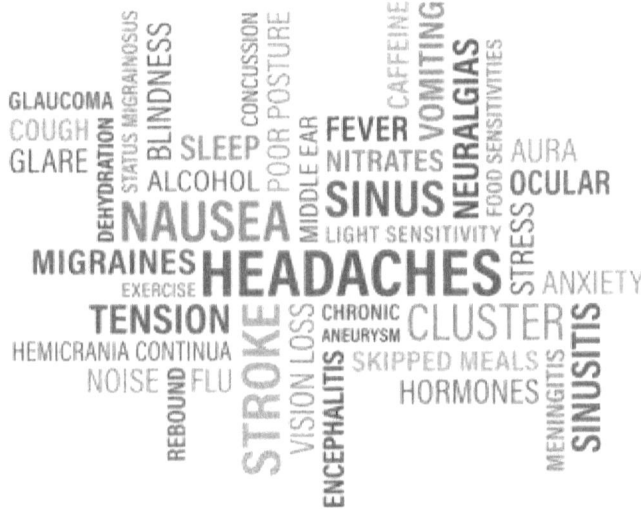

Chapter 252. Pineal Gland, Hypothalamus, and Pituitary

The pineal gland, the hypothalamus, and the pituitary gland are important elements of neurophysiology. These three glands located intracranially, are fundamental elements of body regulation, thanks to their actions that work synergistically towards the orientation of the endocrine and metabolic balance.

Embryology

Pineal gland	Hypothalamus	Hypophysis
From the roof of the third ventricle. The glandular parenchyma forms tubules that are transformed into cells innervated by developing nerves and separated by connective tissue.	In embryonic development, it is derived from the diencephalon, during the first trimester specifically at week 8 of gestation.	It arises within the rostral neural plate. The anterior lobe originates from the bag of Rathke, while the diverticulum originates from the posterior lobe.

Table 214 - 1. Embryology of the pineal gland, hypothalamus and pituitary.

Pineal gland

Also known as the pineal body or epiphysis, it is an uneven endocrine organ with a conical shape, whose relationships are: superiorly the corpus callosum (splenium aspect), superolateral with the choroid plexus of the third ventricle and inferiorly with the inferior and superior colliculi.

Innervation: adrenergic nerves. The sympathetic innervation comes from the superior cervical ganglion, parasympathetic innervation from optic ganglia and pterygopalatine.

Irrigation: derived from the posterior cerebral artery of its choroidal branches.

Venous drainage: internal cerebral vein.

Histology: cells known as pinealocytes and supporting cells. The gland contains a structure known as Corpora arenacea (sand of the brain), which increases calcification with age and is visible on X-rays.

Physiology: The main function is to produce 5-methoxyindole and melatonin. These are antigonadotrophic hormones. Melatonin, on the other hand, helps to modulate the circadian rhythm of sleep, its production is regulated with variations in light (its production increases with darkness and is reduced to light exposure).

Hypothalamus

It consists of the ventral brain region, which is responsible for coordinating the endocrine system by receiving many signals in different brain regions, with which it releases releasing and inhibiting hormones that stimulate the pituitary gland.

Located ventrally in relation to the right and left thalamus, constituting the floor and the lower portion of the lateral walls of the third ventricle. It is connected to the pituitary through the infundibulum.

Hypothalamic regions and irrigation

Region	Irrigation	Description
Anterior or chiasmatic	Branches of the anterior cerebral and anterior communicating arteries.	It extends between the lamina terminalis and the anterior infundibular recess.
Median or tuberal	Irrigated by the posterior communicating artery	Advances towards the anterior column of the cul-de-sac
Posterior or mamillary	Posterior communicating, basilar and posterior cerebral arteries.	It extends to the mammillary bodies.

Hypothalamic nuclei

Core	Function
Anterior hypothalamic nuclei	
Medial preoptic nucleus	Produces gonadotropin releasing hormone GnRH.
Supraoptic nucleus	It produces vasopressin and oxytocin (released from the posterior pituitary gland).
Paraventricular nucleus	Secretes vasopressin and oxytocin. It houses parvocellular neurosecretory neurons which project to the median eminence where axon terminals release growth hormone-releasing hormone (GhRH), corticotropin-releasing hormone (CRH), corticotropin-releasing hormone (CRH), and somatostatin.
Anterior hypothalamic nucleus	Thermoregulation. Regulation of circadian rhythms.

Suprachiasmatic nucleus	It receives afferent information from the retina, projections of the lateral geniculate nucleus and of the superior colliculus. It acts as the dominant regulator of circadian rhythms.
Lateral preoptic nucleus	It mediates the onset of sleep through non-rapid eye movements.
Tuberal hypothalamic nuclei	
Dorsomedial nucleus	Regulates hunger and satiety
Ventromedial nucleus	Regulates hunger and satiety. It intervenes in reactions of fear and aggression.
Arched core	Produces GhRH and dopamine
Posterior hypothalamic nuclei	
Posterior nucleus	Intervenes in thermoregulation
Mamillary nuclei	Components of the limbic and hypothalamic system. They act as a conduit for signals originating from the ipsilateral amygdala of the hippocampus. They transmit these signals to the thalamus through the mamillothalamic tract. They intervene in the recognition memory.
Tuber cinereum	It intervenes in the state of alert through histamine secretion.

Hypophysis

Also known as the pituitary gland, it comprises the predominant anterior lobe, a posterior lobe, and a vestigial intermediate lobe. This gland is located in a bone structure known as the sella turcica of the sphenoid, which is covered by a dural diaphragm.

Anatomy - weighs about 600 mg, with the longest transverse diameter of 13 mm, 6 to 9 mm in vertical height, and about 9 mm anteroposterior. It is located in the sella turcica, a bony structure at the base of the skull.

Irrigation: Superior pituitary arteries, branches of the internal carotid arteries, supply the anterior pituitary, after forming a hypothalamic capillary network. Pituitary portal vessels originate from the infundibular plexuses and the stem and together with the inferior pituitary artery supply the posterior pituitary.

Innervation: The posterior pituitary is innervated by the supraoptic pituitary nerve tracts and the pituitary tube of the posterior stem. Systemic arterial blood supply is preserved by the inferior pituitary arterial branches.

Histology:

Anterior pituitary gland		
Cell	**Express**	**Physiological aspects**
Corticotropes	Proopiomelanocortin peptides (POMC), includes adrenocorticotropic hormone (ACTH).	It stimulates the secretion of the hormones of the adrenal cortex (especially glucocorticoids).
Somatotropes	Growth hormone (GH)	GH receptor dimization (GHR) Activation of the JAK2 tyrosine kinase associated with GHR. Tyrosyl phosphorylation of JAK2 and GHR. Causing:

		Recruitment or activation of signaling molecules (MAP kinases, diacylglycerol, protein C, among others), contributing to GH-induced changes in enzymatic activity, transport function and gene expression causing changes in metabolism and growth, such as: anabolic functions, stimulation of IGF-1 production, among others.
Thyrotropes	Common glycoprotein alpha subunit and thyroid stimulating hormone (TSH, thyrotropin) specific beta subunit.	They stimulate the synthesis and secretion of thyroid hormones. They maintain thyroid structural integrity.
Gonadrotropes	Express alpha and beta subunits of both follicle stimulating hormone (FSH) and luteinizing hormone (LH)	Men: FSH is required for spermatogenesis, while LH stimulates testosterone secretion by Leydig cells. In women: FSH stimulates the growth and development of follicles in preparation for ovulation and estrogen secretion by mature Graafian follicle. LH triggers ovulation and stimulates progesterone secretion by the corpus luteum.
Lactotropes	Prolactin (PRL).	Stimulate the growth and development of mammary glands. Milk production.

		May inhibit pulsatile hypothalamic GnRH secretion.

It also contains supporting cells known as pituicytes or follicle-stelate cells.

Posterior pituitary

Connected by a nervous tract directly to the hypothalamus, this tract is known as the hypothalamic-pituitary nervous tract.

Precursor cell	Express	Physiological aspects
Paraventricular and supraoptic nuclei in the hypothalamus	Oxytocin	Stimulates milk ejection in response to sucking. Stimulates uterine contraction during labor.
	Vasopressin (antidiuretic hormone or ADH).	ADH binds to V2 receptors in the distal tubule and collecting ducts of the kidney, thereby upregulating the expression of the aquoporin channel on the basolateral membrane, increasing water reabsorption.

Bibliographic references

1. Shlomo Melmed, Richard J. Auchus, Allison B. Goldfine, Ronald J. Kowning, Clifford Rosen. Williams Textbook of Endocrinology 14Th edition. ELSEVIER, 2020.

2. Bloise E, Ciarmela P, Dela Cruz C, Luisi S, Petraglia F, Reis FM. Activin A in Mammalian Physiology. Physiol. Rev. 2019 Jan 01; 99 (1): 739-780.
3. Ilahi S, Beriwal N, Ilahi TB. Physiology, Pineal Gland. Stat Pearls Publishing; 2020 Jan

Chapter 253. Neuroendocrinology

Neuroendocrinology is the branch of medicine that is responsible for studying the relationships between the endocrine glands and the nervous system. A fundamental principle of neuroendocrinology is that secretion is regulated by hormones, neurotransmitters or neuromodulators, through specialized cells.

Neurosecretion

It is any neuronal secretory product of a neuron. Neurons are excitable cells, which release neurotransmitters and neuromodulators through their axons at specialized chemical synapses.

Key principle

> **The secretion of hormones from the anterior pituitary gland and the expression of genes encoding these hormones are specifically regulated by releasing and inhibiting factors. These are produced in the hypophysiotropic hypothalamic neurons and are secreted into the bloodstream through the portal vessel system found in the median eminence.**

Neurohumoral or neurosecretory cells: Unique subset of neurons in which axonal terminals are not associated with classical synapses. They secrete directly into the bloodstream.

Hypophysiotropic cells: they comprise secretory neurons in the pituitary portal vessels in the median eminence.

Autonomic nervous system and endocrine control

A fundamental precept in neuroendocrinology is that the nervous system is responsible for modifying and controlling the function of the glands, both endocrine and exocrine. This control is achieved through the action of the anterior pituitary gland and the action of the releasing factor hormones.

In addition, other organs such as the pancreas and adrenal glands receive direct innervation from cholinergic and noradrenergic stimuli, through which they are regulated.

Hypothalamic-pituitary unit

The hypothalamus integrates different sensory and hormonal inputs and in turn provides coordinated responses through motor outputs to key regulatory sites, such as the pituitary gland, cerebral cortex, motor and premotor neurons of the brainstem and spinal cord, as well as limbic system structures and parasympathetic and sympathetic preganglionic neurons. These hypothalamic outputs result in coordinated endocrine, autonomous, and behavioral responses, which allow the maintenance of homeostasis.

Regulation

The pituitary gland receives the regulation of 3 synergistic elements:
- ✓ Hypothalamic inputs (hypophysiotropic hormones or releasing factors).

- ✓ Feedback effect of circulating hormones.
- ✓ Autocrine and paracrine secretions of the gland itself.

Key principle

> Each respective hypothalamic-pituitary axis is maintained through the complex integration of positive and negative feedback loops, which involve the pituitary hormones themselves, descending signals as well as synaptic input from other brain areas to the hypophysiotropic neurons.

The neuropeptides of the hypothalamus are expressed in neurons throughout the brain to modulate the activity of neural circuits and coordinate a set of behavioral greetings that complement the hormonal actions of the hypothalamic-pituitary axes.

On the other hand, in addition to pituitary regulation, the hypothalamus is responsible for regulating fundamental homeostatic functions such as the sleep-wake cycle and thermoregulation.

Bibliographic references

1. Shlomo Melmed, Richard J. Auchus, Allison B. Goldfine, Ronald J. Kowning, Clifford Rosen. Williams Textbook of Endocrinology 14Th edition. ELSEVIER, 2020.
2. Shlomo Melmed. The Pituitary 4th Edition. Academic Press, Elsevier, 2017.

Chapter 254. Oxytocin

It is a non-peptide hormone known for its role in lactation and childbirth, functions from which its name is derived from the Greek (ω κ ν ξ, τ ok ox ξ) which means "rapid delivery". It is made up of 9 amino acids, with a sulfur bridge between the two cysteines.

Indications

FDA approved
Strengthen uterine contractions with the goal of a successful vaginal delivery.
Antepartum situations in mothers with:
Preeclampsia.
Premature membrane rupture.
Maternal diabetes.
Inactive uteri that need stimulation to initiate labor.
Unavoidable or incomplete abortions during the second trimester.
Postpartum period
At the time of extracting the placenta during the third stage of labor.
To control postpartum bleeding.
Stimulate postpartum milk ejection.
Not FDA approved
Treatment of late orgasm.
Induction of sexual arousal.
Treatment of autism.

Mechanism of action

Stored and released from the posterior pituitary gland, but created in the hypothalamus. It has positive feedback loops (oxytocin release leads to actions that cause increased oxytocin release).

It produces the stimulation of uterine contractions in the myometrium by causing G protein-coupled receptors to stimulate an increase in intracellular calcium in the myofibrils of the uterus. When activated, the oxytocin receptor causes many signals that stimulate the uterus to contract and increase intracellular calcium where positive feedback takes place.

It also causes contractions in the myoepithelial cells in the female breasts at the level of the alveolar ducts, as a result, the contractions promote the expulsion of milk. This mechanism is relevant as a reflex mechanism for the ejection of milk through the suckling of the baby on the mother's nipple.

Oxytocin also has vasodilator and antidiuretic effects causing an increase in cerebral, renal and coronary blood flow.

Administration

It is administered intravenously using a drip method.

Postpartum hemorrhage	Induction of labor	Incomplete abortion
10 intramuscular units after delivery of the placenta. Add 10 to 40 U to 1000 ml of non-hydrating IV solution and infuse at the rate required to control atony of the uterus.	0.5 to 1 mUnit / min IV. Titrate 1 to 2 mUnit / min every 15 to 60 minutes until the contraction pattern similar to that found in normal labor is achieved (about 6 mUnit / min). If necessary, you can reduce the dose once you reach the expected frequency of contraction and labor has progressed to 5 or 6 cm of dilation.	10 to 20 m Units / min. Do not exceed 30 units in 12 hours.

Adverse effects
- ✓ Erythema at the injection site.
- ✓ Intensified contractions.
- ✓ More frequent contractions.
- ✓ Nausea and vomiting
- ✓ Stomach pain and loss of appetite
- ✓ Cardiac arrhythmias.
- ✓ Seizures
- ✓ Anaphylaxis.
- ✓ Confusion.
- ✓ Hallucinations
- ✓ Increase in extreme blood pressure.
- ✓ Blurry vision.

Bibliographic references

1. Lee, HJ, Macbeth, AH, Pagani, JH, & Young, WS, 3rd (2009). Oxytocin: the great facilitator of life. Progress in neurobiology, 88 (2), 127–151.https://doi.org/10.1016/j.pneurobio.2009.04.001
2. Ellis JA, Brown CM, Barger B, Carlson NS. Influence of Maternal Obesity on Labor Induction: A Systematic Review and Meta-Analysis. J Midwifery Womens Health. 2019 Jan; 64 (1): 55-67
3. Osilla EV, Sharma S. Oxytocin. [Updated 2020 Aug 11]. In: Stat Pearls [Internet]. Treasure Island (FL): Stat Pearls Publishing; 2020 Jan.

Chapter 255. Melatonin, Serotonin, Dopamine

Melatonin (N-acetyl-5-methoxytryptamine) is a methoxyindole synthesized in the pineal gland. It is secreted during the night and fulfills various beneficial biological effects in the body.

Serotonin or 5-hydroxytryptamine is a neurotransmitter of great importance in the physiology of body systems, because it is responsible for regulating aspects such as behavior, mood, memory, among others. Clinically, it is used as a treatment for psychiatric and neurological disorders.

For its part, dopamine is a neurotransmitter produced by the substantia nigra, the ventral tegmental area and also in the hypothalamus of the brain. Dopamine dysfunction is associated with various nervous system disorders.

Synthesis and biological aspects

Melatonin and Serotonin

Melatonin and serotonin share a common synthetic pathway.

Endogenous production begins with tryptophan, which after several steps is converted to serotonin in other brain regions.

Serotonin is converted to melatonin by regulating the suprachiasmatic nucleus (SCN) of the hypothalamus.

The sympathetic stimulation of the pineal gland (due to information about the conditions of light that travels along the retinohypothalamic tract to the SCN), upregulates the production of the enzyme arylalkylamine N-acetyltransferase (AA-NAT), which converts serotonin into N-acetyl-serotonin, the rate-regulating step for melatonin formation.

Extrapineal sources of melatonin: retina, bone marrow cells, skin, platelets, lymphocytes, Harder's glands, cerebellum, gastrointestinal tract.

Melatonin is regulated by the light-dark cycles.

Dopamine

Its biosynthesis occurs following the enzymatic pathway of norepinephrine.

The initial step for dopamine synthesis is rate-limiting and involves conversion of L-tyrosine to L-DOPA (via the enzyme tyrosine hydroxylase).

The process requires iron and tetrahydrobiopterin as a cofactor, resulting in the addition of a hydroxyl group to the aromatic ring, causing the formation of L-DOPA, which is subsequently converted into dopamine, through the aromatic L-amino acid decarboxylase, which involves removal of the carboxyl group.

Once dopamine is synthesized, it is transported to the synaptic vesicles by means of the vesicular monoamine transporter 2 (CMAT2), to the synaptic terminals.

Biological functions

Melatonin	Serotonin	Dopamine
Adaptation to external and internal changes.	Regulates biological functions such as:	In the CNS it participates in the

Involved in autonomous cardiovascular regulation. Regulation of the immune system: stimulates the production of cytokines, especially IL-2, IL-6 and IL12, improves the immune response of T helper cells. Free radical detoxification. Antioxidant actions (through the action on MT3 receptors which protect the brain from oxidative stress). Its antioxidant function protects the gastrointestinal tract from ulcerations by reducing hydrochloric acid and by increasing the secretion of bicarbonate by the duodenal mucosa. Down-regulation of GnRH gene expression in a cyclical pattern over a 24-hour period.	Cardiovascular function Regulates intestinal motility (gastric emptying, intestinal peristalsis, colonic tone, pancreatic secretion, others). Ejaculatory latency. Bladder control. It could be associated in platelet aggregation processes through receptor-independent transglutaminase-dependent covalent bonding. Regulates the AV node. Vasoconstriction / dilation according to the vascular bed. Uterine vasoconstriction. Contraction of the uterine smooth muscle. Development of the mammary gland. Centrally modulates urination (facilitates protective reflex, role in stress incontinence). Involved in the pathogenesis of pulmonary	regulation of motor functions, affectivity and emotion. In the peripheral nervous system, it modulates cardiac function, gastrointestinal motility, and vascular tone. It is implicated in pathologies such as: Tourette syndrome, attention deficit hyperactivity disorder, schizophrenia, psychosis, Parkinson's disease. Modulates the activity of adenyl cyclase. Regulates neuroendocrine prolactin.

	hypertension. Others.	

Therapeutic indications

Melatonin	Serotonin	Dopamine
Short-term treatment of primary insomnia in people over 55 years of age. Synchronization of circadian rhythms with the environment. Treatment of jet lag. Antioxidant Additive therapy in cancer. Protection against carcinogenesis. Neurodegenerative disorders (Alzheimer's disease).	Selective serotonin reuptake inhibitors are used. Depression. Anxiety. Antiemetic. Appetite suppression (controversial).	It is used to treat low heart rate, hypotension, and cardiac arrest. Low infusion rates, i.e. 0.5 to 2 micrograms / kg x minute: They act on the visceral vasculature and induce vasodilation. Increase urinary flow. Intermediate infusion rates (2 to 10 micrograms / kg / min) They stimulate the contractility of the myocardium. They increase the electrical conductivity of the heart. Cardiac output increases. Higher doses cause vasoconstriction and increased blood pressure. *Indications* Maintenance of blood pressure in: Chronic congestive heart failure. Trauma Renal insufficiency. Open heart surgery. Shock from myocardial infarction or septicemia.

Bibliographic references

1. Berger, M., Gray, JA, & Roth, BL (2009). The expanded biology of serotonin. Annual review of medicine, 60, 355–366.https://doi.org/10.1146/annurev.med.60.042307.110802
2. Berke JD (2018). What does dopamine mean? Nature neuroscience, 21 (6), 787–793.https://doi.org/10.1038/s41593-018-0152-y
3. Tordjman, S., Chokron, S., Delorme, R., Charrier, A., Bellissant, E., Jaafari, N., & Fougerou, C. (2017). Melatonin: Pharmacology, Functions and Therapeutic Benefits. Current neuropharmacology, 15 (3), 434–443. https://doi.org/10.2174/1570159X14666161228122115

Chapter 256. Pineal Tumors

They are a group of neoplasms developed from cells found in and around the pineal gland. Mainly the type of cell found in the pineal gland is the pineal or pinocyte parenchymal cell, which is a specialized neuron that is related to the cones and rods of the retina. The pinocyte is surrounded by a stroma of fibrillar astrocytes, which interact with the adjacent blood vessels forming part of the blood-top barrier.

Statistics and epidemiology

They constitute between 0.4 to 1% of intracranial tumors in adults and about 3 to 8% of brain tumors in children.
The most frequent age range of incidence is between 10 to 20 years of age, with the average being 13 years of age. In adults, the incidence occurs mainly in those over 30 years of age. In boys, they are frequently associated with abnormal pubertal development.

Etiology

Most pineal tumors occur as a result of displaced embryonic tissue as a result of malignant transformation of pineal parenchymal cells or by transformation of adjacent astroglia.
To date, no specific genetic mutations responsible for pineal tumor development have been associated.

Pathophysiological elements

The clinical manifestations occur as a consequence of the anatomical compression of the adjacent structures caused by pineal tumors.
Local infiltration of neural structures could also explain the pathophysiology of clinical manifestations in cases where there are highly invasive tumors.
Histologically, tumors in the pineal region are heterogeneous. They can arise from:
- ✓ Germ cells: choriocarcinoma, germinomas, teratomas, endodermal sinus tumors, mixed germ cell tumors.
- ✓ Pineal parenchyma cells: pineocytoma and pineoblastoma.
- ✓ Bra stroma: gliomas.

Diagnostic criteria

Clinic	The clinical manifestations depend on compression and invasion of adjacent structures by the pineal tumor. Headache, nausea, and vomiting (aqueductal compression). Hydrocephalus Weakness and loss of sensation in the middle of the body (due to invasion of the thalamus). Sleep, thermoregulation and body water disorders (due to hypothalamic invasion). Lethargy. Clouding. Vertical gaze palsy syndrome (superior colliculus involvement).

	Convergence or refractory nystagmus, mydriasis, convergence spasms, anisocoria (greater compression of the periaqueductal gray region). Diabetes insipidus Reproductive abnormalities.
Paraclinical	Tumor markers in cerebrospinal fluid (CSF) and serum. Alpha-fetoprotein Beta-hCG. Cytology. Lactate dehydrogenase isoenzymes (less specific). Placental alkaline phosphatase (less specific). Imaging studies High resolution magnetic resonance imaging with gadolinium.

Treatment options

Surgically removing pineal tumors is difficult depending on their location and the structures adjacent to the gland. However, it can be considered a minimally invasive technique before resorting to other options.

In the case of hydrocephalus, the blockage of CSF flow as a consequence of the enlargement of the pineal gland, makes endoscopic third ventriculostomy considerable. In case of failure, a bypass should be considered.

Most pineal tumors are sensitive to radiation therapy. It is used in patients older than 3 years. Chemotherapy is used only when it is necessary, according to the type of tumor.

Prognosis and monitoring

The 5-year survival for germinomas was 62%, however, the 5-year survival for other malignant tumors was 14%. The spinal metastasis of germinomas ranges between 11%, while for endodermal sinus tumors, the incidence of spinal metastasis is 23%. When a diagnosis is made by intraoperative cytology, the physician should evaluate the presence of spinal metastasis.

The follow-up of children with pineal tumors should be carried out for life since these can reappear locally or distally up to 5 years after the initial diagnosis. Imaging studies should be requested periodically, depending on the results obtained in the biopsy and if the diagnosis of spinal metastasis was established at the time of diagnosis. Similarly, regular tumor marker studies should be requested regularly in these patients.

Bibliographic references

1. Shlomo Melmed, Richard J. Auchus, Allison B. Goldfine, Ronald J. Kowning, Clifford Rosen. Williams Textbook of Endocrinology 14Th edition. ELSEVIER, 2020.
2. Yelamanchi SD, Kumar M, Madugundu AK, Gopalakrishnan L, Dey G, Chavan S, et al. Characterization of human pineal gland proteome. MolBiosyst. 2016 Nov 15. 12 (12): 3622-3632.
3. Awa R, Campos F, Arita K, Sugiyama K, Tominaga A, Kurisu K, et al. Neuroimaging diagnosis of pineal region tumors-quest for pathognomonic finding of germinoma. Neuroradiology. 2014 Jul. 56 (7): 525-34.
4. Arendt J. The Pineal Gland and Pineal Tumors. [Updated 2011 Jan 1]. In: Feingold KR, Anawalt B, Boyce A, et al., Editors. Endotext. South Dartmouth (MA): MDText.com, Inc .; 2000.

Chapter 257. Endocrine - Hypothalamic Syndromes

All those disorders that affect the hypothalamus can cause pituitary dysfunction, behavioral and neuropsychiatric disorders. It can also cause disorders of metabolic and autonomic regulation. However, hypothalamic endocrine syndromes are a group of disorders caused by the alteration of the hypothalamic-pituitary-glandular axis, which depend on the extension of the hypothalamic lesion, the physiological impact and the specific cause.

Epidemiology

Craniopharyngiomas are mainly pediatric tumors that represent between 5% and 15% of intracranial tumors in this age group. Only 25% of craniopharyngiomas occur in patients older than 25 years. Precocious puberty occurs before the age of 9 to 10 in boys and between 7 to 8 years in girls.
About two-thirds of hypothalamic lesions influence human puberty and may be responsible for neurogenic precocious puberty.

Etiology of hypothalamic endocrine síndromes

Hypophysiotropic hormone deficiency
Hypothalamic hypothyroidism.

Craniopharyngioma.
Hypothalamic tumor: infuse me, astrocytoma, teratoma (ectopic pinealoma).
Inflammatory disease: sphenoid osteomyelitis, meningitis and basilar granuloma, sarcoidosis, tuberculosis.
Surgical section of the pituitary stalk.
Hypophysiotropic insufficiency.
Isolated GHRH deficiency

Disorders of the regulation of GnRH secretion	
Female	Male
Precocious puberty: hCG-secreting germinoma, GnRH-secreting hamartoma. Late puberty Neurogenic amenorrhea. Anorexia nervosa. Kallman syndrome. GPR54 (KISS1R) mutation. Functional amenorrhea and oligomenorrhea. Drug-induced amenorrhea.	Early puberty. Fröhlich syndrome. Drug-induced hypogonadism. GPR54 (KISSR1) gene mutation. Kallmann syndrome.

Disorders of the regulation of prolactin regulatory factors
Carbon dioxide narcoidosis.
Drug-induced reflex.
Herpes zoster of the chest wall.
Sarcoidosis
Nipple manipulation.
Postthoracotomy.
Spinal cord tumor.
Psychogenic hypothyroidism.

CRH regulation disorders
Paroxysmal corticotropin secretion (Wolff syndrome).
Loss of circadian variation.
CRH-secreting gangliocytoma.
Depression.

Elements of pathophysiology

Hypothalamic lesions often cause a reduced secretion of most pituitary hormones, however, they can also cause hypersecretion of hormones that are normally regulated with hypothalamic inhibitory control, for example, in PRL hypersecretion, as a consequence of damage to the pituitary stalk.
Each etiology can include different diagnostic elements as a result of the endocrine alteration that it triggers.

Diagnostic criteria and treatments

The etiology of hypothalamic neuroendocrine disorders can cause a wide variety of clinical manifestations and include diverse diagnostic criteria. The age of the patient and his history are fundamental elements at the moment to establish diagnostic suspicion.

Bibliographic references

1. Shlomo Melmed, Richard J. Auchus, Allison B. Goldfine, Ronald J. Kowning, Clifford Rosen. Williams Textbook of Endocrinology 14Th edition. ELSEVIER, 2020.

Chapter 258. Pictures of the Sellar Region

The sellar region is an anatomical area made up of the sella turcica, the pituitary gland, and adjacent structures. Bounded inferiorly by the body of the sphenoid, its upper limit is the posterior aspect of the frontal lobes of the brain, the floor of the third ventricle, and the peduncles of the brain.

This region constitutes the third most frequent site for the development of intracranial tumor lesions. The main neoplasms of the sellar region are pituitary adenomas, although they can include other types of lesions or incidental findings, often without clinical significance.

Magnetic resonance imaging (MRI) is considered a mainstay for the evaluation of sellar pathology, thanks to the high contrast resolution and availability of advanced sequences.

Findings in images of the sellar region

- ✓ Neoplasms
- ✓ Pituitary adenoma.
- ✓ Meningioma.
- ✓ Craniopharyngioma.
- ✓ Chordoma
- ✓ Chondrosarcoma.
- ✓ Schwannoma.
- ✓ Glioma of the optic pathway.
- ✓ Germ cell tumor.
- ✓ Plasmacytoma.
- ✓ Metastasis.

- ✓ Congenital
- ✓ Rathke cleft cyst.
- ✓ Dermoid and epidermoid tumor.
- ✓ Arachnoid cyst.
- ✓ Hypothalamic hamartoma.
- ✓ Vascular
- ✓ Giant aneurysm.
- ✓ Inflammatory or granulomatous disorders
- ✓ Sarcoidosis
- ✓ Lymphocytic hypophysitis.

Images finds from the sellar region

Image	Description
Microadenoma	They are less than 10 mm in diameter. They are located in the pituitary gland. An upward convexity of the upper right pituitary surface is observed, as well as a slight bulge in the suprasellar cistern. There is no compression of the optic chiasm or nerves. On a non-contrast scan, up to 70% of microadenomas can be identified. Giving gadolinium can reduce false negatives by 15 to 30%.
Macroadenoma	They are more than 10 mm in diameter. They are soft and solid lesions that grow from below and then grow upwards. They may have areas of necrosis or hemorrhage as they increase in size. Its configuration is "snowman". It is characterized by the

	enlargement of the sella turcica.
Meningioma 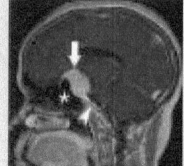 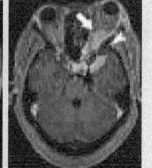	It can be confused with a macroadenoma, however, in a meningioma, there is no diaphragmatic constriction and it presents a uniform enhancement, after the administration of gadolinium. It may have an associated dural tail and pneumosinus dilatans (star). A meningioma that invades the left orbit and the posterior ethmoid can be evidenced in the T1-weighted axial image. The greater sphenoid wing presents hyperostosis and anterior clinoid process (black arrow). The origin of the injury is above the sella turcica.
Craniopharyngioma 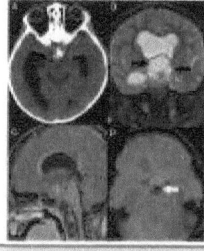	It presents as a large suprasellar mass, with cystic and enhancement components, as well as it can present calcifications. There is evidence of obstructive hydrocephalus.
Trigeminal Schwannoma 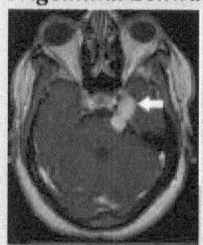	They are benign slow-growing masses which arise from Schwann cells. Image after contrast administration, shows avid enhancement (arrow), which affects the trigeminal ganglion, inside Meckel's cave and in the cisternal segment of the nerve. Its heterogeneity varies according to the presence of cystic, hemorrhagic or calcification changes. It shows hyperintensity in T1 and can be confused with lipomas, although the

	latter suppress the saturated fat sequences.
Rathke cleft cyst 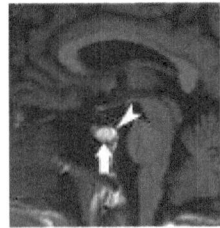	Rathke cleft cysts usually appear in or above the sella turcica. The pituitary gland and optic chiasm may be normal, as well as the carotid artery. Image is T1-weighted. Without the administration of contrast, it shows a hyperintense cyst (arrow), which displaces the pars distalis anteriorly.
Chordoma 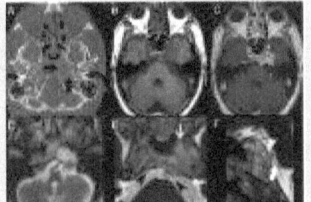	They are the most common lesions of the clivus. The black arrows in image A show an erosive lesion affecting the left petroclival fissure and the carotid duct. Image B shows a T1-weighted axial section, which shows a slightly hyperintense image without contrast. There may be calcifications in this area. Chordomas usually occur in the midline, unlike chondrosarcomas, which usually appear outside the midline.
Germinome 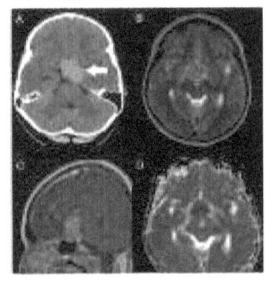	Without contrast, it appears as a hyperdense suprasellar mass. The T2-weighted image in image B shows an isointense or slightly hyperintense mass in the sagittal cortex. The T1-weighted C image shows a heterogeneous enhancement of the mass after the administration of contrast.

Bibliographic references

1. Carlos Zamora, MD, PhD. Mauricio Castillo, MD. Sellar and Parasellar Imaging. Congress of Neurological Surgeons. Neuroradiology review series. Volume 80, N° 1, January, 2017. DOI: 10.1093 / neuros / nyw013.
2. Criales JR, Palacios E, Dimitri IG. Hypophysis and periselar tumors. In: Pedrosa CS. Diagnostic imaging. Treaty of Clinical Radiology. 2 ed. Madrid: McGraw-Hill Interamericana; 2010. p. 1159-73.

Chapter 259. Pituitary Incidentaloma

They are space-occupying lesions located in the sellar area, which are identified by chance or incidentally, at the time of performing a cranial imaging test for the study of another type of pathology not associated with the pituitary. With technological advances in imaging studies, the diagnosis of pituitary incidentalomas has increased in recent years.

Statistics and epidemiology

- ✓ About 10% of autopsy studies present unsuspected pituitary tumors in life.
- ✓ The mean prevalence of pituitary incidentaloma is around 10.7%.
- ✓ The distribution between the sexes is homogeneous.
- ✓ The prevalence of macroadenomas in autopsies is less than 1%.
- ✓ The incidence of incidentalomas is slightly higher in older adults.
- ✓ Magnetic resonance imaging studies in unselected populations have identified microincidentaloma rates between 10 to 38%.

Etiology and pathophysiological elements

The causes that trigger pituitary tumorigenesis are multiple, and in turn various undetected oncogenic abnormalities may be associated.

G protein abnormalities, ras gene mutations, mutations, deletions and rearrangements of the p53 gene have been described. Multiple endocrine neoplasia syndrome has also been associated as a triggering factor for pituitary tumorigenesis, specifically in the development of pituitary adenomas.

According to the type of neoplasia incidentally discovered, the pathophysiological and etiological mechanisms may be diverse.

Diagnostic criteria

By definition, a pituitary incidentaloma is diagnosed incidentally in the absence of clinical manifestations or in the absence of suspected pituitary disorder. The diagnosis is established by imaging studies (CT scan or MRI). However, once an incidentaloma has been identified, patients must be studied thoroughly.

Take a complete medical history and physical examination, including evaluation for hypopituitarism and hormone hypersecretion syndrome. Perform the required biochemical studies.

All patients with a pituitary incidentaloma adjacent to the optic chiasm or optic nerves should undergo a formal visual field (VF) examination.

When the diagnosis has been established by computed tomography, it is recommended that the patient undergo an MRI to obtain a better evaluation of the incidentaloma.

Treatment options

Criteria for surgical therapy of pituitary incidentaloma

Hypersecretion of tumors other than prolactinomas.
VF deficiency due to incidentaloma.
Visual disturbances such as ophthalmoplegia or evidence of

> neurological compromise due to compression of the lesion.
> Injury compressing nerves or optic chiasm.
> Pituitary apoplexy with the presence of visual disturbance.

Other pertinent findings to consider surgical intervention:
- ✓ Incessant headache.
- ✓ Loss of endocrinological function.
- ✓ Clinically significant incidentaloma growth.
- ✓ Injury near the optic chiasm and fertility plan for pregnancy.
- ✓ Follow-up peculiarities

Those patients who do not meet criteria for surgical excision should receive non-surgical treatment, in conjunction with clinical evaluations and relevant tests:
- ✓ Pituitary magnetic resonance image 6 months after the initial examination (in the presence of a macroincidentaloma) or 1 year later (microincidentaloma). In those patients, where no size change is evident, suggest repeating the magnetic resonance imaging annually (for macroincidentalomas) or every 1 or 2 years (for microincidentalomas).
- ✓ Perform clinical and biochemical studies for hypopituitarism 6 months after initial diagnosis. Repeat annually thereafter in patients with macroincidentalomas.

Bibliographic references

1. Freda, PU, Beckers, AM, Katznelson, L., Molitch, ME, Montori, VM, Post, KD, Vance, ML, & Endocrine

Society (2011). Pituitary incidentaloma: an endocrine society clinical practice guideline. The Journal of clinical endocrinology and metabolism, 96 (4), 894–904.https://doi.org/10.1210/jc.2010-1048.
2. Vladimir Vasilev, Liliya Rostomyan, Adrian F Daly, et al. Pituitary 'incidentaloma': neuroradiological assessment and differential diagnosis. European Journal of Endocrinology (2016) 175, R171 – R184

Chapter 260. Hypothalamic Pituitary Dysfunction

The proper function of the hypothalamic pituitary axis can be affected by a number of disorders and conditions, which can lead to hormonal alteration or loss of hypothalamic pituitary function. This can occur as a consequence of a primary disorder or as a result of indirect and distant effects on pituitary hypothalamic hormonal function.

Statistics and epidemiology

The clinically significant incidence of tumors is 20 to 30 per million per year. Tumors that cause hypothalamic pituitary dysfunction are rarely part of type 1 multiple endocrine neoplasia. The incidence of Kallmann syndrome is 1 case per 10,000 people. The incidence of internal carotid artery aneurysm represents 0.3% of all aneurysms.

Etiology

Idiopathic GnRH deficiency	Kallmann syndrome. Prader-Willi syndrome. Laurence-Moon-Biedl syndrome (multiple).
Tissue injury	Trauma Post-surgery Post-radiotherapy
Vascular	Pituitary infarction. Carotid aneurysm.
Neoplasia	Adenoma Craniopharyngioma. Others.

Infiltrator	Sarcoidosis,
	Fungal infection
	Hemochromatosis.
	Tuberculosis.
Drugs	Drug-induced hyperprolactinemia.
	Sex steroids.
Others	Systemic disease
	Malnutrition
	Anorexia nervosa.
	Hypothalamic deficit.
	Pituitary hypoplasia.
	Autoimmune pituitary.

Pathophysiological elements

Alteration of the positive and negative feedback mechanism of the hypothalamic-pituitary axis caused as a consequence of primary or secondary factors.

Diagnostic criteria and treatments

According to the suspected etiology, it is recommended to indicate imaging tests such as computed tomography or magnetic resonance imaging, especially when the presence of neoplasms is suspected. Imaging studies will allow to determine the extent and nature of it.

Complete hormonal biochemical studies should be requested, prioritizing the hormonal function of the anterior part of the pituitary, since it usually presents manifestations of hypopituitarism.

According to the results obtained in the biochemical studies, it can orient specific replacement therapy to the deficiency observed, whenever this is allowed.

Evaluate the PRL concentration, as hypothalamic lesions frequently cause hyperprolactinemia, either from damage to the hypothalamus or as a result of damage to the pituitary stalk.

In the case of a tumor, consider surgical resection whenever possible. Craniopharyngiomas can be managed by limited neurosurgical removal of the accessible tumor and decompression of cysts with subsequent radiation therapy.

Follow-up peculiarities:

Follow up appropriately according to the individualized aspects of your patient based on their general condition and the underlying cause of the hypothalamic-pituitary dysfunction.

Bibliographic references

1. Shlomo Melmed. The Pituitary 4th Edition. AcademicPress, Elsevier, 2017.
2. Lavin N, editor. Manual of endocrinology and metabolism. 4th ed. Philadelphia: Wolters Kluwer / Lippincott Williams & Wilkins Health; 2009. 837 p.

Chapter 261. Polydipsic Polyuric Syndrome

Se is a problem that is often difficult to differentiate in clinical practice, which is defined as the abnormal production of large volumes of urine (more than 3 liters a day in adults and more than 2 L / m2 in children), in in conjunction with the persistent intake of large amounts of fluid. Polydipsic polyuric syndrome encompasses a wide range of disorders.

Statistics and epidemiology

- ✓ Congenital forms represent less than 10% of cases.
- ✓ It can occur in up to 22% of patients who have suffered acute traumatic brain injury or up to 30% of these in long-term follow-up.
- ✓ About 50% of patients with diabetes insipidus of hypothalamic origin have an underlying tumor or a malformation of the central nervous system.

Etiology and pathophysiological elements

Central diabetes insipidus	Hypothalamus or pituitary gland involvement (insufficient vasopressin secretion)
	For example: craniopharyngioma, Sheehan syndrome, trauma, Guillain-Barré syndrome, Sarcoidosis, drug-induced, Alström syndrome, among others.
Nephrogenic diabetes insipidus	Resistance to vasopressin at the renal level.
	Metabolic origin (hypokalemia, hypercalcemia), induced by drugs, kidney disease, systemic diseases

	such as sarcoidosis, vascular disorders, congenital, among others.
Gestational diabetes insipidus	Induced by pregnancy. It occurs as a consequence of increased metabolism of vasopressin induced by placental cysteine aminopeptidase.
Primary polydipsia	Decreased hypothalamic threshold for thirst (dipsogenic DI), psychogenic polydipsia, induced by drugs, among others.

Diagnostic criteria

Clinic	- Increased urinary volume (polyuria). - Persistent increased fluid intake (polydipsia). - Nocturia. - Lethargy, fatigue. - Myalgia. Symptoms in children can be nonspecific and include: - Severe dehydration - Constipation. - Stunted growth - Irritability. - Vomiting - Fever. The following symptoms may also occur in neoplastic causes: - Headache. - Visual disturbances
Paraclinical	✓ Calculation of plasma osmolality: ○ 2 [Na +] + [Glucose] / 18 + [BUN] / 2.8 ✓ Calculation of total 24-hour urine volume. ✓ Baseline values of plasma electrolytes, random

serum and urinary osmolality.
- ✓ Desmopressin test (DDAVP)
- ✓ Baseline Copeptin measurement
- ✓ Greater than 21.4 pmol / L (without prior fluid deprivation): suggests a nephrogenic cause.
- ✓ Less than 21.4 pmol / L (without prior fluid deprivation): copeptin stimulation should be performed (when plasma sodium is greater than 150 mmol (L).

If the posttestimulation result to copeptin is less than 4.9 pmol / L, it suggests a complete or partial central cause.

When the posttestimulation result to copeptin is greater than 4.9 pmol / L, it suggests primary polydipsia.

- ✓ Water deprivation test.

It should be suspended when one of the following conditions is met:

- When the osmolality of the urine reaches the normal reference range.
- When plasma sodium is greater than 154 mEq.
- When urine osmolality is stable in 2 or 3 consecutive hourly measurements (including when increasing plasma osmolality is found).
- When plasma osmolality is greater than 295 to 300 mOsmol / kg.

Treatment options

The underlying cause involves the therapeutic options available for polydipsic polyuric syndrome.

DDAVP, an analog of ADH, can be administered orally, subcutaneously, intranasally, or intravenously. In adults, the dose is 10 mcg per nasal insufflation. 4 mcg can also be used subcutaneously or intravenously. In infants or newborns, the dose is 1 mcg subcutaneously or intravenously for 20 minutes with a maximum dose of 0.4 mcg per kilogram of body weight.

It is essential to replace fluid losses and treat dehydration whenever there are signs or symptoms suggestive of it. Also, correct any electrolyte disturbances present.

Follow-up peculiarities:

The prognosis depends on the cause. Those causes of benign course have a favorable prognosis and follow-up can be established according to the metabolic state of the patient, on the contrary, malignant causes have a reserved prognosis and may require close monitoring.

Postoperative patients should receive a urine density check before starting desmopressin treatment. In addition, the level of serum electrolytes must be measured regularly.

It is essential to properly inform the patient about special measures in case of travel and how to prepare when vomiting or diarrhea occurs in order to avoid dehydration.

Bibliographic reference

1. Christ-Crain M. (2019). EJE AWARD 2019: New diagnostic approaches for patients with polyuria polydipsia syndrome. European journal of endocrinology, 181 (1), R11 – R21.https://doi.org/10.1530/EJE-19-0163

2. Nigro N, Grossmann M, Chiang C, Inder WJ. Polyuria-polydipsia syndrome: a diagnostic challenge. Intern Med J. 2018; 48 (3): 244-253. doi: 10.1111 / imj.13627
3. Ball S. Diabetes Insipidus. [Updated 2018 Jun 13]. In: Feingold KR, Anawalt B, Boyce A, et al., Editors. Endotext [Internet]. South Dartmouth (MA): MDText.com, Inc .; 2000-.

Chapter 262. Central Diabetes Insipidus

It is a polydipsic polyuric syndrome, which consists of an increase in the loss of urinary volume in conjunction with an increase in persistent fluid intake. However, central diabetes insipidus is the clinical manifestation originated as a consequence of a great variety of genetic and structural conditions that alter the hypothalamic or central function associated with the release of vasopressin

Statistics and epidemiology

Familial central diabetes insipidus can occur in about 5% of cases. It can be the result of an acute event (traumatic brain injury) in up to 22% of patients and up to 50% with long-term evaluation.

About 50% of patients with central diabetes insipidus have an underlying tumor or malformation of the central nervous system.

Neurosurgical conditions are the most common causes of central diabetes insipidus. Transsphenoidal or transcranial surgeries cause central diabetes insipidus in up to 50-60% of patients, although most patients recover, however a small number of patients will have permanent diabetes insipidus.

Risk groups or factors

- ✓ Family history of central diabetes insipidus of genetic cause.

- ✓ Craniotomy for large tumors.
- ✓ Transsphenoidal or transcranial surgery.
- ✓ Head injury.
- ✓ Radiotherapy.
- ✓ Immunosuppressed state.

Etiology

Primary	
Genetic	Wolfram syndrome (diabetes insipidus, diabetes mellitus, optic atrophy and deafness). Autosomal dominant. Autosomal recessive.
Developmental syndrome	Septic-optic dysplasia.
Secondary / acquired	
Trauma	Head injury. Post-therapy. Post-surgery.
Vascular	Cavernous sinus thrombosis. Carotid aneurysm.
Inflammatory	Sarcoidosis Lymphocytic hypophysitis. Infundibulo-neurohypophysitis Langerhans cell histiocytosis. Meningitis / encephalitis. Guillain Barre syndrome.
Tumor	Pituitary adenomas. Metastasis. Germinome. Craniopharyngioma.
Infection	Fungal diseases Tuberculosis.
Postpartum	Pituitary apoplexy. Sheehan syndrome.

Pathophysiological elements

It involves the loss of between 80% and 90% of vasopressin production as a result of the destruction of the vasopressinérgic magnocellular neurons of the hypothalamus or as a result of the interruption of the interaxonal transport or processing of vasopressin.

Within the first 24 hours after intracranial surgery, axonal shock can occur in conjunction with the inability of action potentials to spread from the cell body to neurons located in the posterior pituitary.

Subsequently, an antidiuretic phase is entered characterized by the unregulated release of vasopressin by the affected neurohypophyseal neurons. It occurs between 5 to 7 days after surgery and is usually framed with hyponatremia, especially when hypotonic fluids are administered intravenously.

Damaged neurons can suffer gliosis and loss of secretory function, triggering permanent central diabetes insipidus.

Damage to the axons will depend on the regulatory function of vasopressin. When there are remaining intact axons, they may have sufficient vasopressin function to prevent the clinical manifestation of diabetes insipidus.

Diagnostic criteria

Clinical manifestation
- ✓ Polyuria
- ✓ Polydipsia.
- ✓ Nocturia.

✓ Nonspecific symptoms (headache, nausea, vomiting, weakness, myalgia, drowsiness, lethargy, fatigue, among others).

Water deprivation test

Dehydration phase (Step1)	
Process	Intake of all fluids should be restricted from 8:00 am to 4:00 pm The patient should be in a controlled environment. Take baseline and every 2 hour measurements of urine volume, urine osmolality, plasma osmolality, and body weight. The test should be stopped if the patient is unbearably thirsty or when there is a loss of body weight greater than 5% of the initial one.
Analysis	*Central diabetes insipidus (IDH) and nephrogenic (NDI):* Urinary osmolality <300mOsm / kg Plasma osmolality> 290mOsm / kg *Dipsogenic diabetes insipidus (DDI):* Normal plasma and urinary osmolality.
Desmopressin Response Phase (DDAVP) (Step 2)	
***objective*: difference between central diabetes insipidus and nephrogenic diabetes.**	
Process	At 4:00 pm (after step 1) a 1 mcg intramuscular bolus of desmopressin should be administered. Allow fluid intake up to twice the volume of urine output achieved in step 1. Measure urine volume, plasma and urinary olsmolality every hour until 8:00 pm Finally, measure plasma osmolality and serum sodium at 9:00 am the next day.
Analysis	Central diabetes insipidus: Urinary osmolality> 750 mOsm / kg Nephrogenic diabetes insipidus: Urinary osmolarity remains low.

Table 222 - 2.

Other studies

Pituitary function tests.

Cranial magnetic resonance imaging (can be repeated at 12 months, when no structural alteration is evident, but a slow-growing mass is suspected).

Treatment options

Mild forms do not require treatment. When there is symptomatic manifestation of diabetes insipidus, desmopressin can be used:
- ✓ Intranasal spray of 5 to 100 mcg per day.
- ✓ 100 to 1000 mcg tablets per day.
- ✓ Parenteral route at doses of 0.1 to 2.0 mcg per day.

Hyponatremia due to plasma dilution can be avoided by skipping treatment for a short period on a regular basis, that is, skipping one dose per week.

Follow-up peculiarities

Long-term follow-up should be considered. Evaluate family members whenever a family cause is suspected, keeping in mind that the manifestations can be diverse.

Bibliographic references

1. Shlomo Melmed, Richard J. Auchus, Allison B. Goldfine, Ronald J. Kowning, Clifford Rosen. Williams Textbook of Endocrinology 14Th edition. ELSEVIER, 2020.

2. Shlomo Melmed. The Pituitary 4th Edition. Academic Press, Elsevier, 2017.
3. Ball S. Diabetes Insipidus. [Updated 2018 Jun 13]. In: Feingold KR, Anawalt B, Boyce A, et al., Editors. Endotext [Internet]. South Dartmouth (MA): MDText.com, Inc .; 2000-

Chapter 263. Nephrogenic Diabetes Insipidus

It is a pathological process characterized by the excess production of dilute urine that occurs as a consequence of partial or total resistance to the effect of antidiuretic hormone or vasopressin at the renal level.

Statistics and epidemiology

- ✓ More than 90% of cases are recessive and linked to the X chromosome in men.
- ✓ About 200 different V2 receptor mutations have been reported.
- ✓ The incidence of nephrogenic diabetes insipidus caused by AQP2 mutation occurs in 1 in every 20 million births.
- ✓ About 10% of the genetic disorders responsible for nephrogenic diabetes insipidus occur de novo.
- ✓ Most women who carry the V2 X-linked receptor gene mutation are asymptomatic.
- ✓ Severe heterozygous cases occur mainly in males, and rarely in females.
- ✓ Risk groups or factors: Family history.

Etiology or more frequent causes

Genetic	X-linked recessive (V2-R defect).
	Autosomal recessive (AQP2 defect).

	Autosomal dominant.
Idiopathic	
Chronic kidney disease	Polycystic kidneys. Obstructive uropathy.
Metabolic disease	Hypokalemia Hypercalcemia
Drug induced	Demeclocycline. Lithium.
Osmotic diuretics	Mannitol. Glucose.
Systemic disorders	Myelomatosis Amyloidosis

Pathophysiological elements

Renal resistance to vasopressin.
Familial X-linked diabetes insipidus results from loss-of-function mutations in the renal vasopressin receptor.
Autosomal recessive nephrogenic diabetes insipidus is caused by mutations associated with loss of function in the vasopressin-dependent renal water channel, aquuporin 2.

General categories of V2 receptor mutations.

    Type 1: characterized by alteration of binding to vasopressin.
    Type 2: typified by defective transport.
    Type 3: where unstable receptors degrade rapidly.

Diagnostic criteria

Clinic: Polyuria, Polydipsia, Nocturia.
Paraclinical:
    ✓ Water deprivation test and desmopressin test (See Chapter 222).

- ✓ Copeptin test (see Chapter 221).
- ✓ Request kidney biochemical tests.
- ✓ Renal imaging tests required.

Treatment options

- ✓ Adequate water intake.
- ✓ Whenever the underlying cause can be treated, eliminate the causative agent (correction of hypokalemia or stopping lithium administration).
- ✓ It does not respond well to desmopressin, although it may respond to high doses of desmopressin (4 mcg intramuscularly twice daily).
- ✓ Indicate a low sodium diet especially in congenital causes.
- ✓ Indicate thiazide diuretic (can be hydrochlorothiazide at 25 mg / day).

Follow-up peculiarities

Follow-up is carried out annually to evaluate the effectiveness of the treatment based on the reappearance of symptoms, as well as to assess the plasma sodium concentration, so that excessive administration of treatment is avoided.

Bibliographic references

1. Shlomo Melmed, Richard J. Auchus, Allison B. Goldfine, Ronald J. Kowning, Clifford Rosen. Williams Textbook of Endocrinology 14Th edition. ELSEVIER, 2020.
2. Shlomo Melmed. The Pituitary 4th Edition. Academic Press, Elsevier, 2017.

3. Ball S. Diabetes Insipidus. [Updated 2018 Jun 13]. In: Feingold KR, Anawalt B, Boyce A, et al., Editors. Endotext [Internet]. South Dartmouth (MA): MDText.com, Inc.; 2000.

Chapter 264. Primary Polydipsia

Also known as dipsogenic diabetes insipidus, it consists of a polyuria secondary to high and inappropriate fluid intake. It can be the result of a set of systemic pathologies, although it is also associated with psychiatric disorders.

Statistics and epidemiology

About 42% of patients admitted to psychiatric hospitals have some form of polydipsia. At least half of the psychiatric patients with primary polydipsia have no obvious explanation for the polydipsia.

Risk groups or factors
- ✓ Intake of drugs that cause dry mouth.
- ✓ Psychiatric disorders.
- ✓ High fluid intake habit.

Etiology or more frequent causes
- ✓ Compulsively drinking water
- ✓ Affective or psychiatric disorders.
- ✓ Drug-induced.
- ✓ Sarcoidosis of the hypothalamus.
- ✓ Craniopharyngioma.
- ✓ Peripheral disorders that increase renin and / or angiotensin.

Pathophysiological elements

High and persistent fluid intake leads to polyuria adequate to exacerbated intake. However, when the intake exceeds the limit of the renal excretion of free water it can lead to hyponatremia.

Primary polydipsia can be associated with abnormalities related to the perception of thirst:
- ✓ Inability to suppress thirst with low plasma osmolalities.
- ✓ Low thirst threshold.
- ✓ Exaggerated thirst response to osmotic challenge.

Diagnostic criteria

- ✓ The clinical picture is similar to diabetes insipidus and polyuric polyuric syndromes (See Chap. 222, 223), therefore it is recommended to indicate the pertinent tests and studies to rule out nephrogenic or central causes.
- ✓ Ask about the medications the patient is taking, evaluating those that may cause dry mouth. Offer therapeutic alternatives whenever possible.
- ✓ The water deprivation test in primary polydipsia reflects normal urinary and plasma osmolality.
- ✓ Psychiatric evaluation is recommended when it is not possible to identify organic causes that explain the polydipsia.
- ✓ The lack of thirst suppression, after drinking more than 50% of the stimulated levels, is a strong diagnostic indicator.
- ✓ Random urinary osmolality greater than 700 mOsm / Kg confirms the diagnosis of primary polydipsia.
- ✓ Magnetic resonance imaging of the hypothalamic-neurohypophyseal region. When weighted in T1, they

show a classic bright spot, corresponding to the posterior pituitary. In nephrogenic diabetes insipidus it may be absent or present, whereas it may be altered in centrally caused diabetes insipidus.

Treatment options

The therapeutic approach is aimed at reducing excessive fluid intake. Desmopressin (DDAVP) treatment is not recommended due to the high risk of hyponatraemia.

The reduction of fluids should be done in a staggered manner so that the patient can reduce the urinary volume, below the polyuric criterion (50 ml / kg body weight).

Encourage your patients to include measures to reduce dry mouth such as ice chips or hard candy to stimulate saliva flow.

Bibliographic reference

1. Shlomo Melmed, Richard J. Auchus, Allison B. Goldfine, Ronald J. Kowning, Clifford Rosen. Williams Textbook of Endocrinology 14Th edition. ELSEVIER, 2020.
2. Shlomo Melmed. The Pituitary 4th Edition. Academic Press, Elsevier, 2017.
3. Ball S. Diabetes Insipidus. [Updated 2018 Jun 13]. In: Feingold KR, Anawalt B, Boyce A, et al., Editors. Endotext [Internet]. South Dartmouth (MA): MDText.com, Inc .; 2000.

Chapter 265. Syndrome of Inappropriate ADH Secretion

Also known by the acronym SIADH, it consists of a condition characterized by the secretion or unsuppressed release of antidiuretic hormone (ADH), either by the pituitary gland or as a result of non-pituitary sources. It can also occur as a consequence of continuous action on vasopressin receptors.

Statistics and epidemiology

The incidence of SIADH increases with age. When hyponatremia is defined as less than 135 mEq / L, a prevalence between 15 to 38% is observed. SIADH is the most common cause of evolemic hypoosmolality, with a prevalence between 20% and 40% of hypoosmolar patients. Between 10-20% of patients with SIADH do not have significantly elevated plasma vasopressin concentrations.

Risk groups or factors:
- ✓ Family history of hereditary SIADH.
- ✓ Underlying endocrine disorders.
- ✓ Cancer.
- ✓ Polypharmacy.
- ✓ Drugs of abuse.

Etiology and elements of pathophysiology.

Conditions that frequently lead to SIADH		
Etiology		Pathophysiology
Central nervous system disorders	Stroke. Hemorrhage. Infection. Trauma Mental illness and psychosis.	Increased release of pituitary ADH
Neoplasms	Small cell lung cancer (SCLC). Small cell extrapulmonary carcinomas. Head and neck cancers. Olfactory neuroblastomas.	Ectopic production of ADH.
Drugs and drugs	Carbamazepine. Oxcarbazepine. Cyclophosphamide. Selective serotonin reuptake inhibitors. Chlorpropamide. Ecstasy (methylenedioxymethamphetamine). Others	Improves the release or effect of ADH.
Lung disease	Pneumonia (viral, bacterial, tuberculous). Asthma. Atelectasis Severe respiratory insufficiency. Pneumothorax.	Unknown mechanisms.
Hormonal deficiency	Hypopituitarism. Hypothyroidism	They can present with hyponatremia and a picture of SIADH

		correctable with hormone replacement
Exogenous hormonal administration	Exogenous vasopressin (as a therapy for gastrointestinal bleeding). Desmopressin (to treat von Willebrand disease, hemophilia, or others). Oxytocin (to induce labor)	Increase the activity of vasopressin-2 receptors (V2, antidiuretic)
Viral infection	Human immunodeficiency virus (HIV).	Hyponatremia secondary to AIDS, opportunistic infections, adrenal insufficiency or other.
Hereditary SIADH	Gain-of-function mutation in the renal receptor gene V2 (on the X chromosome).	Blockade of renal V2 receptors in a continuous active state, causing excessive water absorption and hyponatremia. In turn, it is resistant to vasopressin receptor antagonists.

Diagnostic criteria

Clinic	The clinical manifestations may be due to hyponatremia, as well as a reduction in osmolality. Nausea and malaise (may appear when sodium is reduced to less than 125 or 130 mEq / L). Headache, lethargy, drowsiness and can lead to seizures when sodium drops more severely. Coma or respiratory arrest (sodium less than 115 mEq / L). There may be muscle cramps, confusion, tremor, asterixis, dysarthria, Cheyne-Stokes breathing, pathological reflexes, irritability, weakness.
Schwartz and Bartter clinical criteria Serum sodium less than 135 mEq / L. Urinary sodium greater than 40 mEq / L (due to ADH-mediated free water absorption from the collecting ducts of the kidneys). Serum osmolality less than 275 mOsm / kg. Urinary osmolality greater than 100 mOsm / kg. Absence of clinical evidence of volume depletion (blood pressure within the reference range, normal skin turgor). Absence of other causes of hyponatremia (liver disease, adrenal insufficiency, heart failure, hypothyroidism, others). Hyponatremia correction due to fluid restriction.	

Treatment options

Correction and maintenance of plasma sodium correction as well as correction of underlying disorders (hypothyroidism, lung infection, among others). The goal of serum sodium correction is to maintain it at levels above 130 mEq / L.

In patients with mild to moderate symptoms, restriction of oral water intake (less than 800 mL per day) may be indicated. In case of persistent hyponatremia, administer sodium chloride as oral tablets or intravenous saline.

Diuretics such as furosemide (20 mg twice daily) can be used.

The correction with saline solution must be done with a 3% hypertonic saline solution whose osmolality is 513 mOsm / kg. This should be used when hyponatremia symptoms are severe or resistant. This is administered as a 100 ml bolus over the first 3 to 4 hours, measuring the sodium level at 2 to 3 hours to adjust the dose.

It should not exceed more than 8 mEl / L per 24 hours or between 0.5 to 1 mEq / L per hour. Faster correction could cause osmotic demyelination of the central nervous system and lead to serious and life-threatening complications such as osmotic demyelination syndrome.

Vasopressin receptor antagonists such as conivaptan (intravenous) or tolvaptan (oral) can be used.

Bibliographic references

1. Shlomo Melmed, Richard J. Auchus, Allison B. Goldfine, Ronald J. Kowning, Clifford Rosen. Williams Textbook of Endocrinology 14Th edition. ELSEVIER, 2020.
2. Lockett J, Berkman KE, Dimeski G, Russell AW, Inder WJ. Urea treatment in fluid restriction-refractory hyponatraemia. Clin. Endocrinol. (Oxf). 2019 Apr; 90 (4): 630-636

Chapter 266. Short Stature

From the clinical point of view, it is defined as short stature, the condition in which the height of a person is in the 3rd percentile according to the average height of the age, sex and population determined by the subject. The diagnosis can be established based on various anthropometric instruments and can be caused by various etiological factors.

Statistics and epidemiology

It is estimated that around 97.5% of the population have normal stature and tall stature, while it is estimated that 2.5% have short stature. However, the prevalence varies according to geographic factors.
In Saudi Arabia, the prevalence of short stature in children is estimated at 11.3% and around 1.8% in adolescents. In Jordan the prevalence of short stature was 4.9%. In Spain, a 1% prevalence of short stature in children due to malnutrition is estimated. A study in India recorded a prevalence rate of 2.86% in school-age children. Around 66.67% of the causes were genetics and constitutional growth retardation.
It can be predominant in men or women according to the population. According to a study in Argentina, the prevalence of short stature was higher in women (16.4%) than in men (8.4).

Etiology

GH-IGF1 axis disorders	GH deficiency	Hypothalamus Congenital disorders. Acquired disorders. Pituitary Congenital disorders (combined pituitary hormone deficiencies, isolated GH deficiency). Acquired disorders (neoplasms such as craniopharyngioma, histiocytosis X).
	Insensitivity to GH	Mutations in GHR signaling proteins and the acid-labile subunit (ALS).
	IGF1 receptor signaling abnormalities	
Growth disorders off the GH-IGF1 axis	Malnutrition	
	Chronic illness	
	Endocrine disorder	
	Osteochondrodysplasias	
	Chromosomal abnormalities	
	Small for gestational age	
	Maternal and placental factors	
Idiopathic short stature		

Pathophysiological elements

Each etiology has precise pathophysiological elements that lead to growth retardation or short stature. Growth disorders can be grouped into:
- ✓ Hypothalamic-pituitary axis disorders (GH deficiency).
- ✓ A disorder that causes deficiency or resistance to the action of IGF1.

- ✓ Growth disorders that especially affect the growth plate or are caused by chronic diseases.
- ✓ Idiopathic short stature (which may have a pathogenic basis on the GH-IGF1 axis or on the growth plate).

Diagnostic criteria

To establish an accurate diagnosis of short stature, a thorough medical interview is required, as well as the use of anthropometric measurements appropriate to the population and other peculiarities associated with the individual (sex, age). The diagnosis may require biochemical tests when there is suspicion of underlying disorders that explain the short stature.

Diagnostic guide

Anthropometric measures:
- ✓ The following measurements should be evaluated based on the age, sex and population of the patient.
- ✓ Measurement of the vertex of the height.
- ✓ Measurement of body weight.
- ✓ Measurement of trunk height and limb length.

Medical history:
- ✓ Evaluation of relevant antecedents (from the gestational period to birth).
- ✓ Appearance of milestones from early childhood to adolescence including the onset of puberty.
- ✓ History of illness.
- ✓ Table of nutritional diet and description of eating habits.

- ✓ Relevant family history associated with family height and development.

Psychosocial aspects: Behavioral changes; and social and family relationships.

Paraclinicals of interest:
- ✓ Biochemical evaluation of growth hormones; and in relation to blood insulin-like growth factor levels.
- ✓ Complete blood count.
- ✓ X-rays (to estimate and correlate bone age in conjunction with chronological age).
- ✓ Indicate additional studies associated with suspected genetic, nutritional, or endocrine disorders, based on the symptoms and patient history.

Treatment options

Mainly, the treatment should be aimed at correcting or treating the underlying condition of the patient that conditions the short stature. Treatment options include:
- ✓ Gonadotropin-releasing hormone analogs (in precocious puberty to allow more time before bone maturation).
- ✓ Low dose androgen therapy such as oxandrolone (increases growth potential).
- ✓ Maternal metformin (increases fetal sensitivity to insulin to enhance development by utilizing glucose).
- ✓ Aromatase inhibitors (reduces the conversion of androgens to estrogens, androstenedione to estrone, and testosterone to estradiol to achieve pubertal delay).

- ✓ Recombinant C-natriuretic peptide (increases growth rate in the treatment of achondroplasia).

Growth hormone treatment

Indication GH deficiency	Dose (mg / kg / week)
Pre-pubertal children	0.16 to 0.35
Puberal	0.16 to 0.70
GH-deficient adults	0.04 to 0.08
Turner syndrome	0.375
Chronic renal insufficiency	0.35
Prader-Willi syndrome	0.24
Idiopathic short stature	0.3 to 0.37
SHOX deficiency	0.35
Noonan syndrome	0.23 to 0.46

Follow-up peculiarities

Follow-up conditions during GH replacement therapy should be carried out in the long term, following the following recommendations:

Parameters	Evaluation
Bone age	Measure at 12-month intervals to assess target height.
Thyroid function test	Measurement at 12-month intervals. It should be measured immediately when identifying reduction in growth rate.
Plasma IGF1 and IGBP-3	Measurement every 12 months. The goal is to keep the IGF1 level within the normal midrange.
Metabolic panel (ESR, CBC, HbA1C).	Perform every 12 months.

Dose adjustment	Based on weight, response to treatment, IGF1 level, comparison with the desired height and pubertal stage.

Bibliographic references

1. Shlomo Melmed, Richard J. Auchus, Allison B. Goldfine, Ronald J. Kowning, Clifford Rosen. Williams Textbook of Endocrinology 14Th edition. ELSEVIER, 2020 ..
2. Lavin N, editor. Manual of endocrinology and metabolism. 4th ed. Philadelphia: Wolters Kluwer / Lippincott Williams & Wilkins Health; 2009. 837 p.
3. Rani D, Shrestha R, Kanchan T, et al. Short Stature. [Updated 2020 Apr 15]. In: StatPearls [Internet]. Treasure Island (FL): StatPearls Publishing; 2020 Jan-.
4. Ergun-Longmire B, Wajnrajch MP. Growth and Growth Disorders. [Updated 2018 Jul 14]. In: Feingold KR, Anawalt B, Boyce A, et al., Editors. Endotext

Chapter 267. GH Deficiency in the Child

It is the most frequent pituitary hormonal deficiency in pediatric age. This can be found in isolation or accompanied by a deficiency of another type of pituitary hormone. GH deficiency in children is associated with abnormally slow growth and short stature while maintaining proper body proportions.

Statistics and epidemiology

Short stature occurs in 2.5% of children. The prevalence of GH deficiency in children is estimated to be around 1 in 4,000 to 1 in 10,000 children. Relative deficit cases are more common. GH resistance is a relatively low cause of growth retardation.

Risk groups or factors:
- ✓ Exposure to more than 30 Gy of radiation at the cranial level.
- ✓ Head injuries.
- ✓ Family history of hypopituitarism.
- ✓ History of brain tumor.
- ✓ Incidental finding of pituitary abnormalities by magnetic resonance imaging.
- ✓ History of organic pituitary alteration.

Etiology or more frequent causes

Structural abnormalities of the pituitary and hypothalamic region (holoprosencephaly, septo-optic dysplasia).
Genetic defects in pituitary development or GH release.

Acquired lesions of the hypothalamic-pituitary region (tumors such as craniopharyngioma, inflammatory infiltrates such as sarcoidosis, histiocytosis, among others, trauma, radiation and chemotherapy.
Idiopathic deficit.
GH neurosecretory dysfunction.

Pathophysiological elements

The synthesis and release of growth hormone is carried out through the intervention of a hypothalamic neuropeptide known as growth hormone releasing hormone or GHRH. This hypothalamic hormone is controlled by neurochemicals which mediate the neuroendocrine control of growth hormone biosynthesis. However, all those functional or hypothalamic developmental abnormalities, as well as genetic or acquired disorders, can cause impaired neuroendocrine control and trigger hypopituitarism, and as a result, impairment of GH synthesis and release. In turn, GH deficiency triggers a set of metabolic and growth disorders, characteristic of the clinical manifestations of the syndrome.

Diagnostic criteria

Clinic	Clinical manifestations and auxology constitute the main factors for diagnosis. Height below the 3rd percentile. Growth speed: Less than 6 cm per year before the age of 4. Less than 5 cm per year between 4 and 8 years. Less than 4 cm per year before puberty. Normal body proportion between the limbs and upper and lower body segments.

	Height less than 1.5 standard deviations (SD) below the mean height of the parents. Height less than 2 SD below average. Other clinical manifestations may occur depending on the underlying cause of the deficiency. Signs of intracranial injury. Signs of multiple pituitary deficiency. Neonatal manifestations / hypoglycemia, prolonged jaundice, craniofacial midline alteration, microcephalus).
Paraclinical	Skeletal maturation (assessed by bone age determination) is greater than 2 years behind chronological age. Measurement of IGF1 and IGFBP-3 levels (they should be interpreted based on bone age rather than chronological age). Growth hormone challenge test. You should not rely on this test as the sole criterion. GH secretion test (can be omitted when a clear risk factor associated with significant GH deficiency is identified). Two tests must be performed: Maximum GH in both tests is less than 10 ng / ml (perform evaluation of the pituitary by MRI, tests in the neonate). GH greater than 10 and height less than -2.25 SD, GH treatment will be considered for idiopathic short stature. Other relevant studies: Thyroid function tests. Neuroendocrinological tests Complete blood count. Creatinine and sedimentation rate. Magnetic resonance Genetic testing (performed when there is a family history associated with GH deficiency). Indicate relevant biochemical studies based on clinical suspicions associated with the underlying cause of growth retardation.

Treatment options

Recombinant GH supplementation, which is indicated for all children with short stature and documented GH deficiency. The dose is administered subcutaneously. Starting dose of 0.16 to 0.24 mg per kg body weight per week.

The increase in height velocity is 10 to 12 cm of growth per year (during the first year), it often decreases, although it remains above the growth rate prior to the start of treatment. It is recommended that GH treatment does not continue beyond achieving growth rate below 2 to 2.5 cm per year.

Follow-up peculiarities

Long-term follow-up should be established with regular assessment of anthropometric measurements and pertinent paraclinics associated with risk factors.

Bibliographic reference

1. Lavin N, editor. Manual of endocrinology and metabolism. 4th ed. Philadelphia: Wolters Kluwer / Lippincott Williams & Wilkins Health; 2009. 837 p.
2. Shlomo Melmed, Richard J. Auchus, Allison B. Goldfine, Ronald J. Kowning, Clifford Rosen. Williams Textbook of Endocrinology 14Th edition. ELSEVIER, 2020.
3. Grimberg A., DiVall SA, Polychronakos C., Allen DB, et al, on behalf of the Drug and Therapeutics Committee and Ethics Committee of the Pediatric Endocrine Society.Hormone and Insulin-Like Growth Factor-I

Treatment in Children and Adolescents: Growth Hormone Deficiency, Idiopathic Short Stature, and Primary Insulin-Like Growth Factor-I Deficiency. Horm Res Paediatr 2016; 86: 361-397.

Chapter 268. GH Deficiency in the Adult

It consists of a clinical condition characterized by a reduction in the body's muscle mass, in conjunction with a reduction in bone mineral density (BMD) in the presence of an increase in visceral adiposity and an alteration of the lipid profile.

Growth hormone (GH) or somatotropin deficiency can cause an increased cardiovascular risk in adults and an increased risk of mortality from cerebrovascular and heart diseases. Growth hormone is produced in the anterior pituitary and is stimulated or inhibited by hypothalamic somatostatin. So GH deficiency in adults can be caused by a group of disorders.

Statistics and epidemiology

About 6,000 adults are diagnosed with GH deficiency each year in the United States.

It is estimated that around 1 in 100,000 people per year is affected with GH deficiency and at least 2 cases per 100,000 people per year when considering patients with GH deficiency beginning in childhood.

Approximately 15-20% of cases occur as a transition from GH deficiency in childhood to adulthood.

The age of onset of acquired GH deficiency in adults often coincides with the finding of pituitary neoplasms. The most common age is usually between the fourth and fifth decade of life.

Risk factors:
- ✓ Cancer.
- ✓ Family history of GH deficiency.
- ✓ Head injury.
- ✓ Intracranial surgery.
- ✓ Head radiation therapy.

Etiology

Causes of growth hormone deficiency in adults.

Acquired:
Pituitary neoplasms: the main causes are due to pituitary adenoma and craniopharyngioma.
Infiltrative diseases (sarcoidosis, tuberculosis, histiocytosis).
Infarction of the pituitary or hypothalamus.
Head injury.
Metastasis.
Pituitary or hypothalamic surgery or radiation therapy.
Congenital conditions:
Genetic abnormalities: GH-releasing hormone receptor gene defects, transcription factor defects (PIT-1, PROP-1, LHX3 / 4, HESX-1, PITX-2).
Structural brain defects: structural abnormalities include agenesis of the corpus callosum, empty sella syndrome, hydrocele, among others.
Idiopathic

Pathophysiological elements

GH is synthesized and secreted by somatotropic cells found in the anterior pituitary. This hormone is responsible for regulating complex physiological processes, among which the control of growth metabolism stands out.

GH is regulated by the stimulation of the GH-releasing hormone, in the same way, ghrelin, a peptide hormone secreted in the stomach, binds to the receptors of the somatotropic cells of the pituitary and stimulates the secretion of GH. For its part, its secretion is inhibited by the hypothalamic peptide known as somatostatin.

Disorders that cause alteration in the synthesis and release of GH can trigger a deficit of this hormone and cause a series of clinical manifestations. Each cause contains specific pathophysiological elements that lead to the deficiency.

Diagnostic criteria.

| Clinic | Some patients are asymptomatic. Memory changes and processing speed as well as attention. Emotional instability. Sleep disorders. Depression and anxiety. Fatigue. Decreased strength. Fibromyalgia Central adiposity. Neuromuscular dysfunction. Decreased sensitivity to insulin. Decreased bone density. Decreased sweating and thermoregulation. Decreased social contact. Reduced libido. Weight gain. Plaques of atheroma in the arteries. Impaired cardiac function. Increase in blood pressure. There may be signs of other pituitary deficiencies. |

Paraclinical	Increase in low-density lipoproteins. Increased inflammation markers such as C-reactive protein. Insulin tolerance test: GH peak measurement of 3 μg / L or less indicates severe deficiency. Optimal limit for GH of 5.1 μg / L. Growth hormone releasing hormone and arginine test combined. Glucagon stimulation test. Growth hormone-releasing peptide 2: a cutoff value of 3 μg / L represents severe GH deficiency, while a value of 5 μg / L defines GH deficiency. Clonidine. Levodopa Arginine plus levodopa. Other auxiliary diagnostic tests can be used such as: IGF-1. IGF-BP3. Magnetic resonance imaging (useful to detect intracranial etiology).

Treatment and follow-up options

Growth hormone replacement treatment

Initial dose between 30 to 60 years: 300 μg / day. This can increase from 100 to 200 μg every 1 to 2 months.

Patients under 30 years of age can obtain greater benefits with higher doses, between 400 to 500 μg / day. The dose may be higher in patients initiating transition from pediatric treatment to adult dose.

The dose in adults over 60 years of age may be lower. The initial dose of these starts between 100 to 200 μg and can be increased according to need, but with smaller increments.

Once the appropriate maintenance dose has been obtained, regular monitoring should be established at 3 to 6 month intervals. In these controls it must be verified that the concentration of IGF-1 is appropriate for the age. In addition, follow-up visits should include a complete clinical assessment and observation of treatment side effects, assessment of lipid profile, fasting blood glucose, determination of cortisol, T4 and TSH. IF indicated, assess bone mineral density.

Bibliographic references

1. Shlomo Melmed, Richard J. Auchus, Allison B. Goldfine, Ronald J. Kowning, Clifford Rosen. Williams Textbook of Endocrinology 14Th edition. ELSEVIER, 2020.
2. Lavin N, editor. Manual of endocrinology and metabolism. 4th ed. Philadelphia: Wolters Kluwer / Lippincott Williams & Wilkins Health; 2009. 837 p.
3. Gupta V. (2011). Adult growth hormone deficiency. Indian journal of endocrinology and metabolism, 15 Suppl 3 (Suppl3), S197 – S202. https://doi.org/10.4103/2230-8210.84865.

Chapter 269. Secondary Adrenal Insufficiency

It refers to the reduction of the stimulation of the adrenal cortex by adrenocorticotropic hormone (ACTH), without alteration of aldosterone levels. The main causes of this disorder are traumatic brain injuries and panhypopituitarism.

Statistics and epidemiology

It occurs more frequently than primary adrenal insufficiency. Secondary adrenal insufficiency is more common in men than in women. The age of diagnosis occurs most frequently in the sixth decade of life. Its prevalence is estimated to be between 150 to 280 cases per million people.

Risk groups or factors
- ✓ Family history of secondary adrenal insufficiency.
- ✓ Head radiation therapy.
- ✓ Intracranial surgery.
- ✓ Intracranial neoplasms.

Etiology and pathophysiological element

Disease	Pathogenic element
Trauma or space occupying injuries	
Pituitary tumor (craniopharyngioma, adenoma, meningioma,	

carcinoma)	
Trauma (injury to the pituitary stalk).	Decreased ACTH secretion
Pituitary surgery or irradiation	
Infections or infiltrative processes (hemochromatosis, meningitis, tuberculosis, others)	
Pituitary apoplexy	
Sheehan syndrome	
Genetic disorders	
Transcription factors associated with pituitary development	
HESX homeobox1	HESX1 gene mutation.
Prader-Willi syndrome (PWS).	Deletion or silencing of genes in the imprinting center for PWS.
Orthodentical Homeobox 2	Mutation of the OTX2 gene.
Congenital proopiomelanocortin deficiency	POMC gene mutation.
LIM homeobox 4	LHX4 gene mutation
SRY (region Y that determines sex) - box 3	SOX3 gene mutation
T-box 19	TBX19 gene mutation.

ACTH deficiency leads to reduced secretion of adrenal cortisol and androgens. However, normal mineralocorticoid production is maintained.

In the early stages, basal ACTH secretion is normal, however, ACTH secretion in response to stress is impaired. As the loss of basal ACTH secretion progresses, atrophy of the zona fasciculata and reticularis of the cortex of the adrenal glands occurs, and as a consequence reduces basal cortisol secretion, preserving the release of aldosterone by the zona glomerulosa.

Diagnostic criteria

Clinic	The clinical manifestations are similar to the primary ones: vomiting, anorexia, weight loss, fatigue, abdominal pain, edema, loss of libido, skin atrophy, stretch marks, muscle atrophy, among others (see Chapter 184).
	However, since there is no increase in ACTH, hyperpigmentation does not occur in the skin.
	Since the zona glomerulosa continues to secrete mineralocorticoids, there is no dehydration or hyperkalemia, and hypotension is mild.
	Hypoglycemia is more common in secondary adrenal insufficiency.
	There may be additional clinical manifestations depending on the underlying cause, for example, in the case of neoplasms, visual defects and headaches may occur.
Paraclinical	You can conduct detailed studies in Chapter 184.
	Baseline morning serum cortisol concentration: low.
	ACTH levels: low or low normal.
	Stimulation test with standard dose of ACTH: level less than 18 or 20 mcg / dl. However, if it is performed in the early stages of the disease, and glandular atrophy has not occurred, it can produce a normal response to stimulation.
	Low-dose ACTH stimulation test.
	Insulin-induced hypoglycemia test.
	Other studies to consider
	MRI of the hypothalamus and pituitary gland.

Treatment options

- ✓ Treatment consists of treating the underlying cause whenever possible.
- ✓ Glucocorticoid replacement therapy (See Chapter 185).
- ✓ Replacement of other hormonal deficits in the anterior pituitary may be necessary.
- ✓ On rare occasions, mineralocorticoid replacement is required (See Chapter 186).

Bibliographic references

1. Shlomo Melmed, Richard J. Auchus, Allison B. Goldfine, Ronald J. Kowning, Clifford Rosen. Williams Textbook of Endocrinology 14Th edition. ELSEVIER, 2020.
2. Nicolaides NC, Chrousos GP, Charmandari E. Adrenal Insufficiency. [Updated 2017 Oct 14]. In: Feingold KR, Anawalt B, Boyce A, et al., Editors.Endotext. South Dartmouth (MA): MDText.com, Inc .; 2000-.

Chapter 270. Secondary Hypothyroidism

It consists of a decrease in thyroid hormones as a result of insufficient stimulation by thyroid stimulating hormone (TSH) in a normal thyroid gland. The term central hypothyroidism is often used to refer to hypothyroidism caused by hypothalamic or pituitary disorders, especially when a clear distinction of the etiologic agent cannot be established, but centrally-caused TSH deficiency has been confirmed.

Statistics and epidemiology

It is estimated that its prevalence is around 1 case per 80,000 people up to 1 case per 120,000 people, being a relatively rare condition. There is no incidence preference between the female and male sex.

Risk groups or factors:

- ✓ Personal history of intracranial surgery.
- ✓ Head injury.
- ✓ Cancer.
- ✓ Infiltrative diseases.
- ✓ Family history of secondary hypothyroidism.
- ✓ Head radiation therapy.

Etiology or more frequent causes

Neoplasms	Pituitary adenoma. Meningioma. Craniopharyngioma.

	Metastasis. Dysgerminoma. Rathke cysts and other cystic mass lesions.
Infiltrative	Sarcoidosis Histiocytosis X. Eosinophilic granuloma.
Traumatic	Radiation. Head injury.
Infectious	Virus. Fungal infections Tuberculosis.
Vascular	Hemorrhage. Pituitary apoplexy. Stem disruption. Aneurysm. Subarachnoid hemorrhage. Sheehan syndrome.
Genetic defects	Pituitary-specific transcription factor defects (HESX1, LHX3, PROP-1, PIT-1). Isolated TRH deficiency. Mutation in the TSH (beta) subunit gene: G29R mutation in axon 2, nonsense mutation in the thyroid stimulating hormone beta subunit gene. Inactivating mutation in the TRH receptor gene. Biologically inactive TSH isoforms.
Transient central hypothyroidism	Sick euthyroid syndrome. Excessive T4 replacement in primary hypothyroidism.
Iatrogenic	Post-external radiation therapy. Post-pituitary surgery.

Pathophysiological elements

Hypothalamic disorders are able to reduce the adequate secretion of TSH and thus alter the production or transport of TRH to the pituitary gland.

Hypothyroidism may be the result of insufficient TSH secreted by the pituitary with an abnormal glycosylation pattern, resulting in decreased biological activity of TSH.

Cases whose etiology is due to congenital disorders are due to structural lesions, for example, midline defects, pituitary hypoplasia, Rathke's bag cysts, or functional disorders in TSH biosynthesis and release.

In adults, however, it is frequently due to the development of pituitary macroadenomas or as a consequence of previous surgeries or pituitary irradiations.

Diagnostic criteria

Clinic	The clinical manifestations are similar to the clinical presentation of primary hypothyroidism, although they tend to be milder (See Chapter 118). Some of these are: Slowdown of body metabolism. Weight gain. Increase in body fat. Retention of liquid and salt. In children: short stature, growth retardation and / or bone maturation. Variations in clinical manifestations associated with the underlying cause may occur.
Paraclinical	Increase in serum cholesterol. Serum T3, T4 and TSH. Measurement of T4 in series. TRH stimulation test: TRH is measured and then serum TSH is measured serially at 20 to 60 meters (the use of 180 tm can be used). The normal response is considered when the TSH value is between 20 and 60 mt of TSH. A flat response is observed in pituitary disease, as well as a delayed response with a value of 60 mt higher than the value of 20 mt as can be observed in hypothalamic disease.

	Other biochemical markers.
	Negative antithyroid antibodies.
	Sex hormone binding proteins.
	Angiotensin Converting Enzyme.
	Carboxyl-terminal telopeptide of type 1 collagen.
	Bone hypoglycemic agent protein.
	Serum soluble IL-2 receptors.
	Imaging studies:
	Magnetic resonance.
	Computed tomography.

Treatment options

Hormone replacement of TRH and TSH is not considered the treatment of choice due to high costs and limited applicability.

Hormone replacement with levothyroxine (treatment of choice). Recommended dose:

Children: starting dose of 10 to 15 µg / kg per day, or 50 µg per day (for infants between 3 and 4.5 kg in weight).

Adults: 1.6 mcg / kg per day.

Older age: 1 mcg / kg per day

Follow-up peculiarities

Infant therapy should be monitored at 4-6 week intervals for the first 6 months, then every 2-3 months for ages 6-24 months.

Follow-up is done every 3 to 6 months starting at 2 years of age.

Bibliographic references

1. Shlomo Melmed, Richard J. Auchus, Allison B. Goldfine, Ronald J. Kowning, Clifford Rosen. Williams

Textbook of Endocrinology 14Th edition. ELSEVIER, 2020.
2. Shlomo Melmed. The Pituitary 4th Edition. AcademicPress, Elsevier, 2017.
3. Gupta, V., & Lee, M. (2011). Central hypothyroidism. Indian journal of endocrinology and metabolism, 15 (Suppl 2), S99 – S106. https://doi.org/10.4103/2230-8210.83337

Chapter 271. Secondary Hypogonadism

Hypogonadism consists of an absolute or relative androgen deficiency state. Secondary or hypogonadotropic hypogonadism occurs due to decreased GnRH or LH production.

Statistics and epidemiology

Prader-Willi syndrome and Angelman syndrome have a prevalence of 1 case per 20,000 people and are characterized by a combination of secondary hypogonadism, hypotonia, and hyposmia, among other manifestations.

The majority of patients with a pituitary base for secondary hypogonadism show an expansive lesion on MRI or have hyperprolactinemia.

Kallman syndrome has a prevalence of 1 in 10,000 men.

Together with primary hypogonadism, it is responsible for 80 to 90% of the causes of male infertility.

Risk groups or factors:

- ✓ Family history of congenital hypopituitarism.
- ✓ Family history of secondary hypogonadism.
- ✓ Personal history of intracranial surgery.
- ✓ Head injury.
- ✓ Infiltrative disease.
- ✓ HIV infection.
- ✓ Morbid obesity.
- ✓ Drug or drug use (opioids, glucocorticoids, medroxyprogesterone acetate, others).

Etiology or more frequent causes

- ✓ Kallman syndrome.
- ✓ Human immunodeficiency virus.
- ✓ Surgery.
- ✓ Head injury.
- ✓ Stress-induced hypogonadism.
- ✓ Hyperprolactinomas.
- ✓ Isolated hypogonadotropic hypogonadism.
- ✓ Pituitary adenomas.
- ✓ Hemochromatosis, thalassemias.
- ✓ Prader-Willi syndrome.
- ✓ Hypopituitarism.
- ✓ Secondary GnRH deficiency (drugs, drugs, toxins, systemic diseases.

Pathophysiological elements

The signaling from the pituitary via LH or from the hypothalamus via GnRH to the testes is inadequate such that it cannot adequately stimulate testosterone production in Leydig cells.

Diagnostic criteria

Clinic	Signs and symptoms associated with androgen deficiency: Reduction of testicular volume. Decreased body hair. Gynecomastia Male factor infertility. Decrease in lean mass. Decreased muscle strength. Visceral obesity.

		Insulin resistance
		Loss of libido
		Decreased sexual activity.
		Erectile dysfunction.
		Decreased nocturnal erections.
		Hot flushes.
		Humor changes.
		Fatigue.
		Sleep disorders.
		Depression.
		Reduction of cognitive function.
		According to the underlying cause, additional clinical manifestations may occur, for example, deficiency of other pituitary hormones, headache, visual disturbances, among others.
	Paraclinical	Screen male patients with HIV infection, end-stage kidney disease, infertility, type 2 diabetes mellitus, osteoporosis, or COPD.
		Androgen deficiency test in older men (ADAM): a 10-item questionnaire designed to identify men with clinical testosterone deficiency.
		Serum testosterone measurements (2 measurements must be taken).
		FSH, LH test.
		Prolactin test.
		TSH and T4.
		Vitamin D.
		Complete blood count.
		Complete metabolic panel (patients often have metabolic syndrome).
		Iron, transferrin.
		Cortisol level.
		Measurement of sex hormone transport globulin.

Treatment options

Treatment consists of administering testosterone replacement therapy: intramuscular injections of testosterone with testosterone enanthate or testosterone cypionate. The dose to be administered ranges from 50 to 100 mg per week. A therapy of 100 to 200 mg every two weeks may also be considered.

Currently, there is an extra long-acting injectable form of testosterone (testosterone undecanoate), which is administered at a starting dose of 750 mg, followed by a second dose at 4 weeks. However, it is not recommended as a first-line treatment.

Follow-up peculiarities

Before treatment (pre-treatment) should be checked Hgb, HCT, DRE (digital rectal exam), two early morning testosterone levels, PSA level.

One month after starting testosterone treatment, a new morning testosterone level study should be requested.

After 3 to 6 months from the start of treatment, the studies indicated in the pre-treatment are performed again, and liver function tests and lipid profile are added.

The follow-up is carried out annually, requesting pertinent biochemical studies.

Bibliographic references

1. Shlomo Melmed. The Pituitary 4th Edition. AcademicPress, Elsevier, 2017.

2. Lavin N, editor. Manual of endocrinology and metabolism. 4th ed. Philadelphia: Wolters Kluwer / Lippincott Williams & Wilkins Health; 2009. 837 p.
3. Shlomo Melmed, Richard J. Auchus, Allison B. Goldfine, Ronald J. Kowning, Clifford Rosen. Williams Textbook of Endocrinology 14Th edition. ELSEVIER, 2020.

Chapter 272. Panhypopituitarism

Panhypopituitarism or hypopituitarism consists of the deficiency of one or more hormones produced by the pituitary gland. That is, hypopituitarism refers to the total or partial insufficiency of the secretion of hormones from the anterior, posterior or both pituitary glands. It can occur as a result of multiple etiologies, either from acquired or congenital causes.

Statistics and epidemiology

Given the diversity of conditions associated with this type of hormonal deficiency, the data are limited in relation to the frequency rate. Among the most common causes, the presence of pituitary tumors stands out.

In the United States, it is considered a rare disorder. It is estimated that in Spain it has a prevalence of 45.5 cases per 100,000 inhabitants.

GH deficiency is estimated to have a prevalence of approximately 9 cases per 1000 people in some pediatric populations. The frequency of congenital TSH deficiency is estimated to be 1 case in every 29,000 live births.

Risk groups or factors:
- ✓ Cancer.
- ✓ Head injury.
- ✓ Infections
- ✓ Family history of congenital hypopituitarism.
- ✓ History of cranial radiation therapy.

Etiology

Congenital	Single or multiple pituitary hormone deficiency	PIT-1, PROP-1, HESX-1, SOX2 mutations.
	Isolated pituitary hormone deficiency	DAX-1, KAL, GH-1, GnRH, TRH receptor mutations. Bardet-Biedl syndromes, Prader-Willi syndrome
Neoplasia	Perhypophyseal tumors	Craniopharyngioma, glioma, meningioma, Rathke cleft cyst, germ cell tumor, metastasis (mainly lung, kidney, breast), Langerhans cell histiocytosis.
	Pituitary adenoma	Working or not working
Infection	Tuberculosis, syphilis, mycosis	
Vascular	Heart attack	Pituitary apoplexy, aneurysm, Sheehan syndrome.
Inflammatory, infiltrative, immunological	Sarcoidosis, lymphocytic hypophysitis, giant cell granuloma, Wegener's granulomatosis, hemochromatosis, CTLA-4 inhibitors.	
Post-radiation	Pituitary, nasopharyngeal, cranial	
Other	Empty sella turcica, cerebrovascular injury, post-surgery.	

Pathophysiological elements

The hypofunction of the pituitary gland can be the result of a disorder of the gland itself, such as occurring due to a hypothalamic disorder. In both cases, the secretion of the pituitary hormones is reduced and according to the type of injury, disorder or extension, a decrease in one or more of the pituitary hormones may occur, causing the organic manifestations attributed to the deficiency:

- ✓ TSH deficiency causes hypothyroidism without a goiter.
- ✓ LH FSH deficiency causes hypogonadism.
- ✓ ACTH deficiencies cause adrenal insufficiency and poor skin pigmentation.
- ✓ PRL deficiency causes absence of puerperal lactation.
- ✓ GH deficiency causes short stature and fasting hypoglycemia.

Diagnostic criteria:

Hormonal deficit	Form of presentation	Clinical presentation
Adrenocorticotrophic hormone	Acute	Weakness, dizziness, nausea, vomiting, fatigue, absence of hyperkalemia. Similar to Addison's disease, but without the lack of hyperpigmentation.
	chronic	Myalgia, hypoglycemia, anorexia, nausea, tiredness, paleness, weight loss.
Thyroid stimulating hormone	Children	Growth retardation
	Adults	Cold intolerance, constipation, weight gain, slow relaxing reflexes, dry skin, fatigue.
Gonadotropins	Children	Delayed puberty
	mens	Altered fertility, decreased muscle mass and strength, decreased libido, decreased bone mass, decreased erythropoiesis, fine wrinkles, testicular hypotrophy, hair

		reduction.
	Woman	Infertility, amenorrhea, oligomenorrhea, loss of libido, fine wrinkles, dyspareunia, breast atrophy, osteoporosis, premature atherosclerosis.
Growth hormone	Children	Short stature, growth retardation, increased adiposity.
	Adults	Increased cardiovascular risk, increased central obesity, reduced lean mass, reduced exercise capacity, impaired psychological well-being
Antidiuretic hormone	Polydipsia, polyuria, including nocturnal presentation.	
Prolactin	Lack of breastfeeding	

Paraclinical

- ✓ Baseline serum hormonal measurements.
- ✓ Dynamic tests for the diagnosis of partial deficiencies.
- ✓ Insulin tolerance test.
- ✓ Modern combined test.
- ✓ Imaging tests (gadolinium-enhancement MRI).

Initial investigation of pituitary function
Adrenocortical axis: measure morning serum cortisol. Thyroid axis: Measure TSH and Free T4. Gonadal axis: Men: testosterone (fasting at 9:00 am), SHBG, albumin, LH and FSH. Women: estradiol, LH and FSH, progesterone (if you are menstruating on day 21). Prolactin

Insulin-like growth factor-1, GH.
Paired osmolality of plasma and urine.

Treatment options

Treatment depends on the cause of the panhypopituitarism, as well as the type of deficiency caused. The main treatment is to address the underlying cause.

Hormone replacement therapy

Hormonal deficiency	Description
ACTH deficiency	Hydrocortisone in doses of 10 mg to 20 mg (morning) and 5 to 10 mg (night).
TSH deficiency	Levothyroxine start with a low dose at 25 ug / day and then increase doses according to need.
FSH / LH deficiency	In women: oral, transdermal or intramuscular estrogen or progesterone replacement therapy. In men: testosterone replacement therapy. Human chorionic gonadotropin therapy can be added to improve fertility.
GH deficiency	If replacement therapy is required, synthetic GH is used and titrated based on IGF1 levels. Long-term follow-up should be established.
ADH deficiency	Intranasal desmopressin.

Follow-up peculiarities

According to the cause and the deficiency triggered, the appropriate follow-up will be established, individualizing the patient according to their particular requirements.

Bibliographic references

1. Shlomo Melmed, Richard J. Auchus, Allison B. Goldfine, Ronald J. Kowning, Clifford Rosen. Williams Textbook of Endocrinology 14Th edition. ELSEVIER, 2020.
2. Lavin N, editor. Manual of endocrinology and metabolism. 4th ed. Philadelphia: Wolters Kluwer / Lippincott Williams & Wilkins Health; 2009. 837 p.
3. Shlomo Melmed. The Pituitary 4th Edition. Academic Press, Elsevier, 2017.
4. Chung TT, Koch CA, Monson JP. Hypopituitarism. [Updated 2018 Jul 25]. In: Feingold KR, Anawalt B, Boyce A, et al., Editors. Endotext [Internet]. South Dartmouth (MA): MDText.com, Inc .; 2000-.

Chapter 273. Sheehan Syndrome

It is also known as postpartum pituitary necrosis. It is the necrosis of the cells of the anterior pituitary gland after a significant postpartum hemorrhage, hypovolemia and shock.

Statistics and epidemiology

It is a rare syndrome in developed countries. In India, a prevalence of around 3% is estimated for women over 20 years of age. Some countries have an incidence of Sheehan syndrome of 5 cases per 100,000 births. In Iceland the prevalence is estimated to be around 5.1 cases per 100,000 women. The chronic form is more common than the acute form.

Etiology

It occurs when the anterior pituitary gland is damaged as a result of significant blood loss during postpartum. As a result of this blood loss, the pituitary gland fails to produce pituitary hormones.

Pathophysiological elements

During pregnancy, pituitary hyperplasia occurs mainly due to the increase in lactotrophic cells in the anterior pituitary gland. This hyperplasia causes an increase in the nutritional and metabolic demand of the anterior pituitary, however, the pituitary glandular blood supply does not increase. Since the pituitary irrigation consists of a relatively low pressure system, it is theorized that in conjunction with significant postpartum hemorrhage, the cells of the anterior pituitary become more vulnerable to ischemia.

As a consequence of ischemia, necrosis of anterior pituitary cells occurs and can lead to selective loss of some pituitary function or to panhypopituitarism with loss of many pituitary functions.

Diagnostic criteria

Clinical manifestation	
Acute form	Chronic form
Nausea and vomiting	Dry Skin.
Hypotension	Daze.
Extreme fatigue	Loss of libido
Hypoglycemia	Lack of breastfeeding.
Lack of growth of shaved pubic hair	Fatigue
Tachycardia	Persistent amenorrhea
Lack of breastfeeding	Nausea and vomiting
	Cold intolerance

Chronic clinical presentation may take months or years after the initial event of hypovolemia and shock before manifesting. However, the acute form is considered dangerous when it occurs if it is not recognized and treated quickly.

Paraclinical
- ✓ Complete blood count with differential count.
- ✓ Basic metabolic profile.
- ✓ Thyroid function tests (TSH, T3 and T4).

- ✓ FSH and LH.
- ✓ Prolactin levels.
- ✓ Cortisol levels.
- ✓ Estrogen level.
- ✓ Growth hormone level.

The finding of an alteration in the hormonal level associated with the anterior pituitary, together with the clinical history of postpartum hemorrhage, could suggest Sheehan syndrome.

Imaging tests: Request an MRI evaluation of the pituitary to confirm the diagnosis. About 70% may have an empty sella turcica and about 30% have a partially empty sella.

Treatment options

The basis of treatment consists of hormone replacement of the deficient hormones as a lifelong treatment. Each hormonal deficiency of the anterior pituitary will be addressed in the corresponding chapter. In rare cases, there may be involvement of the posterior pituitary, so a complete investigation of the recent clinical presentation of the patient is recommended.

Follow-up peculiarities:

According to the hormonal deficiency caused by Sheehan's syndrome, a specific follow-up should be carried out based on the evaluation of the effectiveness of replacement therapy and dose adjustment, as well as the evaluation of side effects to the treatment.

Bibliographic references

1. Shlomo Melmed, Richard J. Auchus, Allison B. Goldfine, Ronald J. Kowning, Clifford Rosen. Williams Textbook of Endocrinology 14Th edition. ELSEVIER, 2020.
2. Shivaprasad C. (2011). Sheehan's syndrome: Newer advances. Indian journal of endocrinology and metabolism, 15 Suppl 3 (Suppl3), S203 – S207.https://doi.org/10.4103/2230-8210.84869
3. Karaca Z, Laway BA, Dokmetas HS, Atmaca H, Kelestimur F. Sheehan syndrome. Nat Rev Dis Primers. 2016 Dec 22; 2: 16092.

Chapter 274. Craniopharyngioma

They are benign tumors of the central nervous system. These neoplasms usually originate in the suprasellar area of the brain and spread to involve the hypothalamus, optic chiasm, cranial nerves, and major blood vessels. They are considered a therapeutic challenge due to their location and ability to infiltrate adjacent structures and can cause significant neuroendocrine dysfunction.

Statistics and epidemiology

- ✓ They have an incidence between 0.5 to 2 cases per million people per year.
- ✓ They can appear at any age. However, it is considered a pediatric disease representing between 5% and 15% of intracranial tumors in this age group.
- ✓ About 25% are diagnosed in people over the age of 25.
- ✓ It has a classic bimodal age distribution.
- ✓ Incidence rate increased between 5 to 14 years and 50 to 74 years.
- ✓ There is no distinction between gender, race, or geographic location.
- ✓ They have a 50% recurrence rate.
- ✓ The 5-year survival is 83 to 96% and the 10-year survival is between 65 to 100%.

Etiology and pathophysiological elements

It presents as adamantinomatous tumors and contains cystic component filled with cloudy fluid with abundant cholesterol as a solid component. It is characterized by organized epithelial cells. Most adamantinomatous craniopharyngiomas present mutations in genes that encode β-catenin (CTNNB1 and APC)

The papillary variety appear in adults and present as solid tumors with less cystic or calcification probability. Papillary craniopharyngiomas have BRAF V600E mutations.

Craniopharyngiomas are the result of modifications or metaplastic changes in remnants of vestigial epithelial cells, which originate in the craniopharyngeal duct or Rathke's bursa during fetal development.

The clinical manifestation develops due to massive intracranial injury and increased intracranial pressure.

Diagnostic criteria

Clinic	Signs of endocrine dysfunction (80 to 90%): the main endocrine deficiency is GH and gonadotropins, another frequent manifestation is TSH and ACTH deficiency and the development of diabetes insipidus. Visual symptoms (62-84%): The most common is temporal hemianopia. Headache (50%). Obesity. Body temperature imbalances.
Paraclinical	Perform pertinent biochemical paraclinical tests to identify endocrine deficiencies. *Magnetic resonance:* it is considered the standard of

> care. Make T1-weighted thin coronal and sagittal slices in the sella turcica and suprasellar regions. The image should be obtained before and after contrast administration.
> Also useful are T2-weighted images with liquid attenuation inversion recovery. These can further delineate the cysts.
> Computed tomography can be used to determine the existence of calcification.
> Craniopharyngiomas have a heterogeneous texture, the combination of solid, calcified and cystic components is a diagnostic clue in imaging modalities.
> Adamantinomatous craniopharyngiomas are large irregular with about 90% calcification and a cystic area. Meanwhile, papillary craniopharyngiomas are mostly solid and rarely present with calcifications or cysts.

Treatment options

The choice of treatment is made based on the characteristics of the tumor (location, invasiveness, proximity to adjacent structures) and the individual characteristics of the patient (age, comorbidities, between thighs). The treatment options are:

Surgery: endoscopic endonasal transsphenoidal approach or transcranial approach. Macroscopic total resection is controversial, according to the higher index of postoperative endocrine deficits.

Radiotherapy: it is used in patients with residual disease or as prevention of recurrences. Conventional external radiation therapy, proton beam, stereotactic radiation therapy, brachytherapy, and radiosurgery can be used.

Intracystic therapy- Used to treat pure cystic craniopharyngiomas. Toxic substances such as bleomycin, alpha interferon, or radioactive isotopes are used to cause tumor fibrosis and tumor sclerosis.

Follow-up peculiarities:

Close postoperative neurologic monitoring should be followed to monitor the cerebrospinal fluid level.

Management of hormonal deficiencies and careful hormonal monitoring, verifying cortisol levels, should be started.

Monitoring and evaluation of postoperative hormonal deficiencies is recommended.

Bibliographic references

1. Shlomo Melmed, Richard J. Auchus, Allison B. Goldfine, Ronald J. Kowning, Clifford Rosen. Williams Textbook of Endocrinology 14Th edition. ELSEVIER, 2020.
2. Kiliç M, Can SM, Özdemir B, Tanik C. Management of Craniopharyngioma. J CraniofacSurg. 2019 Mar / Apr; 30 (2): e178-e183.
3. Lavin N, editor. Manual of endocrinology and metabolism. 4th ed. Philadelphia: Wolters Kluwer / Lippincott Williams & Wilkins Health; 2009. 837 p.

Chapter 275. Non-functioning Pituitary Tumor

They are pituitary tumors, developed from the cells of the pituitary gland but clinically silent because they do not actively secrete pituitary hormones. Among non-functional pituitary tumors, the predominant ones are gonadotropic and corticotropic cell tumors.

Statistics and epidemiology

They comprise between 25% and 35% of tumors of the pituitary gland. The prevalence is variable and is frequently based on autopsies or series of imaging studies (magnetic resonance imaging). The age peak occurs between the fourth and eighth decades of life.

The prevalence of clinically relevant non-functioning pituitary adenomas is estimated to range from 7 to 41.3 cases per 100,000 population.

Etiology and pathophysiological elements

Most non-functional or hormonally silent tumors originate from gonadotrophic cells, are monoclonal tumors and may be associated with genetic mutations, which contribute to tumor development. Associated mutations express mutations in the GNAS regulatory gene, although alterations can also occur in different regions of tumor suppressor genes, such as MEG3. A permissive oncogene of the formation of pituitary adenomas could be responsible for their development.

Non-functioning pituitary tumors present as clinically non-functional masses and not associated with high levels of serum gonadotropins. However, they can express gonadotropin subunits, which can be detected by immunohistochemistry.

Diagnostic criteria

Neurological symptoms	Visual field deficit (61%). Extraocular muscle paralysis (14%). Headache (between 10 to 61%).
Endocrine symptoms	Decreased libido (26). Amenorrhea (10%). Stroke (2 to 12%).
Hormonal deficiencies	GH (36 to 61%). LH / FSH (40%). TSH (36%). ACTH (33%). Diabetes insipidus (2%).
Immunostaining	Gonadotropin subunits (44%). POMC / ACTH (5 to 19%). GH (2 to 4%). PRL (2%). TSH (1%).

Imaging studies and a comprehensive study of pituitary incidentalomas should be performed. In addition, visual field examination and pituitary hormonal tests should be carried out.

Treatment options

Microscopic or endoscopic endonasal transsphenoidal surgery (recommending approach)

Surgery is recommended when patients are symptomatic, that is, visual impairment or in the presence of macroadenomas that threaten vital structures.

Radiotherapy

It is used to reduce the postoperative risk of tumor growth progression. Radiation therapy may be indicated when the tumor mass can expand.

Expectant observation

Due to the slow growth of nonfunctional microadenomas, observational therapy can be initiated. It is estimated that only 10% of microadenomas discovered incidentally will continue to enlarge, however, studies affirm that after 5 years the growth rate may increase. Another 10% of incidentalomas may shrink during the 8-year follow-up.
Therefore, follow-up should be carried out using serial MRI scans 1, 2, and 5 years after initial diagnosis.

Follow-up peculiarities

After treatment for macroadenomas, hormonal tests should be performed every 6 months for 2 years, after which they are followed annually. Hormone replacement treatment is started according to need.

Bibliographic references

1. Shlomo Melmed, Richard J. Auchus, Allison B. Goldfine, Ronald J. Kowning, Clifford Rosen. Williams Textbook of Endocrinology 14Th edition. ELSEVIER, 2020.
2. Shlomo Melmed. The Pituitary 4th Edition. Academic Press, Elsevier, 2017.

Chapter 276. Galactorrheas

It consists of the production of milk from the mammary gland but not related to pregnancy or lactation. Milk production is affected by various hormones such as prolactin, estrogens, and thyrotropin-releasing hormone.

Statistics and epidemiology

The prevalence of drug-induced galactorrhea is increasing, ranging from 30% to 80% of causes in some populations. Prolactinomas are one of the most common secretory pituitary tumors. The clinical presentation of hyperprolactinemia is more obvious in women than in men.

Risk groups or factors
- ✓ Systemic diseases.
- ✓ Family history of multiple endocrine neoplasia.
- ✓ Polypharmacy.
- ✓ Psychiatric disorders (on medication).
- ✓ History of hypothyroidism.

Etiology and pathophysiological elements

Hypothalamic-pituitary causes	Prolactinoma: prolactin-secreting tumor. Non-prolactin-secreting pituitary tumor: interrupts the flow of dopamine from the hypothalamus to the anterior pituitary, reducing prolactin inhibition. Infiltrative disorders.

Non-hypothalamic-pituitary causes	Hypothyroidism: increased TRH stimulates lactotrophs and causes hyperprolactinemia and galactorrhea. Medications: drugs such as risperidone act on D2 receptors in the tuberoinfundibular areas of the hypothalamus and cause hyperprolactinemia. Others like opioids reduce the release of dopamine. Renal failure: decreased renal elimination of prolactin. Chest wall injuries: burns, surgeries, and herpes zoster infections are associated with hyperprolactinemia. Pain signals are theorized to cause decreased dopamine secretion. Idiopathic hyperprolactinemia: cause and mechanism unknown. It usually resolves spontaneously.

Milk secretion is stimulated and synthesized due to the hormone prolactin. This hormone is secreted by the anterior pituitary gland and is regulated by dopamine as an inhibitory signal. Prolactin release is stimulated by TRH and the vasoactive intestinal polypeptide. All factors that disrupt proper prolactin signaling to maintain adequate concentrations can cause hyperprolactinemia and galactorrhea.

Diagnostic criteria

In the table below you will find the diagnostic criteria to evaluate galactorrhea.

Clinic	Milk production in men or women not associated with pregnancy or lactation (or one year after cessation of lactation). Make a careful evaluation of the symptoms associated with hyperprolactinemia (See Chapter 236). Ask about the current use of drugs associated with hyperprolactinemia. Evaluation of galactorrhea should be done with the patient sitting up and leaning forward. Squeeze the areola towards the nipple. Galactorrhea can be white or green in color and is usually bilateral. The presence of bloody discharge is associated with breast tumors and the paraclinical ones should be oriented towards this cause.
Paraclinical	Sudan IV stain for fat drops (confirms milk discharge). Serum prolactin levels (can be up to 5 times higher than normal). Elevation for medications <100 ng / ml (except for antipsychotics that can increase up to 250 ng / ml). Serum thyroxine and TSH concentration. MRI or CT scan.

Treatment options

Guide therapy toward resolution of the underlying cause. Hyperprolactinemia should be treated when there is injury to the pituitary gland or hypogonadism with problematic galactorrhea.

Bromocriptinadosis 2.5 to 15 mg once or twice a day.

Cabergoline 0.25 to 1 mg twice a week.

Microprolactinomas: asymptomatic patients with prolactin concentrations lower than 100 mcg / L or normal imaging studies, can be treated with medical treatment and follow-up. Macroadenomas can be managed with surgical resection and treatment with dopamine agonists.

Follow-up peculiarities

Control of hyperprolactinemia every 3 months.
Follow-up imaging studies (MRI or CT) once a year for at least 2 years.

Bibliographic references

1. Melmed S, Casanueva FF, Hoffman AR, Kleinberg DL, Montori VM, Schlechte JA, Wass JA., Endocrine Society. Diagnosis and treatment of hyperprolactinemia: an Endocrine Society clinical practice guideline. J. Clin. Endocrinol. Metab. 2011 Feb; 96 (2): 273-88
2. Gosi SKY, Garla VV. Galactorrhea. [Updated 2019 Jan 30]. StatPearls Publishing; 2020 Jan-.

Chapter 277. Hyperprolactinemia

The hormone known as prolactin is produced by the anterior pituitary gland from lactotrophs, which are regulated through hypothalamic signals. Hyperprolactinemia consists of the excess increase of prolactin hormone in the blood, exceeding the limit of normality (that is, greater than 5 ng / ml in men and greater than 13 ng / ml in women).

Hyperprolactinemias can be caused by a variety of causes including physiological, pathological, or drug-induced conditions.

Statistics and epidemiology

It occurs in less than 1% of the general population. About 5% to 14% of patients with secondary amenorrhea have hyperprolactinemia.

Prolactinomas represent 40% of all clinically recognized pituitary adenomas.

It is estimated that the average prevalence of a prolactinoma ranges from around 30 cases per 100,000 women and up to 10 cases per 100,000 men. The maximum prevalence in women is 25 to 34 years. The clinical manifestations occur in women earlier than in men.

Risk groups or factors:
- ✓ Polypharmacy.
- ✓ Head injury.
- ✓ Family history of congenital or idiopathic hyperprolactinemias.
- ✓ Systemic disorders

Etiology or more frequent causes

Hypothalamic disease (stem damage)	Cranial irradiation. Granulomas (sarcoidosis, tuberculosis). Infiltrative disorders (histiocytosis). Rathke cyst. Neoplasms (craniopharyngiomas, dysgerminomas, hypothalamic metastases, among others). Cross section of the pituitary stalk (sellar surgery, head injury).
Pharmacological causes	Estrogen therapy. Cholinergic agent (physostigmine). H2 antihistamines (ranitidine, cimetidine). Thyrotropin-releasing hormone. Opioid pain relievers (methadone, apomorphine, morphine, heroin). Antipsychotic / dopamine receptor blocking agents (risperidone, fluphenazine, haloperidol). Antihypertensives (labetalol, methyldopa, verapamil). Dopamine receptor blocking / antiemetic agents (domperidone, prochlorperazine, metoclopramide). Tricyclic antidepressant, serotonin receptor inhibitor (Fluoxetine, Clomipramine, Amitriptyline). Anticonvulsant (phenytoin)
Genetic disorder	Inactivation of the prolactin receptor mutation
Systemic disorder	Pseudocytosis. Primary hypothyroidism. Chronic kidney failure. Hepatic cirrhosis. Polycystic ovary disease. Reflex causes (herpes zoster, chest wall trauma, surgery).
Ectopic production	Carcinoma. Bronchogenic hypernephromas. Prolactinoma.
Idiopathic	

Pathophysiological elements

- ✓ The hypothalamic control of prolactin secretion is inhibited by dopamine and the inhibitory factor prolactin.
- ✓ HRT is a powerful factor capable of stimulating the release of prolactin.
- ✓ In primary hypothyroidism there is a high response to TSH as well as to prolactin.
- ✓ Dopamine antagonists, endothelial growth factor, and vasoactive intestinal peptide are dopamine-releasing factors.
- ✓ Neuroleptic drugs and the like increase prolactin due to its dopamine receptor antagonist property.
- ✓ Atypical antipsychotics antagonize serotonin and dopamine secretions.
- ✓ Prolactin inhibits GnRH, leading to inhibition of LH and FSH.

Diagnostic criteria

Clinical manifestation of hyperprolactinemia	
Woman	**Man**
Menstrual disorders (oligomenorrhea, menorrhagia, amenorrhea). Infertility Galactorrhea. Low bone mass	Hypogonadotropic hypogonadism (secondary): decreased libido, infertility, oligospermia, impotence. Gynecomastia Erectile dysfunction. Galactorrhea (rare). Low bone mass
Caused by space occupying injury effect Visual field defects.	

> External ophthalmoplegic.
> Headache.

Paraclinical
- ✓ Serum prolactin.
- ✓ Thyroid function test.
- ✓ Kidney function test.
- ✓ Insulin-like growth factor-1.
- ✓ Level of hormones FSH, LH, ACTH.
- ✓ Testosterone / estradiol levels
- ✓ Pregnancy test.
- ✓ Imaging studies: magnetic resonance imaging of the pituitary with contrast.

To establish the diagnosis, exclude physiological and pharmacological causes and request neuroradiological imaging of the hypothalamic-pituitary region.

Treatment options

Treatment of hyperprolactinemia depends on the underlying triggering cause. Some general recommendations for the medical treatment of hyperprolactinemias include:

Treatment with dopamine agonists is recommended to reduce prolactin levels, tumor size, and normalize gonadal function in those patients who present with symptoms of prolactin-secreting microadenomas or macroadenomas.

The recommended dopamine agonists are cabergoline and bromocriptine.

Most prolactinomas are treated by medical therapy, however, surgery or radiation therapy is reserved for patients whose medical therapy with dopamine agonists has failed and hyperprolactinemia persists.

Stereotactic radiosurgery with a gamma knife is considered an effective treatment for resistant prolactinomas or in patients intolerant to dopamine agonists.

Follow-up peculiarities

Follow-up will be established based on the underlying cause in relation to the individualized characteristics of the patient and general condition.

Bibliographic references

1. Glezer A, Bronstein MD. Hyperprolactinemia. [Updated 2018 Oct 22]. In: Feingold KR, Anawalt B, Boyce A, et al., Editors. Endotext. South Dartmouth (MA): MDText.com, Inc .; 2000-.
2. Thapa S, Bhusal K. Hyperprolactinemia. [Updated 2020 May 29]. In: StatPearls. Treasure Island (FL): StatPearls Publishing; 2020 Jan-

Chapter 278. Hyperprolactinemia and Pregnancy

Hyperprolactinemia is about elevation of serum prolactin levels above the normal level. Both pregnancy and lactation cause the elevation of prolactin levels in a physiological way. A normal pregnancy can achieve results between 80 to 400ng / ml of serum prolactin. However, pre-pregnancy hyperprolactinemia accounts for about 1/3 of the causes of infertility, although with proper treatment they can achieve pregnancy (see Chapter 236).

On the other hand, prolactin-secreting microadenomas without clinical significance prior to pregnancy, due to gestational changes, may increase in size and require particular management.

Statistics and epidemiology

About 90% of prolactinomas are intersellar. 10% are macroadenomas (greater than 10 mm). Prolactinomas are common among women of reproductive age. The highest incidence rate in women ranges from 25 to 34 years of age. Among women with reproductive disorders, it is estimated that about 15% and 43% with anovulation and galactorrhea have hyperprolactinemia. The risk of prolactinoma enlargement in pregnancy ranges from 4.8 to 32%.

Etiology and pathophysiological elements

In normal pregnancy, the marked increase in estrogen levels improves prolactin synthesis and secretion by stimulating and increasing the size of the lactotrophs. Elevated estrogen causes global pituitary hyperplasia.

Due to the excessive growth of lactotrophs during pregnancy, pituitary neoplasms can be diagnosed during pregnancy and due to the enlargement of the pituitary gland that occurs normally in pregnancy, a woman with prolactinomas may present complications and compressive and functional clinical manifestations.

Other causes associated with hyperprolactinemia have been discussed in Chap. 236, however, because hyperprolactinemia is associated with infertility, it is unlikely that a pregnancy could develop without prior treatment.

Diagnostic criteria

Clinic	Investigate a history of previously treated prolactinomas. The usual clinical manifestations are: Visual disturbances Headache. Diabetes insipidus
Paraclinical	In the case of pre-pregnancy prolactinomas, the size of the tumor must be documented by magnetic resonance imaging. Visual field perimetry. Prolactin levels: may be elevated above the normal range for pregnant women (80 to 400 ng / ml).

Treatment options

According to the clinical manifestations and the size of the prolactinoma, an expectant follow-up can be followed or pharmacological treatment may be indicated to shrink the tumor.

The drug most used during and before pregnancy are dopamine agonists, used to shrink the tumor and improve the probability of pregnancy in women of childbearing age with hyperprolactinemia.

Most used dopamine agonists:
- ✓ Bromocriptine (first choice): requires several daily doses.
- ✓ Cabergoline administered 2 times a week.
- ✓ Quinagolide.

Follow-up peculiarities

The follow-up evaluation is performed every 2 to 3 months, performing a complete clinical examination and evaluating the perimetry of the visual field. Basic follow-up studies of obstetric control should not be neglected.

Bibliographic references

1. Shlomo Melmed, Richard J. Auchus, Allison B. Goldfine, Ronald J. Kowning, Clifford Rosen. Williams Textbook of Endocrinology 14Th edition. ELSEVIER, 2020.
2. Almalki, MH, Alzahrani, S., Alshahrani, F., Alsherbeni, S., Almoharib, O., Aljohani, N., & Almagamsi, A. (2015). Managing Prolactinomas duringPregnancy. Frontiers in endocrinology, 6, 85. https://doi.org/10.3389/fendo.2015.00085

Chapter 279. Prolactinomas

These are prolactin-secreting tumors of the anterior pituitary. These secretory pituitary neoplasms can cause a variety of clinical manifestations due to the effect of prolactin hypersecretion or as a result of the mass effect of the tumor.

Statistics and epidemiology

Prolactinomas have an annual incidence of approximately 30 cases per 100,000 people. About 11% of microadenomas are discovered at autopsies, where at least 46% immunostain for PRL.
The female to male ratio is 20: 1 for microprolactinomas. The maximum age ranges from 25 to 34 years in women. Macroprolactinoma is common in men and women alike.

Risk groups or factors

- ✓ Family history of prolactinomas.
- ✓ Radiation to the head or neck.
- ✓ Family history of MEN1.

Etiology or more frequent causes

- ✓ They arise as monoclonal expansion of the pituitary lactotrophic cells due to somatic mutation.
- ✓ Overexpression of the transforming pituitary tumor gene (PTTG)
- ✓ Mutation of a receptor for fibroblast growth factor 4 (FGF4).

Pathophysiological elements

More than 99% of prolactinomas are benign, well defined, and show no evidence of invasion. However, some prolactinomas could behave aggressively with invasion of adjacent structures, invasive tumors present greater mitotic and pleomorphic activity. Prolactinomas are mostly slow growing and appear sporadically. They usually occur individually.

Diagnostic criteria

Clinical manifestations

Associated with hyperprolactinemia	Associated with tumor mass
Amenorrhea	Visual field disorders.
Infertility	Decreased visual acuity or blurred vision.
Impotence.	
Decreased libido	Pituitary apoplexy.
Premature ejaculation	Headache.
Oligospermia	Symptoms of hypopituitarism.
Galactorrhea.	Hydrocephalus (rare).
Osteoporosis	Seizures (temporal lobe involvement).
	Cranial nerve palsy.
	Unilateral exophthalmos (rare).

A complete medical history should be taken. Prolactinomas can coexist with other triggering causes of hyperprolactinemia, for example administration of neuroleptics.

Paraclinical
- ✓ Serum PRL levels.
- ✓ Serum IGF1 levels (prolactinoma symptoms may be similar in GH-secreting tumors).
- ✓ Magnetic resonance.

Treatment options

The goal of treatment is to normalize the symptoms associated with hyperprolactinemia and reduce or remove the tumor, obtaining relief from the symptoms of a tumor mass.

Medical treatment

Treatment with dopamine agonists is considered the medical treatment of choice.

Bromocriptine: doses of 2.5 to 7.5 mg per day. The starting dose can range from 1.25 mg per day. Withdrawal from doses can promote tumor growth.

Cabergoline: dose of 0.5 to 1 mg twice a week. The starting dose is often 0.25 mg per week.

Radiation therapy

Radiation therapy with linear acceleration has shown effectiveness in reducing and controlling prolactinomas. The usual dose is 4500 to 4600 cGy.

Stereotactic radiosurgery can be effective for resistant prolactinomas or those with dopamine intolerance. Radiation therapy can be used after surgery when there is resistance to medical treatment.

Surgical treatment

The usual treatment to resect prolactinomas is transsphenoidal endoscopic surgery. This is indicated when medical therapy is unsuccessful in reducing PRL levels or failure to reduce tumor size after using medical treatment at maximum dose for several months.

It can also be indicated in women with prolactinomas greater than 3 cm who wish to become pregnant, since prolactinomas can grow during pregnancy.

Chemotherapy

It is indicated in the presence of aggressive prolactinomas that do not respond to other therapies. Temozolomide can be used.

Follow-up peculiarities

Invasive macroprolactinomas require close (weekly) monitoring. Meanwhile, microprolactinomas can be monitored more frequently according to the serum prolactin level and the characteristics of the tumor itself.

Pharmacological treatment can be discontinued in patients with persistent normoprolactinemia for at least two consecutive years.

Long-term follow-up is recommended due to the risk of recurrence of hyperprolactinemia after cessation of treatment.

Follow-up can be done every 3 months during the first year after surgery, subsequently annual follow-up should be performed for at least 5 years, especially in patients with macroprolactinomas.

Bibliographic references

1. Shlomo Melmed, Richard J. Auchus, Allison B. Goldfine, Ronald J. Kowning, Clifford Rosen. Williams Textbook of Endocrinology 14Th edition. ELSEVIER, 2020.
2. Shlomo Melmed. The Pituitary 4th Edition. AcademicPress, Elsevier, 2017.

Chapter 280. Prolactinoma and Pregnancy

In women of childbearing age, prolactinomas are the most common pituitary tumors. Proper treatment allows most pregnant women with prolactinomas to carry a pregnancy to term. This is accomplished through a multidisciplinary team, and watchful waiting is sometimes sufficient for some women.

Effects of pregnancy on prolactinomas

During pregnancy, the pituitary gland undergoes global hyperplasia. This growth begins within the first weeks of pregnancy, causing the pituitary gland to expand to almost 1.2 cm in diameter in the immediate postpartum stage.

This increase in size is accompanied in turn by a concomitant increase in the population of lactotropic cells and their size, as well as a progressive increase in serum prolactin levels.

The mitotic activity that occurs in lactotropic cells, as well as the synthesis of prolactin, is due to the increase in placental estrogens. On the other hand, tumor cells express estrogen receptors, which represents the risk of tumor enlargement during pregnancy.

Microprolactinomas during pregnancy

It consists of tumors smaller than 10 mm in diameter, the course of which tends to be benign in non-pregnant women.

Recommendations

> Stop dopamine agonist therapy as soon as pregnancy is diagnosed.
> Explain to your patients about tumor enlargement during pregnancy.
> Instruct your patients to report symptoms such as headaches or sudden vision changes.
> Schedule visual field perimetry and repeat every 2 months.
> Patients with microprolactinomas, absence of symptoms, and stable visual perimetry can receive watchful waiting.
> Patients with new onset headaches, alterations in the visual fields or alterations in the results of visual perimetry, require urgent evaluation by imaging studies, preferably by magnetic resonance imaging and referral to a specialist. These patients may require surgery during the second trimester of pregnancy or initiate treatment with dopamine agonists.

Macroprolactinomas during pregnancy

They occur less frequently than microprolactinomas. These adenomas are larger than 10 mm in diameter and are associated with increased morbidity among pregnant and non-pregnant women.

Recommendations

> A pregnant patient with Macroprolactinoma should be referred to the neurosurgery or endocrinology service.
> You should explain to your patient about the risk of tumor enlargement during pregnancy and the possible risks.
> Perform visual field perimetry on your patient.
> Evaluate the possible therapeutic options available.
> When it is a relatively small intrasellar tumor or one that extends downward, and does not border the optic chiasm, it can receive a behavior similar to that of a microprolactinoma.
> In the presence of an intrasellar Lorger tumor that adjoins the optic

chiasm, advise your patient to avoid pregnancy until tumor growth is controlled (in women of childbearing age with previously known prolactinoma who wish to achieve pregnancy). In pregnant women with these criteria, treatment with dopamine agonists may be indicated throughout pregnancy when.

Large tumors or refractory to dopamine agonists may require surgical intervention through transsphenoidal pituitary surgery.

Bibliographic references

1. Shlomo Melmed, Richard J. Auchus, Allison B. Goldfine, Ronald J. Kowning, Clifford Rosen. Williams Textbook of Endocrinology 14Th edition. ELSEVIER, 2020.
2. Imran, SA, Ur, E., & Clarke, DB (2007). Managing prolactin-secreting adenomas during pregnancy. Canadian family physician Medecin de famille canadien, 53 (4), 653–658.
3. Glezer A, Bronstein MD. Prolactinomas in pregnancy: considerations before conception and during pregnancy. Pituitary. 2020 Feb; 23 (1): 65-69. doi: 10.1007 / s11102-019-01010-5. PMID: 31792668.

Chapter 281. Thyrotropinomas

Also known as thyrotropin-secreting pituitary adenomas (TSH) or TSH-omas, it is a rare cause of hyperthyroidism caused by autonomous secretion of TSH and refractory to negative feedback from thyroid hormones.

Statistics and epidemiology

It is a rare disorder, which represents about 0.5 to 2% of all pituitary adenomas. The prevalence in the general population is around 1 to 2 cases per million people. Most cases occur between the fifth and sixth decade of life. They occur in equal frequency between men and women.

Risk groups or factors: History of multiple endocrine neoplasia type 1.

Etiology and pathophysiological elements

Several mechanisms are responsible for the pathogenesis of thyrotropinomas, probably these mechanisms interact with each other to trigger cell transformation and promote the proliferation of cells of the pituitary gland. These factors include genetic mutations associated with the development of pituitary tumors, over-activation of proliferative cell signaling pathways, alterations in the hormone regulatory pathway, and insufficient expression of tumor suppressor genes.

This type of tumor can be composed of two different types of cells, a secreting alpha subunit of glucoprotein hormones (alpha-GSU) and another co-secreting alpha-GSU and complete TSH molecules.

Types of thyrotropinomas
- ✓ Pure thyrotropinomas (more common).
- ✓ Thyrotropinomas with associated hypersecretion of other (mixed) pituitary hormones.
- ✓ Mixed TSH / GH-omas.
- ✓ TSH / PRL-omas mixed.
- ✓ TSH / FSH / LH-omas mixed (rare).

Diagnostic criteria

Clinic	The clinical manifestations depend on the type of thyrotropinoma and its hormonal secretion, although it can also cause symptoms associated with the effect of tumor mass. Hyperthyroidism (common). Acromegaly. Multinodular goiter. Hyperprolactinemia. Loss of vision or visual field defects. Loss of function of the anterior pituitary. Headache
Paraclinical	Elevated or not suppressed TSH levels. Elevated levels of free and total T4 and T3. Elevated levels of the algae glycoprotein subunit. Alpha subunit / TSH molar ratio greater than 1 (80% of patients and rule out non-tumor TSH hypersecretion). When secondary hyperthyroidism is chronic, and has previously been treated as primary hyperthyroidism, a euthyroid or hypothyroid state may occur as a result of

thyroid ablation.
Dynamic tests
TRH test.
Ocreotide test.
T3 suppression test.
Circadian TSH secretion.
Imaging studies
Most thyrotropinomas present as large macroadenomas and frequently invade adjacent structures such as the sphenoid and cavernous sinuses. They can extend suprasellarly and compress the optic nerve.
Magnetic resonance imaging and computed tomography are mainly used.

Treatment options

Surgical therapy is the recommended therapeutic option for thyrotropinomas to achieve restoration of normal thyroid and pituitary function. The most commonly used procedures are transsphenoidal or subfrontal adenomectomy.

In severe hyperthyroidism, iopanoic acid can be administered.

Preoperative treatment with somatostatin analogs may help reduce the clinical manifestations of hyperthyroidism and may reduce the size of adenomas.

In case of failure of pituitary surgery and life-threatening hyperthyroid manifestation, total thyroidectomy or thyroid ablation is indicated.

Pituitary radiation therapy or medical treatment with somatostatin analogs may be used when there is a pituitary contraindication to surgery. The recommended dose for radiation therapy is not less than 45 Gy divided to 2Gy per day. It can also be a dose of 10 to 25 Gy in a single dose when a stereotactic gamma knife can be used.

In the presence of mixed PRL / TSH thyrotropinomas, dopamine agonist therapy, especially cabergoline, may be beneficial.

Follow-up peculiarities

- ✓ Follow-up methods have not been clearly established because it is a rare condition. However, the follow-up includes observing the following criteria:
- ✓ Remission of hyperthyroid signs and symptoms, as well as biochemical normalization.
- ✓ Disappearance of neurological manifestations associated with visual impairment due to tumor mass lesion.
- ✓ Normalization of alpha-GSU levels and alpha-GSU / TSH molar ratio.
- ✓ Positive T3 suppression test with undetectable TSH and no response to TRH.

There have been reports of recurrence of thyrotropinomas after healing, however, it is not usual. The patient must be evaluated 2 or 3 times during the first postoperative year and then annually follow-up, through biochemical and clinical studies. Pituitary imaging studies should be performed every 2 to 3 years.

Bibliographic references

1. Shlomo Melmed. The Pituitary 4th Edition. AcademicPress, Elsevier, 2017.

2. Lavin N, editor. Manual of endocrinology and metabolism. 4th ed. Philadelphia: Wolters Kluwer / Lippincott Williams & Wilkins Health; 2009. 837 p.
3. Beck-Peccoz P, Persani L, Lania A. Thyrotropin-Secreting Pituitary Adenomas. [Updated 2019 Jan 11]. In: Feingold KR, Anawalt B, Boyce A, et al., Editors. Endotext [Internet]. South Dartmouth (MA): MDText.com, Inc .; 2000-.

Chapter 282. Gonadotropic Adenomas

Pure gonadotropic adenomas are called pituitary neoplasms capable of secreting gonadotrophic hormones producing supranormal basal serum concentrations of FSH, and less frequently LH. FSH secreted by gonadotropic adenomas has normal or almost normal characteristics, conferring biologically active properties.

Gonadotropic adenomas are considered indistinguishable adenomas from non-functioning pituitary tumors.

Statistics and epidemiology

They are extremely rare. Most of the gonadotropic adenomas confirmed by inhumohistochemistry are hormonally silent (they only present a mass effect).

They represent about 64% of clinically non-functioning pituitary adenomas.

Etiology

They originate from a somatic mutation of a proliferating progenitor cell. It consists of monoclonal adenomas. The growth of adenomas could respond to the effect of an external hormonal stimulation of the hypothalamus.

It is theorized that gonadotropic adenomas could develop as a result of stimulation of gonadotrophic cells due to testosterone deficiency, as occurs in long-standing primary hypogonadism.

Pathophysiological elements

Morphologically identical to non-functioning gonadotropic tumors.

Macroscopically, it is well vascularized, soft, with necrotic or hemorrhagic areas. Microscopically chromophobic cells can be seen which follow a trabecular, sinusoidal or papillary pattern.

They can secrete and stain positively for FSH and LH. They are secretors of the alpha and beta subunits of human chorionic gonadotropin (HCG).

Gonadotropic macroadenomas are capable of producing serum gonadotropin concentrations 10 times higher than normal, although they are frequently or elevated above normal levels.

Diagnostic criteria

Clinic	Women: Pelvic pain (ovarian hyperstimulation). Menstrual irregularities. Infertility Galactorrhea. Mens: Acne. Testicular enlargement. Mass effect: Headache. Visual disturbances
Paraclinical	Women: Normal or fluctuating estrogen. Normal or slightly increased serum FSH. Serum LH suppressed or within normal range. Serum alpha subunit and normal or high inhibin. *Imaging studies:* Pelvic image shows multisept cysts and variable size (anechoic and with low intensity weighted in T1 and T2 in MRI. Pituitary MRI: frequent macroadenomas. Mens: Elevated serum FSH. Serum LH slightly below the reference range, normal or elevated. Alpha and inhibin subunit in normal or increased serum. Increased sperm count.

	Imaging studies: Scrotal ultrasound with evidence of testicular volume enlargement. Pituitary MRI: macroadenomas. FSH response to common TRH. LH beta response to common TRH.

Treatment options

The main treatment consists of surgical excision with the administration of complementary radiotherapy. The approach route is generally made transsphenoidal, rarely a transcranial approach is used. The treatment with dopamine agonists and somatostatin analogues have not shown effectiveness in tumor reduction, therefore they are not recommended as a first line of treatment. Temozolomide therapy may be required.

Follow-up peculiarities

Follow-up is similar to the follow-up for non-functioning pituitary tumors (see Chapter 235). Prioritize follow-up peculiarities based on individual patient qualities.

Bibliographic references

1. Shlomo Melmed. The Pituitary 4th Edition. AcademicPress, Elsevier, 2017.
2. Shlomo Melmed, Richard J. Auchus, Allison B. Goldfine, Ronald J. Kowning, Clifford Rosen. Williams Textbook of Endocrinology 14Th edition. ELSEVIER, 2020.
3. Georgia Ntali, Cristina Capatina, Ashley Grossman, NikiKaravitaki, Functioning Gonadotroph Adenomas, The Journal of Clinical Endocrinology & Metabolism, Volume 99, Issue 12, December 2014, Pages 4423–4433, https://doi.org/10.1210/jc.2014 -2362.

Chapter 283. Cushing's Disease

It consists of a disorder which is characterized by an increase in adrenocorticotropic hormone (ACTH) by the anterior pituitary, which leads to an increase in the excessive release of cortisol by the adrenal glands. This occurs as a result of the presence of a pituitary microadenoma or as a consequence of excessive production of corticotropin-releasing hormone (CRH) by the hypothalamus.

Statistics and epidemiology

It is the second most common cause of Cushing's syndrome. The average incidence of new cases ranges between 2.4 cases per million people per year. The disease is frequently diagnosed between 3 to 6 years after its onset.

The maximum incidence of occurrence is in women between 50 to 60 years of age. The prevalence of glucose metabolic abnormalities and hypertension are significant predictors of morbidity and mortality in untreated cases.

The mortality rate ranges from 10 to 11% of cases.

Risk factors: Family history of Cushing's disease.

Etiology

- Pituitary adenoma: frequently microadenomas (tumors smaller than 5 mm), although 5 to 10% can occur due to macroadenomas. The most frequent mutation involved in the development of this type of adenomas is USP8 (ubiquitin-specific peptidase 8)

- Diffuse corticotropin hyperplasia.

Pathophysiological elements

The USP8 mutation leads to an abnormal expression of growth factors which act with ACTH to increase cortisol.

The increase in serum ACTH causes bilateral adrenal hyperplasia and as a consequence, cortisol production increases, causing alteration in the normal circadian rhythm of cortisol.

Cortisol in high amounts can exhibit mineralocorticoid activity leading to hypokalemia and hypertension through the renin-angiotensin-aldosterone system.

Histopathologically, ACTH-releasing pituitary adenomas are highly positive on periodic acid-Schiff (PAS) staining and basophils on H / E staining. The cells have a large nucleus, with a prominent nucleolus and thick chromatin, as well as granular cytoplasm.

Diagnostic criteria

Clinic	Central obesity (79 to 97%).
	Facial plethora (50 to 94%).
	Glucose intolerance (39 to 90%).
	Red abdominal stretch marks (51 to 71%).
	Ankle edema (27 to 60%).
	Weakness, proximal myopathy (29–90%).
	Low back pain, vertebra collapse or fracture (40 to 50%).
	Dyslipidemia (25 to 60%).
	Arterial hypertension (74 to 87%).
	Renal stones (15 to 19%).

	Psychological changes (31 to 86%). Hyperpigmentation (4 to 16%). Capillary fragility (23 to 84). Headache (0 to 47%). Hirsutism (64 to 81%). Exophthalmos (0 to 33%). Oligomenorrhea or amenorrhea (55 to 80%). Tinea versicolor (0 to 30%). Impotence (55 to 80%). Acne or seborrhea (26 to 80%).
Paraclinical	Free urinary cortisol. Low-dose dexamethasone suppression test. Midnight serum cortisol measurement. Dexamethasone-CRH test. The increase in urinary free cortisol (in two 24-hour urine measurements), in conjunction with the lack of suppression of morning serum cortisol to less than 1.8 µg / dL (measured at 8:00 am), after the administration of 1mg of dexamethasone orally the night before (at 23:00 pm), confirmed hypercortisolism. Other location studies: High-dose dexamethasone suppression test. CRH stimulation test. Bilateral petrous sinus sampling.

Treatment options

The treatment of choice for these adenomas is transsphenoidal surgical resection. The approach can be performed sublabial or endonasal.

Alternatively, pituitary radiation therapy can be used after failed surgery.

External beam pituitary radiation therapy is more recommended in pediatric patients.

Bilateral adrenalectomy can be considered as an immediate reduction in serum cortisol levels. These patients will require glucocorticoid and mineralocorticoid replacement therapy for life.

Follow-up peculiarities

Lifelong follow-up should be established due to the high risk of recurrence of hypercortisolemia, which occurs in about 1/3 of patients after receiving initial treatment. For this, cortisol in nocturnal saliva is used, considered the best predictor of recurrence.

Bibliographic references

1. Shlomo Melmed, Richard J. Auchus, Allison B. Goldfine, Ronald J. Kowning, Clifford Rosen. Williams Textbook of Endocrinology 14Th edition. ELSEVIER, 2020.
2. Dorantes and Martinez. Clinical endocrinology 5th edition, Editorial El Manual Moderno 2016.

Chapter 284. Nelson Syndrome

Also known as post-adrenalectomy syndrome, which is a spectrum of symptoms and signs that originate from an adrenocorticotropin (ACTH) secreting pituitary macroadenoma, after therapeutic bilateral adrenalectomy. These clinical manifestations are associated with local effects of the tumor on adjacent structures, the effects of high serum ACTH concentrations in the skin, and secondary loss of other pituitary hormones.

Statistics and epidemiology

The probability that Nelson syndrome will develop after bilateral adrenalectomy ranges from 8% to 47% in adults and 25% to 66% in children.

The incidence has decreased at present because bilateral adrenalectomy is performed less frequently. The prevalence three years after bilateral adrenalectomy is 38% which increases to 47% at seven years and later reaches a plateau.

About 7% of patients with Cushing's disease are treated with bilateral adrenalectomy.

Risk groups or factors:

Bilateral adrenalectomy.

Elevated serum ACTH levels one year after bilateral adrenalectomy (fasting serum ACTH greater than 154 to 220 pmol / L, is a predictor of Nelson's syndrome one year after bilateral adrenalectomy).

Etiology and pathophysiological elements

Nelson syndrome occurs as a result of bilateral adrenalectomy as a treatment for Cushing's disease.

After bilateral adrenalectomy, cortisol production is drastically reduced, this will produce a negative feedback on the hypothalamus causing an excessive release of corticotropin-releasing hormone (CTRH), which will stimulate the pituitary gland to produce a greater amount of ACTH. It is theorized that this stimulation causes hypertrophy of corticotropic cells and causes a new ACTH-secreting pituitary tumor.

Histopathology

They are monoclonal neoplasms, which present positivity for periodic acid-Schiff and basophilic staining. Its histopathology is similar to that of pituitary adenomas found in Cushing's disease, but with the presence of pleomorphism and mitosis in the corticotropic cells. Nelson syndrome tumors tend to be more invasive. The Ki-67 proliferation index is below 3%.

Diagnostic criteria

Clinic	History of Cushing's disease and bilateral adrenalectomy. Hyperpigmentation of the skin (more intense and darker than other syndromes). There is a prominent black line running from the pubis to the navel. Excessive pigmentation in scars, mucous membranes and areolas. Bitemporal hemianopia and progressive visual loss

	(when the tumors are large). Headache. Weakness. Fatigue.
Paraclinical	Fasting serum ACTH levels (very high). The diagnosis can be confirmed with a 30% increase in the initial ACTH level in 3 consecutive studies. Brain MRI: evidence of a new pituitary tumor or enlargement of a previously known neoplasm.

Treatment options

Surgical excision (microsurgical or endoscopic via the transsphenoidal route).

Fractional radiation therapy or stereotactic radiosurgery (except in patients who received radiation as a treatment for Cushing's disease). Radiation therapy can be used as a prophylactic treatment for Nelson's syndrome, when bilateral adrenalectomy is performed.

Medical treatment (limited): somatostatin analogs (pasireotide and octreotide), sodium valproate, temozolamide, and dopamine agonists (bromocriptine and cabergoline).

Patients with bilateral adrenalectomy require permanent glucocorticoid replacement.

Follow-up peculiarities

After bilateral adrenalectomy, brain MRI monitoring should be performed at regular intervals, especially when elevated ACTH levels are found in plasma or urine.

Bibliographic references

1. Patel J, Eloy JA, Liu JK. Nelson's syndrome: a review of the clinical manifestations, pathophysiology, and treatment strategies. Neurosurg Focus. 2015 Feb; 38 (2): E14
2. Shlomo Melmed, Richard J. Auchus, Allison B. Goldfine, Ronald J. Kowning, Clifford Rosen. Williams Textbook of Endocrinology 14Th edition. ELSEVIER, 2020.

Chapter 285. Acromegaly

It is a disorder caused by the excessive production of growth hormone (GH) in the anterior pituitary. This results in an overgrowth of body tissues, among other metabolic disturbances. Although growth is slow, acromegaly is considered life-threatening.

Statistics and epidemiology

It is estimated that acromegaly has a prevalence which ranges from 28 to 137 cases per million people.
In the United States, more than 3,000 new cases are diagnosed each year. With a prevalence that ranges between 25,000 patients.
In Spain, a prevalence of 3.4 cases per 100,000 people is estimated with an incidence of 0.2.
The preference for occurrence by sex is slightly higher in women than in men.
The age of maximum presentation is generally in the third decade of life.

Etiology

Pituitary tumor: responsible for more than 95% of the causes. It often presents as a benign microadenoma of the pituitary.
Non-pituitary tumor: adrenal neoplasms, tumors and the pancreas are involved in the development of acromegaly as a result of GH production.

Pathophysiological elements

- ✓ Caused by GH-secreting tumors.
- ✓ Elevated levels of GH and IGF1 with manifestations of hypersomatotropism.
- ✓ Increased production of IGF-1 from the liver.

Acral growth shoots caused by the pathological effect of excess IGF-1 after fusion of the growth plates.

The increase in IGF-1 produces general somatic hypertrophy, somatic growth through binding to the IGF-1R receptor, competition with insulin for the insulin receptor, which triggers relative resistance to insulin similar to diabetics.

Diagnostic criteria.

Clinic	Joint pain.
	Pain or numbness in the wrist (carpal tunnel syndrome).
	Snoring and sleep disorders.
	Headache.
	Visual disturbances
	Sexual dysfunction due to erectile dysfunction or low sexual desire.
	Menstrual disorders.
	Hyperhidrosis
	Mandibular enlargement (prognathism).
	Prominent forehead.
	Coarse facial features.
	Macroglossia.
	Thick eyelids.
	Large nose and lower lip.
	Thyroid mass sensation.
	Acromegalic cardiomyopathy.
	Thick and rough skin.

	Skin tags.
	Oily skin.
	Hirsutism and hypertrichosis.
	Galactorrhea.
	Dry atrophied skin.
	Arterial hypertension.
	Heart murmur
	Bibasal crepitus.
	Proximal myopathy.
	Rolling gear.
	Acral enlargement.
Paraclinical	GH suppression tests: 100 g of glucose is administered orally and one hour later serum GH levels are measured. Results lower than 5 ng / ml exclude the diagnosis, on the contrary, those greater than 10 ng / ml suggest acromegaly. *IGF-1 levels* Physiological causes of the increase in IGF-1 such as pregnancy must be ruled out. It can be used to monitor treatment. Growth hormone releasing hormone (GHRH) levels: Greater than 300 ng / ml orient to extrahypophyseal causes. Prolactin level. *Recommended imaging studies:* Head MRI or CT scan: evidence of sella turcica and nearby structures. Skull X-ray: calvaria, thickened or enlarged sella turcica, thick and long jaw, exaggerated ridge, enlarged sinuses. Chest X-ray: barrel rib cage with evidence of long ribs. Hand radiograph: cortical thickening, broad bases in the distal phalanges, osteophytes, cortical thickening, and soft tissue hypertrophy.

Treatment options

Removal of well-circumscribed somatotropic cell adenomas. Transsphenoidal surgery is preferably used by microscopic or laparoscopic techniques.

Medical therapy: it can be used as a complement to surgery or as an alternative when it is not possible. It consists of the administration of somatostatin analogues such as ocreotide or lanreotide. Dopamine receptor agonists such as bromocriptine or cabergoline can also be used. Currently, GH receptor antagonists can be used, which reduce IGF-1 levels without altering GH. This drug blocks the GH hormone at its receptors.

Radiation therapy: used as an adjunct to surgery to prevent remission. Conventional radiation therapy or stereotactic radiosurgery can be used.

Follow-up peculiarities
Close follow-up given the risk of remission. Consider factors associated with remission to establish follow-up as well as considering the individual characteristics of the patient.

Significant predictive factors of biochemical remission in postoperative patients are:

- ✓ Advanced age of the patient.
- ✓ Smaller tumor size.
- ✓ Lower preoperative GH level.

- ✓ Lower preoperative GH level.
- ✓ Imaging studies should be performed 12 to 16 weeks after the surgical procedure to determine the presence of residual tumor.

Bibliographic references

1. Shlomo Melmed, Richard J. Auchus, Allison B. Goldfine, Ronald J. Kowning, Clifford Rosen. Williams Textbook of Endocrinology 14Th edition. ELSEVIER, 2020.
2. Drewes AM, Arlien-Søborg MC, Lunde Jørgensen JO, Jensen MP. [Acromegaly and symptoms of the motor apparatus]. Ugeskr. Laeg. 2018 Nov 12; 180 (46)

Chapter 286. Tall Stature

It consists of a height greater than +2 standard deviations or a height greater than> 2 standard deviations above the target height. Another definition of tall stature is a height above the 97th percentile for sex and age in a defined population.

Statistics and epidemiology

It is estimated that 3 out of 100 children are tall. Tall stature is less common than short stature. Most tall children are healthy, although it may be associated with underlying disorders.

Risk groups or factors: Family history of tall stature.

Etiology and elements of pathophysiology

Family tall stature	Also known as constitutional tall stature (most common cause). Height is above the 97th percentile. The mean parental height above the 90th or 97th percentile. It occurs most often in a girl and her mother. The bone is advanced marginally to moderately (final height is not very high). Physical exam and labs are normal.
Nutrition	Both height and weight are in a higher percentile. Bone age is marginal to moderately advanced.
Hormonal causes	Hyperthyroidism Early puberty. Growth hormone excess. The bone age is moderately advanced.

	Commitment of final adulthood.
Chromosomal causes	Klinefelter syndrome (XXY). Homocystinuria (absence of the enzyme cystathionine beta-synthase). Marfan syndrome (mutation of the FBN-1 gene on chromosome 15q). Sotos syndrome (or cerebral gigantis). Beckwith-weidman syndrome (duplication of the paternal IGF-2 gene and IGF-2 overexpression). Fragile X syndrome. Simpson-Golabi-Behmeles syndrome. Triple X syndrome (XXX, there may be mosaics).

Diagnostic criteria

Clinic	Tall stature is clinically diagnosed by a height above the 97th percentile or more than 2 standard deviations. There may be other manifestations associated with the specific cause: High weight (nutritional causes). Delayed puberty, small firm testes, eunucoid body proportions, and gynecomastia (Klinefelter syndrome). Neonatal hypotonia, macrocephaly, large dolichocephaly, arched palate, among others (Sotos syndrome). Elongated face, protruding ears, intellectual disability, flexible fingers, large testicles, autism (fragile X syndrome). Skeletal, cardiac, kidney, craniofacial abnormalities (Simpson-Golabi-Behmeles syndrome). Elongated limbs, narrow hands, and long, slender fingers. The extension of the arms is greater than the height, the lower segment is greater than the upper segment (Marfan syndrome). Elongated limbs, subnormal intelligence, osteopenia, fatal thromboembolic tendency, lenticular dislocation

	(homocystinuria). Epicantal folds, hypertelorism, upward sloping palpebral fissures, hypotonia, clinodactyly, joint hyperextensibility, congenital hip dysplasia, ovarian failure, among others (triple X syndrome).
Paraclinical	The diagnosis is clinical, however, paraclinical tests are performed to identify the underlying cause of tall stature: Karyotype. Serum prolactin. Serum cortisol level. Thyroid test (T4, TSH). IGF-1 measurement. Serum levels of LH, FSH and testosterone. Evaluation of bone age and prediction of final height. Magnetic resonance imaging of the pituitary. Visual field exam. Glucose suppression test for GH.

Treatment options

Generally, tall stature is not considered a pathological condition, so treatment is not indicated.

The most accepted treatment is the early induction of puberty to achieve a complete fusion of the epiphyses and obtain the final size. For this, testosterone can be used in men and estrogen in women.

Testosterone enanthate is used in men frequently at doses of 250 to 500 mg twice a week for 6 to 9 months.

In women, 17 beta-estradiol is used most often, at doses of 0.2 to 4 mg per day, and a progestin of 10 mg can be added for one week per month.

A somatostatin analog (octreotide) given overnight infusion has been reported to decrease GH secretion. The dose used is between 37.5 to 50 mg one to two times a day subcutaneously.

Bilateral percutaneous epiphysiodesis of the distal femur and proximal tibia and fibula is the most widely used surgical procedure to reduce growth.

Follow-up peculiarities

Depending on the triggering cause of the tall stature, follow-up visits will be established to monitor the specific treatment of the underlying disease state and the risk of associated complications.

Bibliographic references

1. Kumar S. (2013). Tallstature in children: differential diagnosis and management. International Journal of Pediatric Endocrinology, 2013 (Suppl 1), P53.https://doi.org/10.1186/1687-9856-2013-S1-P53
2. Meazza, C., Gertosio, C., Giacchero, R., Pagani, S., & Bozzola, M. (2017). Tallstature: a difficult diagnosis? Italian journal of pediatrics, 43 (1), 66.https://doi.org/10.1186/s13052-017-0385-5

Chapter 287. Pituitary Metastasis

It is a rare pathology that results from the migration of malignant cells from distant regions to the pituitary area. There is no precise serum tumor marker to establish the diagnosis and the imaging methods are not specific for the diagnosis of metastasis and discriminate it from other pituitary tumors. It is a disorder with a poor prognosis.

Statistics and epidemiology

- ✓ They could occur more often in men than women.
- ✓ The average age is approximately 60 years.
- ✓ About 40% may not have a history of malignancy.
- ✓ The median survival after diagnosis is approximately 10 months.
- ✓ It is estimated that about 1.8% of pituitary masses resected by surgery are pituitary metastases.

Risk groups or factors

- ✓ History of malignant tumor.
- ✓ Etiology and pathophysiology
- ✓ Malignant neoplasms in distant structures spread throughout the bloodstream.

Adenocarcinomas, breast cancer, and lymphoma stand out among the most frequent malignancies. The posterior part of the pituitary gland is estimated to be more susceptible to metastasis compared to the anterior.

The mechanism of attraction of metastatic cells to the pituitary gland is unclear. It may be due to the glandular distribution, characteristics of the primary tumor or of the pituitary gland.

Diagnostic criteria

Clinic:

The clinical manifestations are usually multiple and include:
- ✓ Fatigue.
- ✓ Visual disability.
- ✓ Common ocular motor nerve palsy.
- ✓ Diabetes insipidus
- ✓ Gait disturbances.
- ✓ Central obesity.
- ✓ Headache.
- ✓ Hypopituitarism.

Paraclinical

Thyroid hormone levels (can be normal, high, or low).

Enhanced CT scan: May show soft tissue opacity with heterogeneous sellar region and inhomogeneous enhancement.

Magnetic resonance imaging: sellar occupant lesions. There may be isointensity in T1, with a short signal, isointensity in T2 and a long T2 signal, among others.

Treatment options

Treatment is oriented towards microscopic resection with a transsphenoidal approach. Subsequently, the patient must receive treatment with radiotherapy and chemotherapy.

Surgery is also used as a confirmatory element of the diagnosis and helps reduce symptoms.

The use of steroids in high doses before the biopsy of suspicious pituitary masses, as well as the subsequent reduction of them, could mask the diagnosis, resulting in a negative biopsy.

Follow-up peculiarities

Close follow-up should be established due to the poor prognosis of the disease.

Bibliographic references

1. Yi Zhao, Weixun Zhou. Diagnosis, Therapy, and Therapeutic Effects in Cases of Pituitary Metastasis. World Neurosurgery. Volume 117, September 2018, Pages 122-128. DOI:https://doi.org/10.1016/j.wneu.2018.05.205
2. Javanbakht, A., D'Apuzzo, M., Badie, B., & Salehian, B. (2018). Pituitary metastasis: a rare condition. Endocrine connections, 7 (10), 1049–1057. Advance online publication. https://doi.org/10.1530/EC-18-0338

Chapter 288. Pediatric Pituitary Tumor

Around 3.5 to 8.5% of pituitary tumors are diagnosed before the age of 20. It is considered a rare pathology among pediatric patients, representing less than 4% of intracranial tumors. Its annual incidence in children is 0.1 to 4.1 per 100,000 children.

Clinical aspects of pituitary tumors in pediatrics

Epidemiology	Diagnosis	Treatment
Prolactinomas		
It is estimated that at least 50% of intracranial tumors are prolactin-secreting. Predominance in women.	Hyperprolactinemia (prolactin greater than 100 ug / L). Magnetic resonance imaging focused on the pituitary. Campimetry (performed throughout the treatment, when there is initial alteration).	*Dopamine agonists*: bromocriptine, cabergoline (0.5-2 mg / week.) and quinagolide. The dose of cabergoline treatment can be increased from 0.25 by 0.25 mg each week to 1.5 mg / week. Prolactin levels are assessed a month. In case of persistence of hyperprolactinemia, macroprolactinoma intolerant secondary effects, surgical treatment is considered. After 1 year of treatment 2 for macroprolactinoma with normal prolactin levels, the dose of cabergoline is gradually reduced by periodically evaluating the prolactin level.

1559

Cushing's disease		
About 10-15% of Cushing's disease cases occur among children and adolescents. The exogenous cause is the most frequent. The mean age of presentation in pediatric age is 14.1 years.	Growth retardation with predominantly trunk obesity. Fascie on a full moon. Buffalo neck. Fragility. Cutaneous ecchymoses. Vinous red streaks. Myopathy Delay in bone maturation. Midnight plasma cortisol measurement starting at 4.4 ug / dL over 3 days. Cortisoluria greater than 70 ug / m2 / 24h Suppression with high doses of dexamethasone (either at 8 mg at night or over 2 days as 20ug / kg / 6 hours with a maximum of 2mg / 6h).	Adenectomy by transsphenoidal surgery. Periodic evaluation of the cortico-adrenal axis.
TSH-producing tumors		
They represent between 1 to 3% of pituitary adenomas. Extremely rare	Cardiac symptoms (atrial fibrillation, heart failure, palpitations). Tremor.	Transsphenoidal surgery. Beta-blockers, antithyroids, iodine, or somatostatin analogs to achieve thyroid blockage.

in children.	Weightloss. Excessive sweating Insomnia. Fatigue. Exophthalmos or pretibial myxedema. Compressive symptoms (headache, visual disturbances).	Radiotherapy.
Giantism		
GH-secreting adenomas in the pediatric population constitute between 5% and 16% of tumors.	Elevated levels of IGF-1. Lack of GH secretion suppression due to oral glucose overload. Paradoxical response to TRH and RH. Magnetic resonance diagnosis	Transsphenoidal surgery as the therapy of choice. Somatostatin analogs are used to supplement surgery (Octreotide, Lanreotide, Octreotide-LAR). Currently, a GH receptor antagonist (pegvisomant) can be used, which normalizes IGF-1 values by up to 90%.
Non-functioning pituitary tumors		
Most are expressed as macroadenomas. Its mean age of onset in pediatric age is 12.5 years. It occurs more in the male in a ratio of 3 to 1.	Compressive symptoms (headache, cranial nerve palsy, cavernous sinus invasion, obstructive hydrocephalus, liquorrhea). Hormonal deficiencies (GH,	Transsphenoidal surgery.

	adrenal insufficiency, hypothyroidism, hypogonadism). Hyperprolactinemia (involvement of the stem).	

Bibliographic references

1. Chen, J., Schmidt, RE, & Dahiya, S. (2019). Pituitary Adenoma in Pediatric and Adolescent Populations. Journal of neuropathology and experimental neurology, 78 (7), 626–632.https://doi.org/10.1093/jnen/nlz040
2. Alfonso Leal Cerro. Functioning pituitary tumors in pediatric age.10.3266 / RevEspEndocrinolPediatr.pre2014.Apr.222

Chapter 289. Pituitary Tumor and Pregnancy

Pituitary tumors comprise between 10 to 20% of all intracranial tumors. Clinically relevant adenomas have a prevalence of around 1 in 1000 in the general population. However, during pregnancy, a series of physiological changes occur in the endocrine system, and especially in the pituitary gland, which can increase its size 2 or 3 times during pregnancy, mainly caused by hypertrophy and hyperplasia of the lactotrophs, stimulated by the marked increase in estrogen levels. Pituitary tumors represent a challenge for effective management during this period in order to guarantee maternal and fetal well-being.

Pituitary neoplasia	Description	Treatment and management
Prolactinoma (See Chapter 348)	Prevalence about 40% of all pituitary adenomas. Primary cause of hyperprolactinemia. It leads to infertility and gonadal dysfunction. Patients with previously known prolactinomas should receive contraception due to the risk of prolactinoma growth during pregnancy until the tumor is resected.	Dopamine agonist treatment is discontinued upon identification of pregnancy in patients with microadenomas and macroadenomas. Treatment with dopamine agonists is continued when in macroadenomas with suprasellar extension, tumor close to the optic chiasm, or short period of treatment prior to conception. The conduct is close

		monitoring and expectant management. Surgery is indicated in the second trimester of pregnancy.
Acromegaly	In pregnant women with acromegaly, an increase in the plasma level of IGF-1 occurs due to the secretion of placental GH, however, there is no reduction in the autonomic secretion of GH by the adenoma. An immunofluorometric assay without specific interferences for the placental GH variant is required to differentiate it from pituitary GH and establish the diagnosis. There may be improvement in clinical signs and symptoms, mainly during the first trimester of pregnancy. The improvement in IGF-1 can be attributed to the effect of the marked increase in estrogen levels during pregnancy, which inhibits GH signaling, an action mediated by cytokine signaling suppressor proteins causes a state of GH resistance.	Women with acromegaly planning to become pregnant are advised to discontinue current medical treatment for acromegaly at least 2 to 3 months prior to conception. The use of GH receptor antagonists is restricted to exceptional cases of uncomplicated acromegalic pregnant women. Close monitoring of the tumor should be established with visual field tests every trimester and evaluation of compressive symptoms. In the case of macroadenomas, identified during pregnancy or after medical treatment, monthly follow-up visits should be indicated. When there are macroadenomas with a high risk of tumor growth, treatment with dopamine agonists or

		somatostatin analogues should be indicated throughout pregnancy. When there is evidence of tumor growth, second trimester transsphenoidal surgery or medical treatment may be considered. Breastfeeding is contraindicated.
Cushing's syndrome	Pregnancy rarely occurs during the course of Cushing's syndrome, due to the state of hypercortisolism and hyperandrogenism, which suppresses gonadotropic function resulting in amenorrhea and oligomenorrhea accompanied by infertility. Most of the reported cases, Cushing's syndrome is diagnosed during pregnancy and the preconception diagnosis is not established. Only 40% of these cases are associated with an adrenocorticotropic hormone-producing pituitary adenoma. Cushing's syndrome associated with pregnancy increases maternal morbidity in 70% of cases	The treatment of choice is transsphenoidal surgery during the second trimester of pregnancy. Other treatments consist of the administration of medical treatment (metyrapone or ketoconazole) and / or adrenalectomy. However, metyrapone has been associated with hypertension during pregnancy, and ketoconazole has shown teratogenic effects in rats, so they are considered emergency treatments and not routinely indicated. Cabergoline in high doses has shown favorable results.

	and in turn affects the fetal outcome.	
Thyrotropin pituitary adenomas	They represent 0.5 to 3% of pituitary adenomas. Pregnancy is extremely rare and to date, 4 cases have been recorded in the literature. The clinic is associated with symptoms of hyperthyroidism.	Close monitoring. Given the unusual nature of these tumors in pregnancy, there is no established management or strategy for their treatment.
Clinically non-functioning pituitary adenomas	They are not common during pregnancy, because fertility is often impaired. Lactotropic hyperplasia is induced by the absence of an inhibitory effect of dopamine. This occurs in all pregnancies and can cause the tumor to grow and be pushed into the optic chiasm.	The treatment of choice consists of dopamine agonists. Surgery is reserved for cases where no results are obtained with medical treatment or when tumor apoplexy occurs.

Bibliographic references

1. Araujo PB, Neto LV, Gadelha MR. Pituitary Tumor Management in Pregnancy. Endocrinology and Metabolism Clinics of North America. 2015 Mar; 44 (1): 181-97.
2. Nana M, Williamson C. Pituitary and Adrenal Disorders of Pregnancy. [Updated 2019 Apr 16]. In: Feingold KR, Anawalt B, Boyce A, et al., Editors. Endotext [Internet]. South Dartmouth (MA): MDText.com, Inc .; 2000-.

Chapter 290. Cysts of Rathke's Bursa

Also known as the intermediate Pars cyst, it consists of a cystic, intrasellar and epithelial lesion, which derives from the remains of the Rathke bag, which constitutes the embryonic ancestor of the pituitary gland.

Statistics and epidemiology

- ✓ Most cysts occur asymptomatically.
- ✓ It is a rare disorder.
- ✓ In autopsy series, between 12 and 33% have been identified with normal pituitary glands.
- ✓ They are frequently located in the sella turcica, although they can be found in the sphenoid sinus.
- ✓ It usually occurs in children or young adults.
- ✓ It predominates in women.
- ✓ They represent between 6 and 10% of symptomatic sellar and suprasellar lesions.

Etiology and pathophysiological elements

It originates from embryonic remnants of Rathke's pouch, located between the Pars distalis (anterior lobe of the pituitary gland) and the Pars intermedia. So it develops as a cystic lesion between the anterior and posterior lobe of the pituitary.

Unlike craniopharyngiomas, Rathke's bursa cysts do not invade; however, they can expand and cause mass compression.

Histologically, it appears as a thin wall with cloudy and thick fluid. Microscopically it presents tall columnar epithelium of balloon and ciliated cells. They may be filled with oily or mucinous content with squamous cells.

Diagnostic criteria

Clinic	- Large cysts can be associated with hypopituitarism. - Headache - Visual disturbances
Paraclinical	- Radiologically it presents as a cystic or mixed mass. Well defined edges are evident. It erodes or reshapes nearby structures with contrast and can enhance the periphery of the occupational process after contrast administration. - On MRI, it appears as a very bright cystic neoplasm on T1, although it appears less bright or isointense on T2, due to the high protein and / or fat content.

Treatment and follow-up options

Asymptomatic Rathke cysts can maintain expectant therapy with follow-up by serial imaging studies.

Meanwhile, patients with symptomatic Rathke's bursa cysts are managed by surgical decompression. Generally, a transsphenoidal corridor is employed through the use of an operating microscope or endoscope.

The objective of the procedure is to aspirate the contents of the cyst, alleviating the patient's symptoms caused by the mass effect of the cyst. During the procedure, a biopsy sample is obtained from the cyst wall for study.

Bibliographic references

1. Lavin N, editor. Manual of endocrinology and metabolism. 4th ed. Philadelphia: Wolters Kluwer / Lippincott Williams & Wilkins Health; 2009. 837 p.
2. Ramón A Gutiérrez Alvarado, Gerardo Romo Bonilla, Fernando Pacheco. Rathke cyst. EvidMedInvest Health 2013; 6 (3): 95-99.

Chapter 291. Pituitary Granulomas

It is a disorder characterized by the infiltration of immune cells and destruction of the pituitary gland, which triggers varying degrees of dysfunction of the pituitary gland.

Statistics and epidemiology

Its incidence is 1 case per 1,000,000 people, being a very rare disorder. It occurs in equal frequency between men and women. The lymphocytic subtype is observed mainly in women. However, cases have been described more frequently in boys and men.

Sarcoidosis as a pituitary granulomatous process occurs in about 5 to 15% of patients with sarcoidosis. Giant cell granuloma is also a rare cause of hypopituitarism.

Risk groups or factors: History of autoimmune disease; history of infiltrative diseases.

Etiology and pathophysiological elements

Forms of granulomatous disease associated with pituitary failure

- ✓ Sarcoidosis
- ✓ Giant cell granuloma (mainly affects the anterior pituitary).
- ✓ Langerhans cell histiocytosis (presents abnormal dendritic cells, characterized by infiltration of organs, usually there is hypothalamic infiltration).

- ✓ Wegener's granulomatosis (rare).
- ✓ Idiopathic giant cell hypophysitis.
- ✓ Takayasu disease.
- ✓ Cogan syndrome.
- ✓ Crohn's disease.

The infiltration of immune cells can affect the posterior pituitary, the infundibulum and the anterior pituitary. This is known as infundibuloneurohypophysis, although it can also affect both simultaneously known as panhypophysitis. Often in the anterior pituitary the secretory function of hormones is affected.

Lymphocytic infiltration is especially due to cytotoxic T lymphocytes, which cause destruction of the pituitary and replacement with fibrotic material, causing fibrosis. There are also giant cells in granulomatous formation, characteristic of pituitary granulomas.

Hemochromatosis: It is a rare autosomal recessive inherited disorder that causes hypopituitarism due to an infiltration of iron in the anterior pituitary, as a result of an excessive absorption of dietary iron causing an overload of iron.

Diagnostic criteria

Clinic	Clinical manifestations associated with the underlying systemic disorders. Headache. Visual disorders or disturbances. There may be aseptic meningitis (fever, nausea, headache =.

	Symptoms associated with multiple pituitary deficiencies (occurs in about 75% of cases). Thyrotropic and corticotropic cells are most often affected. Granulomas caused by sarcoidosis often include diabetes insipidus and hypopituitarism. It in turn causes systemic evidence of the disease.
Paraclinical	Magnetic resonance imaging: shows symmetrical enlargement of the pituitary gland with suprasellar expansion. Presence of uniform enhancement after gadolinium administration. Also the disease process could cause fibrosis, shrinkage and empty sella turcica. Biochemical tests may show serum ACTH, TSH, and PRL levels below the normal range.

Treatment options

Treatment may comprise conservative treatment or aggressive resection of the mass.

The use of corticosteroids can be considered, although their results are variable, however, good results are observed in the administration of corticosteroids against granulomatosis caused by sarcoidosis.

It is essential to establish the hormone replacement therapy pertinent to the pituitary deficiency that the patient presents.

Follow-up peculiarities: **After remission, recurrence is rare.**

Bibliographic references

1. Shlomo Melmed. The Pituitary 4th Edition. AcademicPress, Elsevier, 2017.

2. Shlomo Melmed, Richard J. Auchus, Allison B. Goldfine, Ronald J. Kowning, Clifford Rosen. Williams Textbook of Endocrinology 14Th edition. ELSEVIER, 2020.
3. Elgamal, ME, Mohamed, R., Fiad, T., & Elgamal, EA (2017). Granulomatous hypophysitis: rare disease with challenging diagnosis. Clinical case reports, 5 (7), 1147–1151. https://doi.org/10.1002/ccr3.1007

Chapter 292. Sellar Arachnoidocele

Also known as the empty sella syndrome (ESS), it consists of a disorder in which the subarachnoid space herniates into the sella turcica, causing compression and flattening of the pituitary, as well as stretching of the pituitary stalk.

This term is used for the radiological finding of "empty sellar space" obtained in magnetic resonance and computed tomography images. It can be partial when less than 50% of the sellar space is occupied by cerebrospinal fluid (CSF) or complete when the CSF occupies more than 50% of this space and the pituitary gland is less than 2mm thick.

Statistics and epidemiology

It is considered a rare entity, with an estimated incidence of between 5.5 and 12% in autopsy studies. In patients undergoing neuroimaging, the incidence reaches around 12%. Studies suggest that in clinical practice it has an occurrence of around 35%.

It has a predilection for the female sex, with a proportion of around 4 or 5 cases in women, compared to 1 case in men, being also more common in obese people. Its maximum incidence ranges between the fourth and sixth decade of life.

Pituitary hormonal dysfunction is more common in men than women with sellar arachnoidocele.

Risk groups or factors:
- ✓ Pituitary surgical history.
- ✓ History of radiotherapy to the head.
- ✓ Obesity.
- ✓ Female gender
- ✓ Pituitary apoplexy.
- ✓ Multiple pregnancies
- ✓ Head injury.
- ✓ Congenital hypopituitarism.

Etiology or more frequent causes

Primary empty sella syndrome (ESP): incompetence of the sella diaphragm and resulting herniation of cerebrospinal fluid in the sella turcica. No predisposing genetic causes have been identified, although it is theorized that it is a condition present at birth.

Secondary empty sella syndrome (SES): result of an intracranial medical procedure (surgery, radiation) or consequence of a pathological process (hemorrhage, infarction) in the pituitary gland.

Pathophysiological elements

Among the mechanisms proposed in the development of sellar arachnoidocele pathology is the incompetence or complete absence of the diaphragm of the sella turcica, temporal expansion followed by regression of the pituitary gland, and chronic intracranial hypertension.

Pathologies that increase CSF pressure are related to PES, for example, brain tumors, intracranial thrombosis, hydrocephalus and idiopathic intracranial hypertension. The causes associated with the development of SES are related to treatments of pituitary adenomas, spontaneous glandular regression, postpartum pituitary necrosis, and lymphocytic hypophysitis.

Diagnostic criteria

Clinic	The physical examination and history are often normal, and endocrine function is generally unimpaired. The most common symptom is a headache. Spontaneous CSF rhinorrhea as well as visual field alterations may occur, however they are unusual manifestations. About 20% of cases have endocrine abnormalities and the clinical manifestations are related to the type of manifest deficiency.
Paraclinical	The diagnosis is often made accidentally by imaging studies. However, the entire pituitary axis should be tested. Common findings: Hyperprolactinemia (occurs in 10 to 17% of cases). GH deficiency (occurs between 4 to 60% of cases). Gonadotropin deficiency (present in 2 to 32% of cases). Adrenocorticotropin, thyroid-stimulating hormone, and antidiuretic hormone deficiency (each occurs in about 1% of cases). All pertinent studies on the pituitary axes and their hormonal function are recommended. Imaging studies: Magnetic resonance. Computed tomography. The typical presentation includes the filling of the CSF

	is in continuity with the overlying subarachnoid spaces, the residual pituitary is flattened against the sellar floor of the enlarged bony sella turcica. The pituitary volume can be evaluated, usually less than 611.21 mm3.

Treatment options

It usually does not require treatment. If there is a deficiency or excess of hormones, the treatment should be personalized and oriented to the characteristics of the individual presentation.

When there is elevated idiopathic intracranial pressure, osmotic diuretics or acetazolamide may be recommended.

Weight loss can have beneficial results in these patients.

Neurosurgical techniques can be used in the presence of rhinorrhea and other causes secondary to sellar arachnoidocele.

Bibliographic references

1. Chiloiro S, Giampietro A, Bianchi A, Tartaglione T, Capobianco A, Anile C, De Marinis L. Diagnosis Of Endocrine Disease: Primary Empty Sella: A Comprehensive Review. Eur. J. Endocrinol. 2017 Dec; 177 (6): R275-R285.
2. Miljic D, Pekic S, Popovic V. Empty Sella. [Updated 2018 Oct 1]. In: Feingold KR, Anawalt B, Boyce A, et al., Editors. Endotext [Internet]. South Dartmouth (MA): MDText.com, Inc .; 2000-.

Chapter 293. Pituitary Apoplexy

It consists of a condition or disorder in which a hemorrhage or heart attack occurs in the pituitary gland. It usually occurs in the presence of pre-existing pituitary adenomas. The term pituitary apoplexy refers to sudden death of the gland, caused by hemorrhage or an acute ischemic infarction.

Statistics and epidemiology

Its incidence ranges from 1.5 to 27.7% of cases of pituitary adenoma. Symptomatic cases have an incidence of 10%. The maximum incidence of dad occurs in the range of 37 to 58 years, with a male to female ratio of 2: 1.

When intratumoral hemorrhage, which does not manifest symptoms, but has been detected through imaging studies, is considered, the incidence can rise to 26%. The apoplexy of the adenomas of the pituitary gland is considered a rare event estimated in a 0.2% annual incidence.

Risk groups or factors:
- ✓ Pituitary macroadenoma.
- ✓ Pituitary tumor.
- ✓ Hypertension or hypotension.
- ✓ Surgery.
- ✓ Heart surgery.
- ✓ Drug's use.
- ✓ Head injury.
- ✓ Radiotherapy.

- ✓ Use of drugs: anticoagulants, estrogen.
- ✓ Major orthopedic procedures.
- ✓ Pregnancy and childbirth.
- ✓ Dengue.
- ✓ Infections
- ✓ Hypophysitis.

Etiology and pathophysiological elements

Pituitary strokes are frequently found, often undiagnosed pituitary adenomas. Stroke occurs as a result of the interaction of pituitary adenomas, predisposing factors that trigger the pathological mechanisms listed below:

The increase in pressure within the bony walls in the sella turcica where the pituitary gland resides, causes the main clinical manifestations. It occurs when suddenly the content of the sella turcica increases due to blood, edema and increased pressure occurs.

Theories on the mechanisms that lead to ischemia and hemorrhage are:

-Compression of the superior pituitary artery and its branches against the diaphragm of the sella turcica, causing ischemia of the anterior pituitary and the tumor.

-Compression of the thin pituitary capillary network.

-Rapid expansion of the tumor that exceeds its vascular supply, resulting in ischemia and necrosis.

Diagnostic criteria

Clinical manifestations
✓ Headache (95%).
✓ Hypotension (cardiovascular collapse) (95%).

- ✓ Diplopia (78%)
- ✓ Vomiting (70%).
- ✓ Visual field defects (64%).
- ✓ Decreased visual acuity. (52%).
- ✓ Hemiplegia (rare).
- ✓ Meningism (rare).

Useful paraclinics to establish the diagnosis

Proof	Expected outcome in stroke
Serum electrolytes	Hyponatremia
Complete blood count	Anemia and thrombocytopenia.
Prothrombin time	Prolonged (probable)
Random cortisol	Often <5 ug / dL.
T4 / FSH	Low / low or normal
Prolactin	Low (less than 1ng / dL).
Visual field tests	Visual defect
Pituitary MRI	Evidence of hemorrhagic infarction in the region of the pituitary. An enlarged sellar or suprasellar mass that is peripherally enhanced and surrounds a hypointense center.
Computed tomography	Sellar / suprasellar mass, associated with intralesional hemorrhage (must be requested first due to its ease of imaging). Subsequently, a study with contrast is performed to delimit the size of the tumor.

Treatment options

Therapeutics should include an assessment by a multidisciplinary team that includes intensive care neurologists, neurosurgeons, neuroophalthmologists, and endocrinologists.

Thorough and careful evaluation of fluid and electrolyte balance (ensure hemodynamic stability and replace corticosteroids).

Intravenous bolus of corticosteroids 100 to 200 mg of hydrocortisone, this should be followed with an additional administration between 50 to 100 mg every 6 hours. Alternatively, a continuous infusion of 2 to 4 mg per hour after the initial bolus can be used. All patients should receive corticosteroids even in the absence of adrenal crisis.

Delay of decompressive surgery may be considered, however, it should be done within a week. If visual symptoms improve or stabilize, watchful or conservative management may be considered.

The necessary measures should be applied to treat the adenoma. The main treatment chosen consists of surgical resection with a transsphenoidal approach.

Follow-up peculiarities:

About 80% of patients have residual hypopituitarism after a pituitary apoplexy. However, not all patients present with signs of hypopituitarism immediately. In addition, there is a risk of tumor regrowth and recurrent stroke.

Therefore, a follow-up should be established every 3 to 6 months, including evaluation of imaging studies (pituitary magnetic resonance), until the anatomy stabilizes. Follow-up is continued annually for 5 years.

One month after discharge, it is recommended to reassess hormonal biochemical studies and indicate hormone replacement therapy whenever necessary.

Bibliographic reference

1. Shlomo Melmed, Richard J. Auchus, Allison B. Goldfine, Ronald J. Kowning, Clifford Rosen. Williams Textbook of Endocrinology 14Th edition. ELSEVIER, 2020.
2. Shlomo Melmed. The Pituitary 4th Edition. AcademicPress, Elsevier, 2017.
3. Rajasekaran, S., Vanderpump, M., Baldeweg, S., Drake, W., Reddy, N., Lanyon, M., Markey A., Plant, G., Powell, M., Sinha, S., Wass , J. UK guidelines for the management of pituitary apoplexy. ClinEndocrinol (Oxf) 2011 Jan 74 (1); 9-20. PMID 21044119

Chapter 294. Hypophysitis

It is an autoimmune inflammatory disorder, which occurs during or shortly after delivery. Cases have also been reported after menopause. It is a rare cause of hypopituitarism, which can occur as a primary or idiopathic cause or as a secondary cause due to lesions in the sella turcica, systemic diseases or the administration of drugs.

Statistics and epidemiology

- ✓ About 57% of cases have been documented in association with pregnancy.
- ✓ Most of the time, it occurs in the last month of pregnancy or during the first 2 months after delivery.
- ✓ At least 15% of the cases have been identified in men.
- ✓ About 20% of patients have diabetes insipidus.

Risk groups or factors: **History of autoimmune disease**

Etiology or more frequent causes

Primary hypophysitis	Isolated Associated with autoimmune diseases (polyglandular autoimmune syndrome, autoimmune thyroiditis, diabetes mellitus 1, others).
Secondary hypophysitis	*Drugs:* Immune checkpoint inhibitors. Alpha interferon.

	Ribavirin.
	Sellar and parasellar disease
	Germinome.
	Rathke cleft cyst.
	Craniopharyngioma.
	Pituitary adenoma.
	Systemic diseases
	Granulomatosis with polyangiitis.
	Sarcoidosis
	Crohn's disease.
	Takayasu syndrome.
	Thymoma
	Infections:
	Tuberculosis.
	Cytomegalovirus, Herpes virus.
	Mycosis
	Toxoplasma gondii.
	Others.

Pathophysiological elements

It presents a pituitary infiltrate by lymphocytic cells and plasma cells, which can be found in isolation or in association with other endocrinopathies.

Circulating antipituitary antibodies can occasionally be found, in conjunction with the presence of an isolated deficiency of pituitary hormones. This could involve an autoimmune process selectively targeting pituitary cells.

Histopathological forms of primary hypophysitis
- ✓ Lymphocytic hypophysitis.
- ✓ Granulomatous hypophysitis.
- ✓ Xanthomatous hypophysitis.
- ✓ Plasmacytic hypophysitis, related to IgG4.

- ✓ Necrotizing hypophysitis.
- ✓ Mixed forms.

Diagnostic criteria

Clinic	Short-term natural history. Presence of secondary adenohypophyseal cell atrophy with evidence of resulting empty sella turcica. Headache. Visual field alteration. Clinic associated with hyperprolactinemia. Clinic associated with pituitary hormone deficiency.
Paraclinical	Hyperprolactinemia. Erythrocyte sedimentation rate is usually elevated. Magnetic resonance imaging: shows a pituitary mass indistinguishable from a pituitary adenoma. There is evidence of suprasellar, intrasellar, and pituitary stalk enlargement. Attenuated GH and ACTH responses to hypothalamic hormone challenge tests. Pathological criteria for diagnosis: Islands of cells of the anterior pituitary, surrounded by diffuse lymphocytic infiltrates (T cells and B cells). Presence of plasma cells in 53% and eosinophils in 12%, there may also be mast cells.

Treatment and follow-up options

If there is no evidence of visual field disturbances due to compression and the diagnosis has been convincingly established, surgical therapy should be discontinued and replacement for pituitary hormone deficiencies started.

Due to the often spontaneous resolution of the hypophysitis, the inflammatory mass will be followed expectantly.

Transsphenoidal or endoscopic surgical resection may be recommended when there are clinical manifestations of compression or confirmation of the tissue diagnosis is necessary. However, viable pituitary tissue should be preserved in view of the frequent spontaneous resolution.

Bibliographic references

1. Shlomo Melmed, Richard J. Auchus, Allison B. Goldfine, Ronald J. Kowning, Clifford Rosen. Williams Textbook of Endocrinology 14Th edition. ELSEVIER, 2020.
2. Dorantes and Martinez. Clinical endocrinology 5th edition, Editorial El Manual Moderno 2016.

Chapter 295. Surgery of the Pituitary

Pituitary surgeries are often indicated for the excision of massive lesions that cause central pressure effects, including primary correction of hormonal hypersecretion, visual compromise, primary correction, or functional removal of the tumor in patients who do not respond to medical conventional medication. Additionally, sellar lesions of unusual characteristics may require diagnostic tissue evaluation, and wide excision is sometimes required.

General description

Transsphenoidal approach
Prevents invasion of the cranial cavity, excluding the risk or need to manipulate brain tissue. The pituitary can be clearly distinguished from the tumor tissue, since this approach allows an operative field with good visibility and internal illumination. Morbidity and mortality: minimal risk. Hospitalization time: 3 days. Benefit: allows the tumor tissue to be clearly distinguished, facilitating microdissection and removal of small tumors. The ventral sphenoid approach does not involve the cranial fossa either.
Endoscopic surgical technique
It allows approaching the sellar region, through an endonasal approach or an approach through the base of the skull. Lesions are reached through transposition of the pituitary to reach the lesion. It allows to obtain results similar to the traditional transsphenoidal approach in experienced hands.

Craniotomy
It is indicated when rare invasive suprasellar masses are found, which extend towards the middle or frontal fossa, extensive posterior clival invasion or when it extends towards the optic nerves. The hourglass configuration (suprasellar extension contained by a small diaphragmatic opening), often requires a transcranial approach.

Occasionally, the removal of pituitary masses requires a combination of a surgical approach between intracranial and transsphenoidal surgery.

However, the surgical technique of choice for the resection of most pituitary masses is the transsphenoidal surgical approach.

Transsphenoidal surgery

Primary indications
General
Compression of the visual tract or central nervous system. Tissue histology requirement for diagnosis. Tumor recurrence after surgery or irradiation. Personal decision. Desire for immediate pregnancy with macroadenoma. Relief of compressive hypoparathyroidism caused by present, residual or recurrent tumor tissue. Intolerance or resistance to medical therapy. Cerebrospinal fluid leak. Pituitary hemorrhage.
Specific
TSH-secreting adenoma. Cushing's disease. Acromegaly. Prolactinoma. Nelson syndrome.

Clinically non-functional macroadenoma.
Side effects
Transient
Narcolepsy Pulmonary embolism Local abscess. Diabetes insipidus Meningitis. Aranoiditis. Epistaxis. Damage to the arterial wall. Local hematoma. Loss of cerebrospinal fluid and rhinorrhea. Postoperative psychosis. Inappropriate ADH secretion.
Permanent (occurs in 10% of cases)
Nasal septum perforation. Vascular occlusion. Diabetes insipidus Central nervous system damage (encephalopathy, hemiparesis, oculomotor paralysis). Visual loss Inappropriate ADH secretion. Total or partial hypopituitarism.
Causes of mortality associated with surgery (occurs in 1% of interventions).
Pneumocephalus Cerebrospinal fluid leak. Vascular damage Hypothalamic injury, brain. Seizure. Related to anesthesia. Postoperative meningitis. Acute cardiopulmonary disease.

After the procedure, patients should be kept at rest with the bed at an angle of 30 to 45 degrees. Serum and urinary osmolality should be measured, together with serum electrolytes every 6 hours postoperatively.

Bibliographic references

1. Shlomo Melmed, Richard J. Auchus, Allison B. Goldfine, Ronald J. Kowning, Clifford Rosen. Williams Textbook of Endocrinology 14Th edition. ELSEVIER, 2020.
2. Shlomo Melmed. The Pituitary 4th Edition. AcademicPress, Elsevier, 2017.

Chapter 296. Radio and Pituitary Chemotherapy

The treatment of pituitary masses or lesions frequently uses surgical therapeutics or medical treatments to improve the compressive symptoms caused by the pituitary hormonal imbalance.

However, radiotherapy and pituitary chemotherapy are usually used as an adjunct to surgical therapy, when the approach is not possible or in the presence of rare or malignant pituitary masses, among others.

Radiotherapy

The principle of radiotherapy in the treatment of pituitary masses consists of administering high-energy ionizing radiation to deep tissues, using megavoltage techniques to provide maximum necrotizing radiation in the pituitary gland injury, avoiding exposure to adjacent normal structures. .

Fractional approaches: up to 5000 rads (50 Gy) are administered in 180 rads daily fractions for 5 to 6 weeks.

They can be administered through stereotactic radiosurgery or through robotic surgery with cobalt-60 Gamma Knife or Cyber Knife or also with linear accelerator.

Radiosurgery is the most appropriate technique for the treatment of intraselar and cavernous lesions distant from the optic nerves.

Pituitary irradiation

Indications	Side effects
Pituitary adenoma (Cushing's disease, non-functional adenoma, adjuvant treatment for acromegaly, prolactinoma). Resistance to surgery and medical treatments. Nelson syndrome. Invasive non-adenomatous sellar mass. Rumor recurrence. Recurrence of hormonal hypersecretion.	Hypopituitarism. Visual loss Optic neuritis. Brain necrosis. Temporal lobe deficit. Cognitive dysfunction.

Chemotherapy

It is usually used as the last option in the treatment of benign, malignant or metastatic pituitary lesions which, despite prior administration of first-line treatments, no significant clinical improvement is achieved.

Indications

Salvage therapy for stone-like pituitary adenomas or carcinomas that progressively grow despite multiple efforts for removal through surgical resection, medical treatment (dopamine agonists or somatostatin analogs), and radiation therapy without achieving complete remission.

Chemotherapeutic agents most used in pituitary treatment

- ✓ Temozolomide.
- ✓ Lomustine.
- ✓ 5-flurouracil.

- ✓ Cisplatin
- ✓ Carboplatin
- ✓ Etoposide.

Temozolomide

The success is variable, however, currently the most used is temozolomide, due to its high response rate and the favorable profile of its side effects.

Temozolomide dose: 150 to 200 mg / m2 / day orally for 5 days every 4 weeks.
Side effects:
Sickness.
Constipation.
Fatigue.
Teratogenic.
Reduced fertility (azoospermia and premature ovarian failure).
Potential complications (they are late and often permanent).
Myelodysplastic syndrome.
Myelogenous leukemia.

Bibliographic references

1. Shlomo Melmed, Richard J. Auchus, Allison B. Goldfine, Ronald J. Kowning, Clifford Rosen. Williams Textbook of Endocrinology 14Th edition. ELSEVIER, 2020.
2. Lin, AL, Sum, MW, & DeAngelis, LM (2016). Is there a role for early chemotherapy in the management of pituitary adenomas ?. Neuro-oncology, 18 (10), 1350–1356. https://doi.org/10.1093/neuonc/now059

Part VIII. Gonadal Conditions

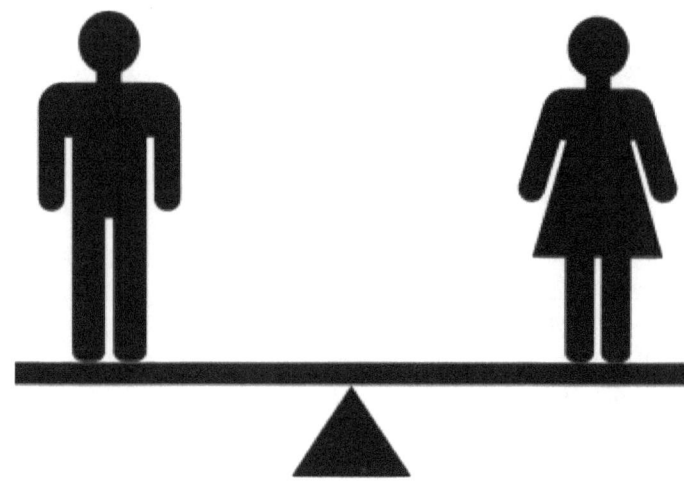

Chapter 297. Endocrinologic Gynecology

The hypothalamus, the pituitary gland, the ovaries and the endometrium, through coordinated functions, allow cyclical and predictable menstruations, characteristics of regular ovulation, to be possible. In addition, the proper functioning of the endocrine glands, such as the adrenal and thyroid glands, intervenes in endocrine gynecological functions.

Endocrinological gynecology encompasses the deep knowledge associated with the functions and interactions between the hypothalamus, the pituitary, the uterus and the ovaries and their relationship with other systems, so that it allows establishing precise diagnoses of reproductive disorders and proposing precise therapeutic strategies.

Central nervous system-hypothalamus-pituitary-gonadal axis and target organs

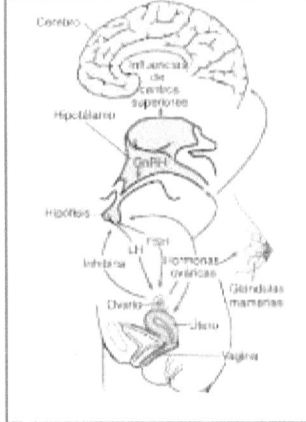	**Central Nervous System:** Pulsatile secretion of gonadotropin-releasing hormone (GnRH). Negative feedback effect of various factors (such as ovarian steroids), regulate hypothalamic GnRH secretion in portal vessels. Norepinephrine, serotonin, dopamine, and opioids produced in the brain, may intervene in the regulation of GnRH release by ovarian hormones, among other stimuli.

	In response to GnRH, follicle-stimulating hormone (FSH) and luteinizing hormone (LH) are secreted by the anterior pituitary.
	Ovaries:
	LH and FSH promote ovulation and in turn stimulate the release of sex hormones such as estradiol and progesterone from the ovaries.
	Activin and follistatin are produced in the ovary and pituitary and appear to regulate pituitary FSH secretion by autocrine or paracrine (non-endocrine) pathways. Follistatin suppresses the action of activin, while activin stimulates the production of FSH.
	Target organ of the reproductive system (vagina, uterus, breasts):
	Estrogens and progesterone are found circulating in the bloodstream almost totally bound to plasma proteins. However, the biologically active sex hormones are in their free state and are the ones that stimulate the target organ.
	The action of sex hormones is inhibitory but they can stimulate gonadotropin secretion.
	Estradiol induces the growth of the endometrium.
	Progesterone limits the estrogenic effect, improving differentiation.
	The detachment of the functional layer of the endometrium follows the withdrawal of estrogen or progesterone.

The normal function of the female reproductive system depends on coordinated actions that result in regular menstruation every 24 to 35 days. Any condition in any of these tissues or dysfunction of other systems that intervene secondary to these reproductive structures, can cause anovulation and irregular uterine bleeding.

Reproductive functions

Features
Hypothalamus: Produces gonadotropin-releasing hormone.
Anterior pituitary: Gonadotrophic cells synthesize both LH and FSH.
Ovary (generation of a fertilizable egg and preparation of the endometrium for implantation):   Periodic release of oocytes.   Production of steroid hormones, progesterone and estradiol.
Endometrium: *Functional layer:* prepared for blastocyst implantation. It is the site of proliferation, secretion and degeneration.   *Basal layer:* provides regenerative endometrium after menstrual loss of function.

Bibliographic references

1. Shlomo Melmed, Richard J. Auchus, Allison B. Goldfine, Ronald J. Kowning, Clifford Rosen. Williams Textbook of Endocrinology 14Th edition. ELSEVIER, 2020.

Chapter 298. The Ovaries

The ovaries are a pair of endocrine organs located intraperitoneally, typically in the lower, left, and right abdominal quadrants, respectively. They constitute the female gonads, which play a fundamental role in reproduction and hormonal production.

Embryology

The ovaries originate from the intermediate mesoderm. They are differentiated in the medulla and have a layer of germinal epithelium on the surface.
The dorsal endoderm of the yolk sac is responsible for producing immature egg precursor cells, these will migrate to the posterior intestine and then to the gonadal crest which will be formed in week 4 of gestation. During this process, the ovary is called the oogonia, which will continue to mature inside the connective tissue layer until it becomes granulosa cells.
Once the follicle reaches two layers of granulosa cells, another layer morphologically distinct from somatic cells, the theca cells, differentiates from the ovarian stroma.
The ovaries will descend during embryological development to locate in their abdominal location. The proper ovarian ligament originates from the remnant of the governmental.

Anatomy

Description
They are oval bodies with a length of 2 to 5 cm and a width of 1.5 cm. They are 0.5 to 1.5 cm thick.
They are located near the posterior and lateral pelvic wall, attached to the posterior surface by the broad ligament through the peritoneal fold (mesovarian).
Its posterior relationship is the ureter and the internal iliac artery, while its anterior relationship is the medial umbilical ligament.
Ovarian structure:
External cortex: contains the follicles and the superficial germinal epithelium.
Central medulla: consists of a stroma and a hilum around the area of attachment of the ovary to the mesovarium.

Irrigation	Sewer system	Innervation
Ovarian artery (originating in the abdominal aorta) Uterine artery.	*Venous drainage:* Left ovarian vein (drains into the left renal vein). Right ovarian vein (drains into the inferior vena cava). *Lymphatic drainage:* Para-aortic lymph nodes	*Sympathetic innervation:* Ovarian plexus (renal plexus origin). Superior ovarian nerve. *Innervation for sympathetic:* Uterine plexus (arises from pelvic splanchnic nerves).

Ovarian Histology and Physiology

The outermost portion is called the tunica albuginea, covered by only a layer of superficial cuboidal epithelium known as the germinal epithelium. For their part, the oocytes are enclosed in complexes called follicles, which are found in the inner part of the cortex located as incrustations in the stroma.

During each cycle, a dominant follicle is recruited for ovulation. This pre-ovulatory follicle becomes a corpus luteum after ovulation. In the absence of pregnancy, the corpus luteum regresses to transform into the corpus albicans.

Stromal tissue is made up of connective tissue and interstitial cells, which are derived from mesenchymal cells, it is presumed that these have the capacity to respond to LH or hCG with the production of androstenedione. The medullary and central segment of the ovary is derived mainly from mesonephric cells.

Follicle

The follicle is considered as the key functional unit of the ovaries, in relation to the development of germ cells, as well as the production of steroids. It takes about 85 days to reach the pre-ovulatory state, however the average time for the selected follicle to develop to the point of ovulation is 10 to 14 days.

If a follicle is not recruited, a process known as atresia occurs in which the oocyte and granulosa cells within the basal lamina die and are replaced by fibrotic tissue.

Ovulation

- ✓ Increased level of circulating estradiol as the middle of the cycle approaches.
- ✓ The LH and FSH are then increased to a lesser extent, triggering ovulation of the dominant follicle.
- ✓ In each menstrual cycle, a follicle ovulates and gives rise to a corpus luteum.

- ✓ LH (or its substitute hCG), is essential to stimulate the rupture of the mature follicle.
- ✓ Rapid follicular enlargement occurs followed by a bulge of the follicle from the surface of the cortex of the ovary.
- ✓ The enlargement is followed by the rupture of the follicle, as well as the extrusion of an egg-cumulus complex into the peritoneal cavity.
- ✓ Ovulation occurs between 34 to 36 hours after the onset of the LH surge.
- ✓ After ovulation, the dominant follicle reorganizes to become the corpus luteum.

Bibliographic references

1. Shlomo Melmed, Richard J. Auchus, Allison B. Goldfine, Ronald J. Kowning, Clifford Rosen. Williams Textbook of Endocrinology 14Th edition. ELSEVIER, 2020.
2. Li YY, Guo L, Li H, Li J, Dong F, Yi ZY, Ouyang YC, Hou Y, Wang ZB, Sun QY, Lu SS, Han Z. NEK5 regulates cell cycle progression during mouse oocyte maturation and preimplantation embryonic development. Mol. Play Dev. 2019 Sep; 86 (9): 1189-1198.

Chapter 299. Disorder of Sex Development

Disorders of sexual development, also known as sexual dysgenesis, are those conditions in which the chromosomal, gonadal or anatomic sex presents atypical characteristics. It is a disorder of sexual development and can be the result of a wide range of pathologies, and therefore requires a multidisciplinary team with experience in this type of pathology, where the endocrinologist plays a key role.

Statistics or epidemiology

In the neonatal period, about 1 in 4500 live births have atypical genitalia. The most common etiology is congenital adrenal hyperplasia, followed by androgen insensitivity and mixed gonadal dysgenesis.

Klinefelter syndrome occurs in 1 in 500 or 1 in 1000 live-born males. Turner syndrome occurs in 1 in 2,500 live-born females.

Risk factor's:
- ✓ Maternal exposure to androgens during pregnancy.
- ✓ Exposure to contraceptives during pregnancy.
- ✓ Maternal exposure to soy.
- ✓ Consanguinity between parents.
- ✓ History of previous neonatal deaths.
- ✓ Family history (siblings) with primary amenorrhea and XY karyotype.

Etiology and pathophysiological elements

The sexual development of mammals is produced by two sequential stages:

Sex determination (initial phase):
Guided by inherited sexual complements at the time of conception.

Sex differentiation:
Characterized by hormonal secretion and other factors by the differentiated gonad, which guide genital development and maturation (external and internal). The secretion of testosterone in conjunction with the anti-Mullerian factor by the Leydig and Sertoli cells, stimulate the development of the internal male organs and the reciprocal regression of the female sexual organs. On the contrary, the absence of these hormones leads to the development of the female sexual organs.

There is a wide set of genes, which are involved in the orchestration of sexual determination and differentiation. The mutation of any of the genetic factors involved in sexual development could lead to atypical genitalia.

Overview of the most relevant genetic factors in sexual development

Gen	Description
Gen SRY	It is the main regulator of male sexual differentiation. The expression causes the translation of the SRY protein that is involved in testicular development.
Gen SOX9	Its expression follows the SRY gene. It is responsible for the differentiation of Sertoli cells.

Gen DHH	It is involved in testicular differentiation.
DAX / NROB1	It is considered as a positively regulated anti-testicular factor in the ovary.
Gen WT1	It encodes a transcription factor which is involved in the development of the kidneys and gonads. The mutation of this gene causes congenital syndromes that involve abnormal genitourinary development.
Wnt4 and Wnt 7a	Wnt4 causes the suppression of male sexual differentiation and ovarian androgen production.

The loss of genes involved in male sexual development could result in a male with undervirilized characteristics or 46 XY with a female phenotype.

The external male genitalia need the presence of dihydrotestosterone for the normal phenotype to develop properly, therefore, resistance or deficiency to this hormone causes undervirilized genitalia.

On the other hand, the exposure of the female genitalia to an excess of androgens (due to endogenous production or exogenous administration), causes the virilization of the female genitalia.

During early fetal development, a common developmental angle is shared in both males and females until week 7 of development, after which different genetic pathways follow. Inheritance of XY chromosome 46 leads to expression of the SRY gene found on the Y chromosome.

Control switch for male sexual development.
Its appearance causes important effects to be triggered, which result in male gonadal formation.

Mutations in this gene lead to 46 XY gonadal dysgenesis. Its translocation and expression in individuals with 46 XX, results in male or atypical genitalia.

The SOX9 gene is the second most important gene in male sexual determination. Its mutation causes autosomal dominant campomelic dysplasia, manifested as atypical or female external genitalia. Duplication of this gene leads to male or atypical genitalia in a 46 XX baby.

Diagnostic criteria

Clinic history
Description of factors of maternal exposure to androgens (Danazol, and others), during the current pregnancy.
Maternal history of virilization during pregnancy.
Evidence of risk factors.

Clinical examination
It should be performed with the patient supine in a frog's leg position.
Take a careful and detailed assessment
The size of the penis or clitoris, the number of perineal orifices, the presence of testicles in the labial or inguinal region should be documented.
The average length of the stretched penis in a term neonate is 2.8 to 4.2 cm. While the mean length of the clitoris in full-term girls ranges from 3.3 to 6.5 mm (> 9 mm is defined as clitoromegaly).

Clinical Features of Sex Chromosome Disorders of Sex Development

Condition	Karyotype	Gonad	Internal genitalia	Features	
Klinefelter syndrome	47, XXY and variants	Hyalinized testes	No uterus	Small testicles. Azoospermia. Hypoandrogenemia. Tall stature with longer leg length. Language delay. Obesity. Learning difficulty Breast tumors Impaired glucose tolerance. Varicose veins	
Turner syndrome	45, X and variants	Streaks of gonads or immature ovary.	Uterus	*Childhood:* Shield chest. Knitted collar. Heart defects Coarctation of the aorta. Short stature. Kidney and urinary abnormalities. Ulna worth. Hypoplastic nails. Scoliosis. Otitis media and hearing loss. Ptosis and amblyopia. Nevus. Visuospatial learning disability. Autoimmune thyroid disease.	*Adulthood:* Pubertal insufficiency. Hypertension. Primary amenorrhea. Dilation and dissection of the aortic root. Sensorineural hearing loss. Colon cancer. Thyroid disease Increased risk of CVD. Diabetes mellitus and glucose intolerance. Osteoporosis. Inflammatory bowel disease
Mixed gonadal dysgenesis	45, X / 46, XY and variants	Dysgenetic testis or gonad	Variable	Increased risk of gonadal tumors. Features of Turner syndrome may be present. Short stature.	

1606

| Ovotesticular Sex Development Disorder | 46, XX / 46, XY chimerism | Testicle, ovary, or ovotestis | Variable | Increased risk of developing gonadal tumors (probable). |

Table 253 - 1. Characteristics of the DSD. Source: Williams Textbook of Endocrinology 14Th edition. Elsevier, 2020 (Modified).

Paraclinical

- ✓ Karyotype (Generally performed in peripheral leukocytes).
- ✓ Fluorescent in situ hybridization (FISH) for the SRY gene.
- ✓ Measurement of 17 Hydroxyprogesterone.
- ✓ Dehydroepiandrosterone measurement.
- ✓ Measurement of 17-hydroxypregnolone.
- ✓ Measurement of 11-deoxycortisol.
- ✓ Testosterone analysis after stimulation.
- ✓ Gonadotropin measurement.
- ✓ Imaging studies (ultrasound and magnetic resonance imaging) allow to delineate the anatomy and visualize gonads, uterus and vagina.
- ✓ Vaginoscopy can be considered when it is required to specify the vaginal anatomy.

Treatment options

Treatment includes various strategies that are oriented according to:

Initial stabilization.
Evaluate for congenital adrenal hyperplasia, which may present as a life-threatening salt-wasting crisis.

Accurate diagnosis and decisions about the parenting gender.
Delay diagnosis when there is no clear evidence of the disorder. Refer the case to a center experienced in the management of disorders of sexual development when necessary.
Gender assignment comprises three considerations:
Functional and anatomical capacity of the genitalia (size and fertility potential).
Causes of ambiguous genitalia.
Family values and wishes.

Planning of surgical intervention and hormonal treatment.
According to the causal disorder of the atypical genitalia, surgical and hormonal therapy is conducted, also considering the decision on the parenting gender. They will be addressed in the corresponding chapter.
All patients and parents should receive psychosocial support and education associated with the disorder of sexual development.

Follow-up peculiarities
Follow-up is long-term, and requires guidance from a pediatric endocrinologist during childhood and adolescence and an adult endocrinologist at the time of transition to adulthood.
The disorder has a good prognosis, although it is associated with considerable psychosocial morbidity.

Bibliographic references

1. Shlomo Melmed, Richard J. Auchus, Allison B. Goldfine, Ronald J. Kowning, Clifford Rosen. Williams Textbook of Endocrinology 14Th edition. ELSEVIER, 2020.
2. Lavin N, editor. Manual of endocrinology and metabolism. 4th ed. Philadelphia: Wolters Kluwer / Lippincott Williams & Wilkins Health; 2009. 837 p.
3. Lee PA, Houk CP, Ahmed SF, Hughes IA., International Consensus Conference on Intersex organized by the Lawson Wilkins Pediatric Endocrine Society and the European Society for Pediatric Endocrinology. Consensus statement on management of intersex disorders. International Consensus Conference on Intersex. Pediatrics. 2006 Aug; 118 (2): e488-500.

Chapter 300. Normal Puberty

Puberty is about the stage of life that, through dramatic physiological and psychological changes, leads to adulthood. Clinically, the onset of puberty is estimated, when secondary sexual characteristics appear, especially the breasts, in the case of women and in the case of men, testicular enlargement, as well as the growth of pubic and axillary hair in both sexes.

Clinical features of normal puberty

Tanner Stages

Scale	Female (Breast development)	Male (External genitalia)	Pubic hair (same in men and women)
Stage 1	Mammary glandular tissue is not palpable	Testicular volume less than 4 ml or axis length less than 2.5 cm.	Hairless
Stage 2	Palpable mammary bud below the areola. First female pubertal sign.	4 to 8 ml or 2.5 to 3.3 cm long. First pubertal sign in males.	*Mens:* Long, downy hair can appear in the months after testicular growth. *Women:* long, downy pubic hair. Close to the lips
Stage 3	Palpable breast tissue outside the	Testicular volume	Evidence of sparse terminal hair.

	areola. no evidence of areolar development.	between 9 to 12 ml or 3.4 to 4 cm long.	Increases the amount and pigmentation of the hair.
Stage 4	Areola raised above the contour of the breast, forming the "double shovel" appearance.	Testicular volume between 15 to 20 ml or length between 4.1 to 4.5 cm.	Terminal hair, which fills the entire triangle that covers the pubic region.
Stage 5	The areolar mound recedes towards the contour of a sinus. Hyperpigmentation of the areola, development of papillae and protrusion of the nipple are evident.	Testicular volume greater than 20 ml or 4.5 cm long.	Terminal hair, which extends beyond the inguinal crease to the thighs.

Average ages

On average, the range for the development of normal puberty is between 8 to 13.5 years. Afro-descendant girls can see development of female sexual characteristics, around the age of 8 to 9 years.

In Caucasian girls, the age of onset can be 7 years on average, but in Afro-descendant girls it can start around 6 years.

The uterus grows to 16 years of age.

Menarche occurs in most girls in stage 4, one to three years after thelarche.

The development of armpit hair and facial hair (men) often occurs in stage 4.

Most males reach maximum growth rate during stage 5.
Acne, armpit hair, and body odor occur during the onset of puberty.

Endocrine aspects of normal puberty

GnRH neurons are the main building block for the onset of puberty.
Puberty begins with pulsatile GnRH secretion. It is currently known that the KISS1 and neurokinin B genes are associated with the regulation of GnRH release.
Once GnRH levels are increased, LH and FSH increase in the anterior pituitary.
The beginning of puberty is preceded by an increase in the levels of androgens secreted by the adrenal glands.
The initiation of the production of DHEA and DHEA-S leads to adrenochemia.
During this process, adrenal androgens are increased, while cortisol remains stable.
The linear growth observed in puberty is due to the pulsatile increase in the secretion of growth hormone.
Increased insulin-like factor 1 is also present.

Bibliographic references

1. Shlomo Melmed, Richard J. Auchus, Allison B. Goldfine, Ronald J. Kowning, Clifford Rosen. Williams Textbook of Endocrinology 14Th edition. ELSEVIER, 2020.

2. Beccuti G, Ghizzoni L. Normal and Abnormal Puberty. [Updated 2015 Aug 8]. In: Feingold KR, Anawalt B, Boyce A, et al., Editors. Endotext [Internet]. South Dartmouth (MA): MDText.com, Inc .; 2000

Chapter 301. Precocious Thelarchy

Precocious thelarche is the unilateral or bilateral growth of the female mammary glands, prior to 8 years of age and in the absence of other pubic signs, such as pubic hair, accelerated growth, or significantly advanced bone age.

Statistics and epidemiology

It is considered the most common disorder associated with puberty. It has an incidence that ranges from 1.6 to 8.9%. About 10% of girls with precocious thelarchy progress to true precocious puberty.

Etiology and pathophysiological elements

Neonatal thelarchy "breast intumescence"	Non-neonatal thelarchy
It occurs as a result of the transfer of maternal hormones during pregnancy. It can be accompanied by milk secretion which disappears after 2 weeks, in the case of males and in the case of girls, persist for several months.	Most occur before 2 years of age, although a second group can occur between 6 and 8 years. The pathophysiological and etiological elements are not clear at present, although different hypotheses have been postulated: Partial and transient activation of the hypothalamic-pituitary-gonadal axis with excessive secretion of follicle-stimulating hormone. Obesity. Presence of endocrine disruptors (phytoestrogens). Increased sensitivity of breast tissue to

	estradiol. Increased production of estrogens from precursors of adrenal origin. Transient estradiol secretion from an ovarian cyst.

Diagnostic criteria

Clinic	The diagnostic is fundamentally clinical. Take a detailed medical history as well as a complete physical exam. Evaluate the growth rate, it is usually normal in these patients. The bone age is not advanced. Record the age of appearance of the breast bud and describe the details of growth (unilateral or bilateral, evolutionary changes in size and breast consistency, among others). Ask the child's representative about possible exposure to drugs such as cimetidine, contraceptives, or phytoestrogens such as soy milk and derivatives. Take an appropriate anthropometric measurement. Check for armpit or pubic hair. *Findings:* Normal growth curve. Absence of pubertal signs. Pink areola. Genital mucosa corresponding to the prepubertal one. Difference between bone and chronological age less than 1 year.
Paraclinical	Gonadotropin value and LH-RH test correspond to prepubertal ones. Pelvic ultrasound can evaluate the presence of ovarian cysts. Carpal X-ray.

Treatment and follow-up options

The behavior in girls with precocious thelarchy is monitoring and periodic observation. Follow-up should be done every 4 to 6 months in order to rule out progression towards precocious pubarche that requires studies or specific treatment.

Consider exploring underlying causes in persistent early thelarche after 2 years of age or with mammary Tanner greater than III.

Bibliographic references

1. Khokhar A, Mojica A. Premature The larche. Pediatric Ann. 2018 Jan 1; 47 (1): e12-e15. doi: 10.3928 / 19382359-20171214-01. PMID: 29323691.
2. Martínez-Aedo Ollero MJ, Godoy Molina E. Precocious puberty and variants of normality. Diagnostic protocol pediatr. 2019; 1: 239-52.ISSN 2171-8172.

Chapter 302. Precocious Adrenarche

It is the term used for the maturational increase in the production of adrenal androgens, which can be visualized biochemically as an increase in the secretion of adrenal androgen precursors, especially dehydroepiandrosterone (DHEA) and its sulfate (DHEAS). Clinically, it occurs in girls and boys resulting in the development of pubic and armpit hair and apocrine body odor in adults.

Statistics and epidemiology

It can occur in boys and girls before 8 to 9 years of age. It is the most common cause of precocious puberty.

Risk groups or factors:
- ✓ Obesity.
- ✓ Polycystic ovarian syndrome.
- ✓ Metabolic syndrome.
- ✓ Insulin resistance
- ✓ History of low birth weight.
- ✓ Small for gestational age.

Etiology and pathophysiological elements

Premature adrenochemia is considered a variant of normal adrenochemia. However, it is associated with a moderately increased risk of polycystic ovary syndrome, insulin resistance, and metabolic syndrome in adulthood.

Currently, it has been associated with a history of small for gestational age and low birth weight.

Development milestones

After birth, a remodeling of the adrenal cortex occurs, which begins to consist of continuous bands of cells of the zona glomerulosa and fasciculata. Reticular cell islands appear at around 3 years of age, and finally fuse at 6 or 8 years of age, where biochemical adrenochemia begins. This process continues to expand from adrenochemia to early adolescence, peaking around 13 years of age.

In early adrenochemia, an early maturation of the adrenal cortex occurs with a biochemical adrenochemia between approximately 5 to 6 years of age.

Considerations for the differential diagnosis associated with causes of precocious puberty

Idiopathic premature adrenochemia (constitutional)
Congenital adrenal hyperplasia
21 hydroxylase deficiency.
11 beta-hydroxylase deficiency.
3 beta-hydroxysteroid dehydrogenase deficiency.
Cushing's disease.
Glucocorticoid resistance (glucocorticoid receptor inactivating mutations).
Apparent cortisone reductase deficiency (caused by inactivation of hexose-6-phosphate dehydrogenase).
Apparent DHEA sulfotransferase deficiency due to genetic inactivation caused by PAPSS2 mutation.
Exogenous, endogenous or autonomous androgen excess.
Exogenous treatment with testosterone.

Diagnostic criteria

Clinic	Start before 8 or 9 years of age. Appearance of pubic hair. Appearance of armpit hair. Adult body odor. Acne or comedones. Greasy hair. Moderate increase in growth rate and skeletal age (consistency between bone age and chronological age). They tend to be taller (compared to their peers). Overweight (common).
Paraclinical	The diagnosis requires that other causes be excluded, for example, excess androgens. DHEA level measurement. DHEAS level. Serum insulin level (usually hyperinsulinemia). Pelvic ultrasound (prepubertal findings). Testosterone (slightly elevated at times). Metabolic panel.

Treatment and follow-up options

This condition is considered benign, however, follow-up studies should be carried out especially in those children who present risk factors such as obesity. Follow-up consultations should be carried out in the long term to clarify the causes of the metabolic changes detected in these patients and indicate early preventive measures and control of body weight.

Bibliographic references

1. Oberfield, Sharon E et al. "Approach to the girl with early onse tofpubi chair." The Journal of clinical endocrinology and metabolism vol. 96.6 (2011): 1610-22. doi: 10.1210 / jc.2011-0225.
2. Martínez-Aedo Ollero MJ, Godoy Molina E. Precocious puberty and variants of normality. Protocdiagn ter pediatr. 2019; 1: 239-52. ISSN 2171-8172.
3. Utriainen P, Laakso S, Liimatta J, Jääskeläinen J, Voutilainen R. Premature adrenarche - a common condition with variable presentation. Horm Res Paediatr. 2015; 83 (4): 221-31. doi: 10.1159 / 000369458. Epub 2015 Feb 7. PMID: 25676474.

Chapter 303. Pubertal Gynecomastia

It is a benign condition that occurs in men during the pubertal stage, characterized by the proliferation of the glandular elements of the breast, and which results in a concentric enlargement of one or both breasts.

Statistics and epidemiology

Gynecomastia occurs in about 30% of men. It is a condition that is self-limiting in 75 to 90% of affected adolescents. It has a spontaneous regression in 1 to 3 years. Pathological gynecomastia is rare in adolescents.
Risk factor's: Family history of pubertal gynecomastia.

Etiology and biological elements

E2 levels increase faster than testosterone during early puberty, this leads to an increased estrogen / androgen ratio. This results in a relative and transitory imbalance between sex hormones, leading to gynecomastia.
Most of the cases of men with pubertal gynecomastia present self-limited enlargement which recedes concomitantly with the progression of puberty and the increase in testosterone levels.
For this reason, this condition requires treatment only in a small group of subjects, who have persistent gynecomastia despite having passed the usual time for its regression.

Histological types of gynecomastia

Florida	Fibrous	Intermediate
Characterized by ducal hyperplasia and proliferation. With loose and edematous stroma.	It contains more stromal fibrosis and fewer ducts.	It has characteristics of the previous two.

Diagnostic criteria

Clinic	The medical history and physical examination comprise the most relevant elements of the evaluation in a patient with pubertal gynecomastia. During gynecomastia (enlarged breasts in men), it can occur simultaneously: Mastalgia. Bleeding or discharge from the nipple. The physical exam should evaluate: Voice change. Increase in height. Testicular size. Development of body and facial hair. Penis size and development. Increase in muscle mass. Search for testicular masses. The diagnosis is fundamentally clinical, however, the presence of gynecomastia among prepubertal men warrants more investigations to detect endocrinopathies.
Paraclinical	When there is suspicion of endocrinopathies, the pertinent laboratory studies are: Luteinizing hormone serum level. Testosterone and serum estradiol level.

	Follicle stimulating hormone level.
	Serum prolactin.
	Dehydroepiandrosterone.
	Human chorionic gonadotropin.

Treatment options

Observation and reassurance is considered the safest and most reasonable treatment. However, consider the psychological and emotional aspects associated with gynecomastia. Treatment is indicated in gynecomastias that do not regress over time.

Medical treatment: indicated to correct hormonal imbalance. The strategies can be:
- ✓ Block the effects of estrogens in the breast (by raloxifene, tamoxifen or clomiphene).
- ✓ Administer androgens (via danazol).
- ✓ Inhibit the production of estrogens (testolactone or anastrozole).

Surgical treatment: indicated in non-obese patients with persistent breast enlargement without regressing for an observational period of 12 months, or with pain or tenderness in the breasts that is not relieved by medication or significant psychosocial discomfort. See Chapter 297.

Bibliographic references

1. Lemaine, V., Cayci, C., Simmons, PS, & Petty, P. (2013). Gynecomastia in adolescent males. Seminars in plastic surgery, 27 (1), 56–61. https://doi.org/10.1055/s-0033-1347166

2. Soliman AT, De Sanctis V, Yassin M. Management of Adolescent Gynecomastia: An Update. Acta Biomed. 2017 Aug 23; 88 (2): 204-213. doi: 10.23750 / abm.v88i2.6665. PMID: 28845839; PMCID: PMC6166145.

Chapter 304. Precocious Puberty

Precocious puberty has traditionally been defined as the development of secondary sexual characteristics before the age of 8 in girls and before the age of 9 in boys.

Associated terminology:
- ✓ Thelarche: development of the breasts (estrogenic response).
- ✓ Pubarche: development of pubic hair (androgenic response).
- ✓ Adrenoche: initiation of adrenal androgen production, which contributes to pubarche.

Statistics and epidemiology

There are currently limited studies that describe trends and prevalence associated with precocious puberty. It is estimated that around 0.2% of women have some form of precocious puberty, while men have around 0.05%.

The main cause is of idiopathic origin. It occurs predominantly in girls in about 20 to 23 cases per 10,000 girls, as opposed to boys, where 5 cases occur per 10,000 boys.

In Spain, it is estimated that the annual incidence occurs between 0.02 and 1.07 cases per 100,000 person. The incidences and prevalence could vary according to the population, however, there is a predominance of female cases.

Risk groups or factors:
- ✓ Exposure to androgens or estrogens.
- ✓ Fetal development abnormalities.
- ✓ Family history of precocious puberty.
- ✓ History of head trauma.
- ✓ Intracranial neoplasms.
- ✓ Irradiation to the skull.

Etiology and pathophysiological elements

Central precocious puberty (GnRH-dependent or premature activation of the hypothalamic GnRH pulse generator)
Represents true pubertal development or complete isosexual precocity. It can be diagnosed in the presence of the appearance of any manifestation of sexual maturation in Caucasian girls under 7 years of age and in Afro-descendant girls under 6 years of age (currently controversial age limits).
Idiopathic true precocious puberty.   Central nervous system (CNS) tumors.   Hypothalamic astrocytoma.   Optic glioma associated with type 1 neurofibromatosis.   Other CNS disorders: Brain abscess.   Encephalitis.   Cranial irradiation.   Vascular injury   Hydrocephalus   Trauma to the head.   Sarcoid or tuberculous granuloma.   Developmental abnormality, including hypothalamic hamartoma of tuber cinereum.   Arachnoid cyst.   Myelomeningocele.

Static encephalopathy.
True precocious puberty due to gain of function mutations:
In the KISS1R / GRP54 gene.
In the KISS1 gene.
True precocious puberty after delayed treatment for congenital virilizing adrenal hyperplasia or other chronic exposure to sex steroids.

Peripheral precocious puberty or incomplete isosexual precocity (independent of hypothalamic GnRH)

Female	Males
Peutz-Jeghers syndrome. Ovarian cyst Estrogen-secreting ovarian or adrenal neoplasm.	Gonadotropin-secreting tumors. HCG-secreting CNS tumors (such as teratomas, germinomas, or chorioepitheliomas) Cortisol resistance syndrome. Virilizing adrenal neoplasia. Leydig cell adenoma. Congenital adrenal hyperplasia (CYP11B1 and CYP21 deficiency). Increased secretion of adrenal or testicular androgens. HCG-secreting tumors found outside the CNS (Hepatoma, choriocarcinoma, teratoma). Familial testotoxicosis (sex-limited autosomal dominant pituitary gonadotropin-independent germ cells and Leydig cells early maturation).
Both genders Iatrogenic or exogenous sexual precocity (including inadvertent exposure to estrogens in cosmetics, drugs, or food). Hypothyroidism McCune-Allbright syndrome.	
Variations in pubertal development Macroorchidism. Adolescent gynecomastia in children. Premature isolated menarche. Premature thelarchy.	

Premature adrenarche.	
Contrasexual precocity	
Feminization in men	Virilization in women
Chorioepithelioma. Testicular neoplasia (Peutz-Jeghers syndrome). Late-onset adrenal hyperplasia. CYP11B1 deficiency. Adrenal neoplasia. Increased extraglandular conversion of circulating adrenal androgens to estrogens. Iatrogenic (exposure to estrogens).	Aromatase deficiency. Virilizing adrenal neoplasia (S. de Cushing). Virilizing ovarian neoplasia (arerenoblastoma). Congenital adrenal hyperplasia (CYP21 deficiency, CYP11B1 deficiency, βHSD deficiency). Cortisol resistance syndrome. Iatrogenic (exposure to androgens).

Table 254 - 1. Source: Williams Textbook of Endocrinology 14Th edition. ELSEVIER, 2020 (Modified).

Testotoxicosis consists of an unusual autosomal dominant disorder, whose clinical phenotype is reserved for males. It is caused by a mutation that activates the germ line of the LH receptor gene leading to the activation of Leydig cells and elevated levels of testosterone.

Diagnostic criteria

Clinic	*In women:* Increased development of the breasts. *In males:* Increase in testicular volume (greater than 4 ml). *Both of them:* Increased linear growth. Acne.

1628

	Muscle changes Changes in body odor Development of pubic and armpit hair. *Neurological symptoms:* Headache. Increased head circumference. Seizures Visual and cognitive changes. Diabetes insipidus Others: Decreased growth rate. Abdominal pain (ovarian pathology). *Clinical examination:* The accelerated progression of puberty at an appropriate age should be studied. Anthropometric data (height, weight, growth rate as a function of cm / year) and the exact BMI must be properly documented. In girls: Tanner accurate breast staging. In children: use an orchidometer to determine testicular volume (volume greater than 4 ml confirms the diagnosis. In both girls and boys with pubic hair and body odor in the absence of increased testicular volume or breast development, investigation of peripheral causes should be promoted.
Paraclinical	Bone age Measurement of LH, FHS (when baseline prepubertal LH is> 0.3 IU / L suggests a central cause, while levels below 0.3 suggest peripheral causes). Testosterone measurement Dehydroepiandrosterone sulfate measurement. 17 OH progesterone levels. Thyroid function tests. HCG levels. GnRH stimulation test (gold standard for the diagnosis of central causes).

	Pelvic ultrasound (to detect ovarian tumors or cysts in women).
	Testicular ultrasound (reveals nonpalpable Leydig cell tumors in males).
	Magnetic resonance imaging (rule out hypothalamic lesion).

Treatment and follow-up options

Central precocious puberty	Peripheral precocious puberty
It depends on the age of the child, when symptoms progress rapidly or bone age is significantly advanced, it should be treated. *Goals:* Preserve adult height and alleviate associated psychosocial stress. *Therapeutic options* GnRH agonists: Leuprolide acetate administered every 3 months is frequently used. Follow-up should be done periodically as puberty progresses evaluating the rate of growth and skeletal maturation.	Treatment is geared toward eliminating the source of sex steroids. Options: Surgery: used to treat gonadal and adrenal tumors. Eliminate exogenous sources of sex steroids. Glucocorticoids. McCune-Allbright syndrome can be treated by blocking estrogen synthesis using aromatase inhibitors (letrozole, anastrozole), in conjunction with a selective estrogen receptor modulator (tamoxifen). Familial precocious puberty: A combination of androgen antagonist such as spironolactone is often used in conjunction with an aromatase inhibitor (testolactone or anastrozole).

Bibliographic references

1. Shlomo Melmed, Richard J. Auchus, Allison B. Goldfine, Ronald J. Kowning, Clifford Rosen. Williams Textbook of Endocrinology 14Th edition. ELSEVIER, 2020.
2. Kiess W, Hoppmann J, Gesing J, Penke M, Körner A, Kratzsch J, Pfaeffle R. Puberty - genes, environment and clinicalissues. J. Pediatr. Endocrinol. Metab. 2016 Nov 01; 29 (11): 1229-1231.
3. Haddad NG, Eugster EA. Peripheralprecociouspubertyincludingcongenital adrenal hyperplasia: causes, consequences, management and outcomes. BestPract. Res. Clin. Endocrinol. Metab. 2019 Jun; 33 (3): 101273.

Chapter 305. Delayed Puberty

Delayed, late puberty or sexual infantilism is the delay of puberty in men and women. In women, the evidence of delayed puberty is the lack of development of the breasts at 13 years of age and a delay of more than 4 years of thelarche and completion or absence of development of menarche at 16 years of age. For its part, in men it is defined as the lack of testicular enlargement at 14 years of age or an interval of more than 5 years between testicular enlargement and the end of puberty.

Puberty is directly associated with the development or maturation of the hypothalamic-pituitary-gonadal (HPG) axis, however, the manifestations of adrenochemia such as the development of axillary or pubertal hair and body odor are the result of the secretion of adrenal androgens, for therefore, a boy may manifest signs of adrenochemia independent of puberty and may be diagnosed as delayed puberty.

Statistics and epidemiology

The most common cause of delayed puberty is constitutional delay of puberty and growth (CDPG).
CDPG is more common in males, affecting about 63% of males, while it only affects 30% of females.
CDPG affects about 53% of adolescents under 18 years of age in the United States with delayed puberty.

About 19% of the causes of delayed puberty are hypogonadotropic hypogonadism.

Risk groups or factors:
- ✓ History of craniopharyngiomas.
- ✓ History of radiotherapy to the skull.
- ✓ Head trauma
- ✓ Eating disorders.
- ✓ Malnutrition.
- ✓ Chronic illness.

Etiology and pathophysiological elements

Idiopathic (constitutional) delay in growth and puberty (delayed activation of the hypothalamic LRF pulse generator)
Hypogonadotropic hypogonadism: sexual infantilism related to gonadotropin deficiency
CNS disorders
Tumors
Craniopharyngiomas. Astrocytomas. Hypothalamic and optic gliomas. Germinomas. Pituitary tumors (MEN1, prolactinoma).
Other causes
Lymphocytic hypophysitis. Langerhans histiocytosis. Postinfectious lesions of the CNS. Vascular abnormalities of the CNS. Head trauma Radiotherapy. Congenital malformations (especially those associated with craniofacial

anomalies).

Isolated gonadotropin deficiency

Kallmann syndrome (with or without anosmia or hyposmia).
Prohormone convertase 1 deficiency (PCI).
Isolated LH or FSH deficiency.
LHRH receptor mutation.
Congenital adrenal hypoplasia (DAX1 mutation)

Idiopathic and genetic forms of multiple pituitary hormone deficiencies (including PROP1 mutation).

Various disorders

Laurence-Moon and Bardet-Biedl syndrome.
Prader-Willi syndrome.
Gonadotropin functional deficiency.
Cystic fibrosis.
Sickle-cell anaemia.
Chronic systemic disease.
Chronic kidney disease
Chronic gastroenteric disease.
Acquired immunodeficiency syndrome.
Malnutrition.
Anorexia nervosa.
Psychogenic amenorrhea.
Altered puberty.
Bulimia.
Gaucher disease.
Mellitus diabetes.
Hypothyroidism
Exercise amenorrhea: altered puberty and late menarche in athletes and ballet dancers.
Cushing's disease.
Hyperprolactinemia.
Use of marijuana.

Hypergonadotropic hypogonadism

Males	Female
Seminiferous tubular dysgenesis syndrome and variants	Gonadal dysgenesis syndrome and variants (Turner syndrome).

(Klinefelter syndrome) Trauma or surgery. Other forms of primary testicular failure: Chemotherapy. Radiotherapy. Anorchia and cryptorchidism. Sertoli only syndrome. Testicular steroid biosynthetic defects. LH receptor mutation.	XX and XY gonadal dysgenesis Aromatase deficiency. Other forms of primary ovarian failure: Radiotherapy. Chemotherapy. Galactosemia. Autoimmune oophoritis. Resistant ovary. Type 1 glycoprotein syndrome. FSH receptor mutation. Polycystic ovary disease. Noonan-Others syndrome.

Table 255 - 1. Etiology and pathophysiological elements of delayed puberty. Source. Williams Textbook of Endocrinology 14Th edition. Elsevier, 2020 (Modified).

Diagnostic criteria

Clinic history

Ask about the history of the current disease, and carefully examine the patient so that you can assess for breast development, testicular enlargement, armpit or pubertal hair, body odor, or acne. Distinguish between the development of adrenache and pubarche.

Fatigue or weight loss can signal an underlying chronic illness (sickle cell anemia, depression, or malnutrition).

Evaluate the patient's history (asthma, cystic fibrosis, vaccination status, surgical, among others).

Research the medications or treatments the patient took previously (emphasizing radiotherapy or chemotherapy treatments).

Assess the patient's social environment and developmental milestones.

Describe the anthropometric data of the patient (height, weight, BMI) and evaluate the growth curve and establish a goal of the expected adult height based on the height of the biological parents.

Paraclinical
- ✓ Complete blood count.
- ✓ Complete metabolic panel.
- ✓ Thyroid tests (T4 and TSH).
- ✓ Erythrocyte sedimentation rate (when chronic inflammatory disorders are suspected).
- ✓ Measurement of LH and FSH.
- ✓ Estradiol level (women)
- ✓ Total testosterone (men).
- ✓ GnRH stimulation test (not usually included in initial evaluation).
- ✓ Bone age (x-ray of the wrist and hand).
- ✓ Abdominal ultrasound (evaluate the ovaries and uterus in case of suspected Turner syndrome).
- ✓ Testicular ultrasound (useful to identify cryptorchidism or testicular mass).
- ✓ Brain MRI (when there is a history or suspicion of craniopharyngioma).
- ✓ Request additional pertinent paraclinics, based on clinical manifestations and suspected diagnosis.

Treatment options

Specific treatment will be approached based on the underlying cause of delayed puberty.

CDPG patients:
Treatment is usually oriented in relation to the goals of the patient and the parents. A short-term treatment with low doses of testosterone in men or estrogen in women may be considered. Treatment can improve sexual maturation, mental well-being, and improve growth rate.

Men: An oral or intramuscular form of testosterone can be used (although the IM route is recommended to avoid liver toxicity.

Women: oral administration is the most widely used therapeutic option.

Follow-up peculiarities
During treatment, patients should be closely monitored for signs of pubertal development (testicular enlargement and breast development).

Bibliographic reference

1. Bozzola M, Bozzola E, Montalbano C, Stamati FA, Ferrara P, Villani A. Delayed puberty versus hypogonadism: a challenge for the pediatrician. Ann Pediatr Endocrinol Metab. 2018 Jun; 23 (2): 57-61
2. Shlomo Melmed, Richard J. Auchus, Allison B. Goldfine, Ronald J. Kowning, Clifford Rosen. Williams Textbook of Endocrinology 14Th edition. ELSEVIER, 2020.

Chapter 306. Turner Syndrome

Also known as congenital ovarian hypoplasia syndrome, it was initially described by Henri Turner in 1938. It consists of a common sex chromosomal abnormality that occurs when one of the X chromosomes is partially or completely missing.

Statistics and epidemiology

It is seen in about 1 in 2,000 to 2 in 2,500 live female births. It occurs in a similar way in different countries and populations. The statistic is not accurate because there are mild undiagnosed forms.

The prevalence of Turner syndrome at birth has decreased, due to the termination of pregnancy by mothers with fetuses with Turner syndrome diagnosed by prenatal ultrasound. About 99% of 45, X conceptions abort spontaneously; 1 in 15 spontaneous abortions have a 45, X karyotype.

Etiology and pathophysiological elements

Turner syndrome occurs as a result of a deletion or non-functioning of an X chromosome in women. About 50% of patients with this syndrome have a monosomy X (45, X0), while the other half have a mosaic chromosomal component (45, X with mosaicism).

Chromosomal abnormalities leading to non-functional X chromosome:

Isochromosome Xq: presence of two copies of the long arm of the chromosome connected head to head.

Xp or Xq deletion: deletion of part of the short arm of the X chromosome.

Ring chromosome: absence of part of the ends of the long and short arms of the X chromosome:

Monosome X is a non-hereditary random event, which occurs during the formation of reproductive cells in the parent the individual. An error in cell division known as nondisjunction occurs resulting in reproductive cells with an abnormal number of chromosomes. When an atypical reproductive cell is involved in the genetic makeup of a child, each cell will possess only one X chromosome.

The characteristic short stature occurs due to the loss of a gene which contains homeobox and is located in the pseudoautosomal region (PAR1) of the short arms of the X (p22) and Y (p11.3) chromosomes, which encodes a osteogenic factor.

Diagnostic criteria

Clinic	New born:
	Congenital lymphedema of the hands and feet.
	Webbed neck.
	Nail dysplasia.
	Narrow and high arched palate.
	Fourth metacarpals or short metatarsals.
	As they grow:
	Short stature.
	Shield chest with widely spaced nipples.
	Webbed neck.
	Low hairline at the base of the neck.

	Ulna worth.
Madelung deformity of the wrist and forearm.
Normal intelligence or specific cognitive deficit (problems with visuospatial organization, memory and attention).
During adolescence:
Delayed puberty or primary amenorrhea.
Strip gonads.
Increased risk of cardiovascular malformations:
Aortic anomaly.
Elongated transverse aortic arch.
Venous pulmonary abnormality.
Hearing abnormalities:
Hearing loss due to recurrent otitis media.
Kidney abnormalities:
Malformations in the collecting system
Positional anomalies.
Horseshoe kidneys.
Eye abnormalities:
Myopia or hyperopia.
Squint.
Amblyopia.
Epicanthic folds.
Ptosis.
Hypertelorism
Red-green color blindness.
Others:
Increased risk of autoimmune disorders.
Increased risk of gonadoblastoma.
Infertility (common).
Paraclinical	Prenatal:
Chorionic villus sampling.
Amniocentesis.
Prenatal ultrasound:
Increased nuchal translucency.
Nuchal cystic hygroma.
Coarctation of the aorta and / or left heart abnormalities.

	Brachycephaly
	Horseshoe kidney.
	Polyhydramnios, oligohydramnios, or non-immune hydrops.
	Genetic testing with karyotype analysis (peripheral blood in neonates).
	Adolescence:
	Elevated FSH levels.
	Elevated levels of anti-Mullerian hormone (AMH).
	Second karyotype (used for skin, buccal mucosa cells or bladder epithelial cells): it is indicated when the first initial karyotype test is normal in a patient clinically suspected of Turner syndrome.
	Electrocardiogram.
	Echocardiogram or cardiac magnetic resonance.
	When diagnosing Turner syndrome, indicate pertinent studies to evaluate other associated anomalies, such as renal and cardiac anomalies, among others.

Treatment and follow-up options

Treatment options are individualized according to the clinical manifestations caused by Turner syndrome.

Short stature
Although there is no evidence of growth hormone deficiency, patients respond well to GH therapy. This therapy is indicated when stature less than 5% of the estimated height for age is evidenced.
During GH therapy, patients should be encouraged to monitor the condition of the spine, and each follow-up visit should be evaluated for the presence or absence of scoliosis. Some patients may require orthopedic surgery
Continue GH therapy until the patient reaches adulthood and no longer has growth potential.
Cardiac disorders
At the time of diagnosis of Turner syndrome, the patient should be evaluated by a cardiologist and request an electrocardiogram (evaluate prolonged QT interval).

Stop drugs that prolong the QT interval.
In the presence of coarctation of the aorta, corrective surgery should be indicated.
Aortic dilatation should be monitored by echocardiography or cardiac MRI on a regular basis.
To reduce the risk of aortic dilation and dissection, keep your blood pressure within the normal range. Use beta-blockers as first-line treatment or an ACE inhibitor as a second option.
Hearing loss
Due to the high risk of hearing loss, monitor hearing function regularly with serial audiological evaluations.
Follow-up is done for life every 3 years in children and every 5 years in adults.
Ovarian failure
Estrogen replacement therapy (starts at 11 to 12 years when there is no evidence of beginning of breast development).
Almost all patients with Turner syndrome require estrogen therapy even if they have spontaneous puberty, due to the high incidence of primary ovarian failure in this syndrome.
The starting dose ranges from 1/10 to 1/8 of the dose usually used in adults. It can be progressively increased every 6 months to simulate the gradual increase in normal puberty until the dose is obtained in adults.
Osteoporosis and fractures
A decrease in bone mineral density frequently develops.
Treatment with estrogens, calcium, and vitamin D supplements can reduce the risk of osteoporosis.

Bibliographic references

1. Shlomo Melmed, Richard J. Auchus, Allison B. Goldfine, Ronald J. Kowning, Clifford Rosen. Williams Textbook of Endocrinology 14Th edition. ELSEVIER, 2020.
2. CH, Sas TCJ, Mauras N. Estrogen Replacement in Turner Syndrome: LiteratureReview and

PracticalConsiderations. J. Clin. Endocrinol. Metab. 2018 May 01; 103 (5): 1790-1803.
3. ShankarKikkeri N, Nagalli S. Turner Syndrome. [Updated 2020 Aug 10]. In: StatPearls Publishing; 2020.

Chapter 307. Primary Amenorrhea

Primary amenorrhea is defined as failure to initiate menstruation at the age of 14 years and in the absence of secondary sexual characteristics. Also included in this definition is the absence of menarche at 16 years of age regardless of the development of secondary sexual characteristics or normal growth.

Epidemiology

Incidence is estimated to occur in less than 1% in the United States. There has been no evidence of variation in the general prevalence of primary amenorrhea according to population group or ethnic origin. About 43% of cases of primary amenorrhea are caused by gonadal dysgenesis.

Etiology or more frequent causes

Anatomical defects (partial and complete dysgenesis, Muller's agenesis, imperforate hymen or transverse vaginal septum, isolated absence of the vagina or cervix).
Elevated FSH levels (ovarian failure).
Hyperprolactinemia (inhibition of gonadotropin-releasing hormone secretion).
Hypothalamic amenorrhea (hypothalamic functional disorder)
Polycystic ovary syndrome (hyperandrogenism, polycystic ovaries, ovulatory dysfunction).

Pathophysiological elements

The development of the menstrual cycle corresponds to a set of coordinated hormonal changes, which control the ovaries and the endometrium to stimulate the growth of a follicle and release an ovum, while the endometrium is prepared for implantation in case of the occurrence of the fertilization.

For normal menstrual function to occur, the proper functional and anatomical state of the structures that are involved in this menstrual process such as the uterus, ovaries, adrenal glands, and hypothalamus is required. An alteration in any of these levels can cause the absence of bleeding.

Diagnostic criteria

Clinic	Begin the evaluation by including a complete medical history and physical examination. Absence of menstruation at 14 years without development of secondary sexual characteristics or absence of menstruation at 16 years with or without development of secondary sexual characteristics. Evaluate Tanner scale to determine pubertal development. Cyclical abdominal pain and pubertal development can lead to an imperforate hymen or other anatomical alteration. History of anosmia, headache, galactorrhea, visual disturbances, are indicative of central nervous system disorders. Goiter or thyroid nodule could suggest thyroid disorders as an underlying cause. Record anthropometric data and describe traits of sexual infantilism, in conjunction with short stature leading to

	sexual dysgenesis. Other clinical manifestations are indicative of the underlying cause.
Paraclinical	The diagnosis of primary amenorrhea is clinical. Paraclinical tests should be performed based on the clinical manifestations that suggest the underlying cause: Pregnancy test. Pelvic ultrasound (uterine presence or absence). Serum FSH levels (low levels indicate hypogonadotropic hypogonadism, high levels indicate ovarian failure) Serum LH levels. Measurement of thyroid hormones. Karyotype (the presence of the Y chromosome in conjunction with elevated serum testosterone levels, orients towards androgen insensitivity, on the contrary, a normal karyotype with an elevated FSH suggests 17-hydroxylase deficiency). ACTH stimulation test. Ultrasound or MRI.

Treatment options

Congenital anomalies	Imperforate hymen: crossed incision to open the vaginal opening. Transverse septum: surgical removal. Hypoplasia or absence of cervix (in the presence of a functional uterus): probable hysterectomy, preserving the ovaries. Short or absent vagina: progressive dilation.
Gonadal failure and hypogonadotropic hypogonadism	Cyclical estrogen therapy It can be started with daily conjugated estrogens or estradiol. Do not use high doses in the presence of short stature to prevent the epiphyses from closing

	prematurely. 17-lpha-hydroxylase deficiency: initiate replacement therapy with corticosteroids (dexamethasone or hydrocortisone).
Other causes	Craniopharyngioma: surgical resection by craniotomy or transsphenoidal approach. Germinomas: radiation therapy. Hyperprolactinemia: dopamine agonists. Kallmann syndrome: hormone replacement therapy. Y chromosome (gonadal dysgenesis): removal of gonads to prevent neoplasms.

Follow-up peculiarities

Follow up specifically according to the underlying cause. Primary amenorrhea is not life threatening, however, it can cause complications.

Bibliographic references

1. Shlomo Melmed, Richard J. Auchus, Allison B. Goldfine, Ronald J. Kowning, Clifford Rosen. Williams Textbook of Endocrinology 14Th edition. ELSEVIER, 2020.
2. Practice Committee of American Society for Reproductive Medicine. Current evaluation ofamenorrhea. Fertile. Steril. 2008 Nov; 90 (5 Suppl): S219-25.

Chapter 308. Oligomenorrhea and Secondary Amenorrhea

Oligomenorrhea is defined as the presence of irregular or inconsistent menstrual blood flow in women, which does not correspond to physiological periods of menstrual disturbances such as menarche, postpartum or the perimenopausal period. Oligomenorrhea is considered a menstrual cycle of more than 35 days or 4 to 9 menstrual cycles in a year.

On the other hand, secondary amenorrhea is determined, when a woman has had her menarche and subsequently passes 6 months or more without menstrual bleeding.

Oligomenorrhea and secondary amenorrhea are clinical manifestations associated with chronic anovulatory disorders, one of the most common gynecological problems in clinical practice.

Statistics and epidemiology

The prevalence of secondary amenorrhea is around 2–5%. The prevalence of oligomenorrhea is 13.5% in the general population. Around 11 to 44% of dancers and between 6 to 60% of athletes, have oligomenorrhea at some point in their life.

Polycystic ovary syndrome accounts for 4 to 10% of oligomenorrhea in women of childbearing age.

Etiology and pathophysiological elements

Disorders that predispose to anovulation lead to disorders of secondary amenorrhea and oligomenorrhea. This can occur as a result of a hormonal alteration that causes irregularities in the menstrual cycle, physical damage to the endometrial integrity preventing its growth or the obstruction of the outlet for menstrual blood. According to the triggering causes, the pathophysiological mechanisms are diverse and they will be indicated in the corresponding chapter.

Physiological causes of secondary amenorrhea:
- ✓ Pregnancy (secondary amenorrhea).
- ✓ Lactation.
- ✓ Pathological causes:
- ✓ Polycystic ovary disease.
- ✓ Prolactinoma.
- ✓ Cushing's syndrome.
- ✓ Thyroid disorders.
- ✓ Hypothalamic amenorrhea (diet, stress, vigorous exercise, chronic disease).
- ✓ Asherman's syndrome.
- ✓ Pelvic inflammatory disease.
- ✓ Androgen-secreting ovarian tumor.
- ✓ Mellitus diabetes.
- ✓ Pelvic inflammatory disease.
- ✓ Drugs (antiepileptics, antipsychotics, side effect of oral contraceptives).
- ✓ Adrenal hyperplasia.
- ✓ Ovarian failure
- ✓ Anatomical alterations.

Diagnostic criteria

Clinic	To pinpoint the diagnosis, include an accurate and detailed history of menstruation, including cycle length, age and date of menarche, duration of menstruation, number of pads used per day, interval between two cycles, and regularity of previous cycles. Describe the presence of additional symptoms (hot flashes, night sweats, headache, signs of virilization, galactorrhea, changes in bowel habits, among others). Ask about the menstrual pattern before oligomenorrhea. Ask about drug or drug use. The physical examination must be complete prioritizing in: External examination: In case of secondary amenorrhea, investigate development of abnormal secondary sexual characteristics, such as clitoromegaly or hirsutism. Rectovaginal Exam: Evaluate vaginal walls and palpate for any anatomical abnormalities or obstructions (exam with gloved finger lubricated with anesthetic gel), examine masses or tenderness. Vaginal speculum exam: Assess for discharge, signs of inflammation, or growths. Abdominal examination - Inspect for ascites, masses, and tenderness. Look for groin adenopathies.
Paraclinical	Pregnancy test FSH levels (increased suggest primary ovarian failure, if low in conjunction with low estradiol, suspect hypothalamic-pituitary dysfunction). Prolactin levels (elevated levels are associated with prolactinoma). TSH levels. LH levels (FSH / LH ratio helps identify polycystic ovarian disease). Free testosterone levels (elevated in congenital adrenal hyperplasia and polycystic ovarian disease). 17-OH measurement.

	Estrogen-progesterone provocation test. Nocturnal suppression test with dexamethasone (performed when Cushing syndrome is suspected). Pituitary MRI (confirms the presence of prolactinoma). Ultrasound of the abdomen and pelvis (evidence of polycystic ovaries, pelvic inflammation or ascites). Computed tomography (useful to evaluate adrenal or adrenal masses).

Treatment options

The treatment options available depend on the underlying cause or disorder responsible for the oligomenorrhea or primary amenorrhea.

Changes in lifestyle: especially when the cause is due to hypothalamic-pituitary anovulation (stress, malnutrition, others). Weight loss is useful for the treatment of polycystic ovaries, as well as metformin treatments.

Hormone therapy: Oral contraceptives are used as hormone replacement therapy to restore the regularity of the menstrual cycle, for example in polycystic ovarian disease.

Specific medical treatments: depending on the cause, for example, antithyroid drugs are indicated to patients with hyperthyroidism.

Surgical management: in adrenal or adrenal tumors, prolactinoma removal, thyroidectomy, among others. In the case of Asherman's syndrome, hysteroscopic lysis of adhesions is performed.

Follow-up peculiarities

Follow up promptly for the underlying cause. Assess the risk of infertility and take steps to reduce the risk. Untreated oligomenorrhea can increase the risk of endometrial hyperplasia and endometrial cancer.

Bibliographic references

1. Shlomo Melmed, Richard J. Auchus, Allison B. Goldfine, Ronald J. Kowning, Clifford Rosen. Williams Textbook of Endocrinology 14Th edition. ELSEVIER, 2020.
2. Hennegan J, Brooks DJ, Schwab KJ, Melendez-Torres GJ. Measurement in the study of menstrual health and hygiene: A systematic review and audit. PLoS ONE. 2020; 15 (6): e0232935.

Chapter 309. Premenstrual Syndrome

Premenstrual syndrome (PMS) is a set of physical, behavioral or mood symptoms that occurs in a cyclical pattern, prior to menstruation and then disappears after the menstrual period in women of reproductive age.

This comprises a syndrome of multiple and diverse clinical manifestations whose intensity can vary from mild to even interfere with the daily routine of the patient. When the symptoms are mild or a discomfort, premenstrual syndrome is determined, however, when the symptoms (especially psychiatric ones), are associated with an anxiety greater enough to intervene in daily activities and interpersonal relationships, it is called premenstrual dysphoric disorder (PMDD), although some literatures may attribute the name PMDD to both conditions.

Statistics and epidemiology

They can affect all women of childbearing age from menarche to menopause. About 70 to 90% of women of childbearing age complain of premenstrual discomfort. About 1/3 of women with premenstrual symptoms have symptoms that are severe enough to qualify the diagnosis of PMS.

American women with PMDD can experience about 6.4 severe symptoms in each menstrual cycle.

Risk factor's:
- ✓ Women of reproductive age.

- ✓ Past traumatic events.
- ✓ Smoking
- ✓ Obesity.

Etiology and pathophysiological elements

Currently the etiology is not well defined and is poorly understood. Some theories suggest that it is the result of an aberrant response of central neurotransmitters to normal changes in gonadal steroids during the menstrual cycle. However, no theory has been corroborated and they lack universal acceptance.

Recent evidence suggests that reproductive hormone release patterns are normal in PMS / PMDD, although patients are more sensitive to cyclical variations in hormone levels, which predisposes them to experience the symptoms associated with this syndrome.

Diagnostic criteria

Clinical manifestations
Mood
Feeling sad, depressed, hopeless, or worthless.
Increased irritability or anger (manifested in frequent interpersonal conflicts).
Mood lability (mood swings, for example feeling suddenly sad).
Anxiety or feeling nervous.
Behavior
Fatigue, lack of energy.
Decreased interest in usual activities.
Feeling out of control or overwhelmed.
Concentration problems.
Appetite changes
Changes in sleep pattern.
Somatic

Headache.   Swelling or tenderness in the breasts.   Muscle or joint pain   Feeling bloated
Symptomatic expression pattern: Symptoms are experienced from a few days before the start of menstruation to 2 weeks before it. Most women experience intensification of symptoms 6 days before and may be worse 2 days before menstruation.

Currently, it is included in the Diagnostic and Statistical Manual of Mental Disorders 5th Edition (DSM-5), as a different entity in depressive disorders. According to the following diagnostic criteria:

Criterion A: **At least 5 of the following 11 symptoms must be present (including 1 of the first 4 listed):**
Markedly depressed mood, feelings of hopelessness, or self-critical thoughts.   Marked anxiety, tension, feelings of being "excited" or "on edge".   Marked affective lability.   Irritability or persistent and marked anger or increase in interpersonal conflicts.   Decrease in interest in usual activities (hobbies, friends, work, among others).   Subjective feeling of difficulty concentrating.   Lethargy, easy fatigue, or marked lack of energy.   Marked appetite change (cravings for specific foods or overeating).   Insomnia or hypersomnia.   Subjective feeling of being overwhelmed or out of control.   Other physical symptoms such as breast swelling or tenderness, headache, muscle or joint pain, feeling of bloating or weight gain.
Criterion B: symptoms severe enough to significantly affect or interfere with social, occupational, school, or sexual functioning
Criterion C: symptoms discreetly associated with the menstrual cycle

and should not be explained by an exacerbation of symptoms of other disorders, for example, a panic disorder, major depressive disorder, dysthymic disorders or a personality disorder. Although symptoms may overlap with these disorders.	
Criterion D: Criteria A, B and C corroborated by prospective daily ratings for 2 or more consecutive symptomatic menstrual cycles.	

Assessment scales

Premenstrual symptoms detection tool: it consists of a questionnaire with 19 elements, which allow to qualify the severity of premenstrual symptoms.

Calendar of premenstrual experiences (COPE): consists of an instrument that brings together 22 symptoms grouped into 4 categories (mood reactivity, fluid retention, autosomal / cognitive, appetite).

Visual analog scale (VAS).

Information system for measuring results reported by the patient (PROMIS).

Daily problem severity log (DRSP).

Paraclinical

They are not required to establish a diagnosis of PMS, however, a complete blood count and / or a sensitive TSH measurement may be requested, in case anemia, leukemia, thyroid dysfunction or another disorder that simulates the symptoms of PMS is suspected.

Treatment options

Non-pharmacological methods	Exercise (they stimulate the production of beta-endorphins, which improves symptoms). Dietary modification (ingestion of carbohydrates or complex proteins increases the availability of

	tryptophan, thereby increasing the level of serotonin). Stress management through relaxation techniques.
Pharmacological method	Serotonin reuptake inhibitors (clomipramine, citalopram, escitalopram, fluoxetine, and others). Benzodiazepines.
Ovulation suppression	Hormonal therapies (used for very severe premenstrual syndromes, the goal is to block the hypothalamic-gonadal cycle). Danazol. Oral contraceptives.

Follow-up peculiarities

It is recommended to track the symptoms associated with premenstrual syndrome, for at least 2 consecutive cycles, evaluating other possible causes. Perform the paraclinics that you consider pertinent in relation to atypical clinical manifestations of the premenstrual syndrome that occur during the evaluation.

Bibliographic references

1. Bertone-Johnson ER, Hankinson SE, Willett WC, Johnson SR, Manson JE. Adiposity and the development of premenstrual syndrome. J WomensHealth (Larchmt). 2010 Nov; 19 (11): 1955-62.
2. Mishra S, Elliott H, Marwaha R. Premenstrual Dysphoric Disorder. [Updated 2020 May 28]. In: StatPearls. Publishing; 2020 Jan.

Chapter 310. Dysfunctional Uterine Bleeding

Currently known as abnormal uterine bleeding (AUS), it is a term used to describe irregularities or alterations in the menstrual cycle and that involve the frequency, duration, regularity and volume of flow outside of pregnancy.

It can be classified as acute abnormal uterine bleeding that occurs as excessive bleeding and requires immediate intervention to stop blood loss and chronic dysfunctional uterine bleeding, which refers to menstrual bleeding irregularities with high incidence in the previous 6 months.

Statistics and epidemiology

It is estimated that it has a prevalence in women of reproductive age between 3 to 30% worldwide. The highest incidence occurs at menarche and perimenopause.

About 1 to 2% of women with anovulatory bleeding can develop endometrial cancer.

Abnormal uterine bleeding is a common diagnosis, accounting for 5-10% of cases in the outpatient setting.

Risk groups and factors

- ✓ Polycystic ovarian disease.
- ✓ Hypothyroidism
- ✓ Polypharmacy.
- ✓ Von Willebrand disease.
- ✓ Coagulopathies.
- ✓ Alcoholism.
- ✓ Smoking habits.
- ✓ Obesity.

Etiology or more frequent causes

According to the International Federation of Obstetrics and Gynecology (FIGO), the acronym PALM-COEIN is useful for classifying the causes of SUA. The first part (PALM) describes structural disorders, while the second part (COEI) refers to non-structural ones. Finally, the N represents "Not otherwise classified" pathologies.

Structural	
P	Polyp
TO	Adenomyosis
L	Leiomyoma
M	Malignancy and hyperplasia.
Non-structural	
C	Coagulopathy
OR	Ovulatory Dysfunction
AND	Endometrial Disorders
I	Iatrogenic
N	Not otherwise classified (rare pathologies such as arteriovenous malformations, myometrial hyperplasia and endometritis).

Pathophysiological elements

Under normal conditions, progesterone levels are low during the end of the menstrual cycle, which causes the breakdown of enzymes in the functional endometrial lining. This degradation causes the loss of blood and the shedding that constitutes menstrual bleeding.

On the other hand, the functioning of thrombin, platelets and the vasoconstriction of the endometrial arteries, allow the control of blood loss.

However, any structural or functional uterine alteration causes this regulatory mechanism leading to abnormal or dysfunctional uterine bleeding.

These patients may have constant estrogen levels that are not recycled, but remain stimulating the growth of the endometrium. This proliferation without periodic shedding, causes the endometrium to exceed the blood supply causing the tissue to break and detach from the uterus causing irregular scarring.

Diagnostic criteria

The diagnosis is made through a complete evaluation of the physical examination and a detailed medical history, prioritizing the registration of menstrual history.

Menstrual history
Age of menarche.
Date of the last menstrual period.
Frequency, regularity, volume of menstrual flow and duration of menstruation.
Common <24 days, normal 24 to 38 days, rare> 38 days.
Regular variation +/- 2 to 20 days, irregular variation greater than 20 days.
Duration: long> 8 days, normal 4 to 8 days, shortened <4 days.
Volume: heavy> 80 ml, normal 5 to 80 ml, light <5 ml (measured according to the frequency of change of medical devices per day).
Intermenstrual and postcoital bleeding.
Sexual and reproductive history
Obstetric personal history (number of pregnancies, mode of delivery).
Desire for fertility.
Current contraceptive method.
History of sexually transmitted infections.
Pap smear history.

Other symptoms and systemic manifestations:
- ✓ Pain.
- ✓ Weightloss.
- ✓ Download.
- ✓ Anemia.
- ✓ Bleeding disorder
- ✓ Endocrine disorders.
- ✓ Intestinal or urinary symptoms.

Paraclinical
- ✓ Urine pregnancy test.
- ✓ Complete blood count.
- ✓ Ferritin.
- ✓ Coagulation panel.
- ✓ Thyroid function test.
- ✓ Liver function tests (against suspicion of a disorder that alters the hepatic metabolism of estrogens associated with SUA).
- ✓ Gonadotropin levels.
- ✓ Prolactin levels.
- ✓ PAP test.
- ✓ Endometrial sampling (biopsy): This is done in women at high risk for cancer over the age of 35 and in younger women at extreme risk for endometrial hyperplasia or carcinoma.
- ✓ Transvaginal ultrasound (useful to demonstrate uterine shape and size and evidence of leiomyomas, adenomyosis, ovarian abnormalities, and endometrial thickness).
- ✓ MRI (not the first line in women with SUA).

- ✓ Hysteroscopy and Sonohysterography: they are useful to observe endometrial polyps.

Treatment options

The therapeutic options for abnormal uterine bleeding depend on the etiological factors involved, the desire for fertility, the patient's clinical stability, and the presence of other medical comorbidities.

Acute abnormal uterine bleeding	Replacement of intravenous fluids and blood products (assess hemodynamic status of the patient). Hormonal methods (first line of medical treatment). Intravenous conjugated equine estrogen. Combined oral contraceptives. Oral progestins. Foley tube tamponade of uterine hemorrhage. Intranasal, subcutaneous, or intravenous desmopressin (SUA secondary to von Willebrand disease).
Chronic abnormal uterine bleeding.	
Leiomyomas (fibroids)	Uterine artery embolization. Endometrial ablation. Hysterectomy. Levonorgestrel-releasing intrauterine device (recommended by the American College of Obstetricians and Gynecologists regardless of the age of the patient and in conjunction with progestin in the device). GnRH agonists. Systemic progestogens. Tranexamic acid and NSAIDs.
Malignancy or hyperplasia	Surgery. Adjuvant treatment. Progestins in high doses (when there is impediment to surgery).

	Radiotherapy.
Coagulopathies	Tranexamic acid. Desmopressin
Ovulatory dysfunction	Lifestyle modification. Specific endocrine therapy (for example, cabergoline for hyperprolactinemia and levothyroxine for hypothyroidism).

Bibliographic references

1. Committee. The two FIGO systems for normal and abnormal uterine bleeding symptoms and classification of causes of abnormal uterine bleeding in there productive years: 2018 revisions. Int J Gynaecol Obstet. 2018 Dec; 143 (3): 393-408.
2. American College of Obstetricians and Gynecologists. ACOG committee opinion no. 557: Management of acute abnormal uterine bleeding in non pregnant reproductive-agedwomen. Obstet Gynecol. 2013 Apr; 121 (4): 891-6.
3. Shlom oMelmed, Richard J. Auchus, Allison B. Goldfine, Ronald J. Kowning, Clifford Rosen. Williams Textbook of Endocrinology 14Th edition. ELSEVIER, 2020.

Chapter 311. Polycystic Ovarian Syndrome

Polycystic ovarian syndrome (PCOS), also known as Stein-Leventhal syndrome, is the most common endocrine pathology among women of reproductive age, characterized by chronic anovulation associated with excess androgens of ovarian origin and adrenal.

Statistics and epidemiology

It occurs between 5 to 10% of women of childbearing age, although the incidence varies according to the diagnostic criteria. According to ultrasound studies, the incidence of PCOS ranges from 25 to 30%.

The prevalence in Great Britain ranges between 8 and 20%. The prevalence in Mexico is approximately 6%, while in Brazil it is around 8%; in Spain it is around 6.55%. Heritability occurs in 70% of cases.

Risk groups or factors:
- ✓ Family history with PCOS.
- ✓ Obesity.
- ✓ Metabolic syndrome.
- ✓ Reproductive age.

Etiology

PCOS is considered as a multifactorial disease, where there is a set of susceptible genes and which can contribute to the pathophysiology of the disease in conjunction with predisposing environmental factors for the expression of PCOS such as obesity and insulin resistance. Fetal exposure to androgens may be listed as an environmental factor in some literature.

Etiological theories of PCOS
- ✓ Hypothalamic -pituitary dysfunction (impaired primary gonadotropin secretion).
- ✓ Ovarian and adrenal hyperandrogenism.
- ✓ Primary peripheral insulin resistance disorder.

Pathophysiological elements

- ✓ Hyperandrogenic state with anovulation.
- ✓ Dysregulation of androgen secretion with excessive 17-OH-P response to gonadotropin stimulation.
- ✓ About 3% of patients have isolated adrenal hyperandrogenism.
- ✓ Functional ovarian hyperandrogenism (hyperandrogenism, oligoanovulation, polycystic ovarian morphology).
- ✓ Excess insulin sensitizes the ovary to the action of luteinizing hormone, by interfering with the LH homologous desensitization process during the normal ovulation cycle, and by intrinsic imbalance of regulatory systems within the ovary.
- ✓ Overexpression of steroidogenic enzymes and proteins associated with androgen synthesis in theca cells. Anomaly at the level of steroidogenic enzymatic activity (especially P450c17).

The excessive amount of androgens improves the recruitment of the primordial follicles in the growth group. Simultaneously, early luteinization begins, impairing the selection of the dominant follicle, resulting in macroscopic and classic histological changes of PCOS (cystic follicles).

Diagnostic criteria

Clinic	A complete medical history is essential and should cover all aspects associated with ovarian function. History of ovulatory dysfunction (oligomenorrhea or amenorrhea, irregular uterine bleeding). Pubertal onset. History of cyclical and predictable menses makes the diagnosis of PCOS unlikely. Associated common manifestations: Hirsutism Acne. Alopecia. Seborrhea. Clitoromegaly. Infertility Acanthosis nigricans.
Criteria for defining SOP	
Declaration of the National Institutes of Health (1990).	Hyperandrogenism and / or hyperandrogenemia. Oligoovulation. Exclusion of related disorders.
Statement European Society for Human Reproduction	It includes two of the following conditions, in addition to the exclusion of associated disorders: Oligoovulation or anovulation (abnormal uterine bleeding, amenorrhea). Clinical and / or biochemical signs consistent with

and Embryology / American Society for Reproductive Medicine (2003).	hyperandrogenism (hirsutism, high total or free serum testosterone). Ultrasound diagnosis of polycystic ovaries.
Criterion suggested by the Androgen Excess Society (2006).	Hyperandrogenism: hyperandrogenemia and / or hirsutism. Ovarian dysfunction: polycystic ovaries and / or oligoanovulation. Exclusion of other disorders due to excess androgens or associated.

Paraclinical:
- ✓ Free (elevated) testosterone levels.
- ✓ Metabolic panel.
- ✓ Morning cortisol level.
- ✓ Prolactin levels.
- ✓ TSH levels.
- ✓ Fasting oral glucose tolerance test.
- ✓ Glucose 2 hours after a 75g oral glucose load.
- ✓ Urine pregnancy test.
- ✓ Progestin challenge test (after pregnancy test to confirm anovulation. If uterine bleeding does not follow progestin challenge, it is recommended to rule out pregnancy again, as well as other causes of chronic anovulation).
- ✓ LH and FSH levels.
- ✓ ACTH stimulation test (to rule out other pathologies).
- ✓ Serum levels of DHEAS (increased to 8 μg / ml in about 50% of patients with PCOS).

- ✓ Endometrial biopsy (in the initial study).
- ✓ Morphology of the polycystic ovaries.
- ✓ Morphological evaluation is more accurate by transvaginal ultrasound.
- ✓ Normal ovarian size limit is 10 ml.
- ✓ Presence of at least 12 to 25 follicles of 2 to 9 mm throughout the ovary or due to an increase in the size of the ovary to more than 10 ml.

Treatment options

Modification of the lifestyle.	Exercise. Decrease in body weight. Change of nutritional habits (low carbohydrate diets can be used).
Hormonal contraceptives	Oral contraceptives, vaginal patch or rings: Progestin component. Ethinylestradiol 20 mcg dose combined with a progestin such as desogestrel or drospirenone.
Metformin	According to the Endocrine Society, it is recommended to start treatment with metformin in all patients with PCOS who have diabetes mellitus or glucose intolerance, where lifestyle modifications did not offer significant improvement.
Infertility treatment	Clomiphene citrate (first line). Estrogen modulators (letrozole). Metformin (adjuvant).
Treatment for hyperandrogenism	Oral contraceptives as the first line of treatment (See Chapter 263).

Follow-up peculiarities

The goal of treatment is to reduce the risk of complications by improving your lifestyle. A consultation by a multidisciplinary team that includes physical therapy and dietetics is recommended because the first line of treatment is lifestyle change.

Emphasize among your patients the need for regular physical exercise, and suggest support groups to help reduce stress and increase confidence. PCOS is considered a chronic pathology, and regular follow-up should be performed, supervising the development of possible pathologies associated with this syndrome such as cardiovascular disorders, gestational diabetes, pre-eclampsia, premature births, among others.

Bibliographic references

1. Shlomo Melmed, Richard J. Auchus, Allison B. Goldfine, Ronald J. Kowning, Clifford Rosen. Williams Textbook of Endocrinology 14Th edition. ELSEVIER, 2020.
2. Teede HJ, Misso ML, Costello MF, Dokras A, Laven J, Moran L, Piltonen T, Norman RJ., International PCOS Network. Recommendationsfromtheinternationalevidence-basedguidelinefortheassessment and managementofpolycysticovarysyndrome. Clin. Endocrinol. (Oxf). 2018 Sep; 89 (3): 251-268.
3. Misso ML, Tassone EC, Costello MF, Dokras A, Laven J, Moran LJ, Teede HJ., International PCOS Network. Large-ScaleEvidence-BasedGuidelineDevelopmentEngaging the International PCOS Community. Semin. Play Med. 2018 Jan; 36 (1): 28-34

Chapter 312. Adolescents with Polycystic Ovaries

It corresponds to the syndrome that presents with variable combinations of menstrual irregularity, acne, hirsutism and obesity, which can be diagnosed during adolescence and with a history in early childhood. The diagnosis of polycystic ovarian syndrome (PCOS) during adolescence is challenging and controversial due to the coexistence of normal pubertal physiological changes, similar to the symptoms of PCOS.

Statistics and epidemiology

It affects between 8 to 13% of women of reproductive age, occurring between 6 to 18% among adolescents. According to the WHO, adolescence is the period between 10 and 19 years of age.

Aetiopathogenic considerations

Currently the pathogenesis is not well understood, however, it is likely that the etiopathogenic aspects of PCOS have their origin in the interaction between environmental and genetic factors.

Theories about its etiology include:
- ✓ Alteration in the secretion of neuroendocrine gonadotropins.
- ✓ Hyperandrogenism.

- ✓ Insulin resistance
- ✓ Hyperinsulinemia
- ✓ A combination of some of the above.
- ✓ The etiologic and pathophysiologic aspects have been described in Chap. 268.

Diagnostic criteria

Irregular menstrual cycles and ovulatory dysfunction

Post menarche time	Definition of irregular menstrual cycles
<1 year after menarche	The normal pubertal transition may present irregular menstrual cycles.
1 to 3 years after menarche	<21 days or > 45 days
> 3 years after menarche	<21 days or > 35 days or less than 8 cycles per year
> 1 year after menarche	> 90 days for any cycle
	Primary amenorrhea at 15 years or more than 3 years after thelarchy.

Endocrine Society Diagnostic Criteria for PCOS in Adolescents (2015)

Abnormal uterine bleeding pattern
Abnormal for age or gynecological age.
Persistent symptoms for 1 or 2 years.
Evidence of hyperandrogenism
Persistent increase in testosterone levels.
Moderate to severe hirsutism.
Moderate to severe hirsutism or moderate to severe inflammatory acne vulgaris.

Ultrasound in adolescents for the diagnosis of PCOS

Due to the various physiological changes that occur in adolescents, ultrasound investigation is not a first-line investigation in this age group; however, ovarian dysfunction should be investigated based on oligomenorrhea and / or biochemical evidence of anovulation.

Recommended laboratory tests for adolescents with clinical manifestations of PCOS

FSH, LH, and estradiol (especially in adolescents with amenorrhea).
Total or free testosterone level.
SHBG
17-Oh progesterone.
TSH.
Prolactin level.
DHEAS
Insulin fasting.
Lipidic profile.
Fasting blood sugar

Treatment options

Lifestyle interventions
Nutritional modifications.
Weightloss.
Physical exercise.
Combination of the above.
Local therapies (hirsutism)
To be
Electrolysis.
Others
Medical treatment
Metformin: in lean patients, it can be started at low doses (850 mg), while in obese or overweight patients, it is used at high

doses (1.5 to 2.5g)
Anti-androgens (spironolactone, Finasteride, Flotamid).
Oral contraceptives (products with low androgenic or antiandrogenic effects).
Combination therapy

Follow-up peculiarities

Plan long-term follow-up checks. Patients must be accompanied during adolescence and in the transition to adulthood, especially fertility treatment.

Bibliographic references

1. Ramezani Tehrani, F., & Amiri, M. (2019). Polycystic Ovary Syndrome in Adolescents: Challenges in Diagnosis and Treatment. International journal of endocrinology and metabolism, 17 (3), e91554.https://doi.org/10.5812/ijem.91554
2. Peña, AS, Witchel, SF, Hoeger, KM et al. Adolescent polycystic ovary syndrome according to the international evidence-based guideline. BMC Med 18, 72 (2020). https://doi.org/10.1186/s12916-020-01516-x

Chapter 313. Hydroxyprogesterone

17-hydroxyprogesterone (17-OHP) is an intermediate steroid in the adrenal biosynthetic pathway from cholesterol to cholesterol, which is the substrate of the steroid 21-hydroxylase. Therefore, a hereditary deficiency of 21-hydroxylase, causes very high serum 17-OHP concentrations, meanwhile, the absence of cortisol synthesis causes an increase in adrenocorticotrophic hormone.

Steroid synthesis

In the adrenal glands, the synthesis of cortisol and aldosterone from cholesterol occurs.

It begins by capturing cholesterol in the mitochondria through the action of the steroidogenic acute regulatory protein (StAR).
This is followed by a side chain cleavage of an enzyme of cytochrome P-450 (now CYP11A1), to release pregnenolone.
Pregnenolone and cholesterol possess β-hydroxyl groups at carbon 3 (C3) and double bonds at C5 to C6 (5-ene).
Pregnenolone can be hydroxylated at C17 by 17 alpha-hydroxylase (CYP17A1) in the smooth endoplasmic reticulum of the adrenal zona fasciculata. This produces 17-hydroxypregnolone, which, by the action of 3β-hydroxysteroid dehydrogenase and 5,4-isomerase (HSD3B2), is transformed into the steroid hormone 17-OHP (17-hydroxy 4-pregnene-3.20 - dione) with carbonyl at C-3 and C4 to C5 double bond (4-ene).
This 17-OHP, becomes 11-deoxycortisol by the enzyme hydroxylase C-21.
The 11-deoxycortisol then migrates to the mitochondria for 11-hydroxylation by 11 beta hydroxylase producing cortisol in the zona fasciculata.
In the outer zona glomerulosa, pregnenolone is converted into

progesterone, deoxycorticosterone, aldosterone, and corticosterone, through actions of CYP21A2, HSD3B2 and then CYP11B2, which has 18-hydroxylase and aldosterone synthetase activity.

Clinical utility of 17-hydroxyprogesterone

Serum 17-OHP is a laboratory test used for the diagnosis of congenital adrenal hyperplasia (CAH), associated with the deficiency of the enzyme 21-hydroxylase, due to genetic disorders frequently male.

The 17-hydroxyprogesterone test is indicated as a diagnosis and follow-up treatment for congenital adrenal hyperplasia.

17-OHP Analysis

The immunoassay is the most widely used technique for measuring steroids.
Chromatographic methods of measurement of 17-OHP include:
LC with ultraviolet detection.
Gas chromatography coupled with mass spirometry.
GC with tandem mass spectrometry.
LC-MS / MS.

Reference findings of 17-OHP with RIA and GC-MS, baseline and after stimulation with ACTH (Supraregional Trial Service)

Group	RIA (serum) nmol / L (60 min of ACTH stimulation)	GC-MS (serum) nmol / L (30 min of ACTH stimulation)	LC-MS / MS

Infants (no stress)	<13	<5 (<8)	
Infants (stressed)	<40		
Adult men	2 to 9 (3 to 30)	1.2 to 5 (3 to 10)	1.2 to 7.6
Adult women (in the follicular phase)	2 to 6	1 to 4.5 (2 to 8)	0.4 to 3.6
Adult women (in the luteal phase)	> 6	1.0 to 6 (2 to 10)	1.2 to 7.6
Patients with untreated 21-hydroxylase deficiency	Often greater than 100	>> 100	
Patients with NC-CAH	(63 to 470)	<5 to 200 (60 to 600)	
Heterozygous carriers	(6 to 44)	*(5 to 50)*	

Table 325 - 2. 17-OHP reference values. Source: Honor JW. 17-Hydroxyprogesterone in children, adolescents and adults. Ann Clin Biochem. 2014 Jul; 51 (4): 424-40.

Bibliographic references

1. Rodríguez A, Ezquieta B, Labarta JI, Clemente M, Espino R, Rodriguez A, et al. Recommendations for the diagnosis and treatment of patients with classic forms of congenital adrenal hyperplasia due to 21-hydroxylase deficiency. Annals of Pediatrics. 2017 Aug; 87 (2): 116.e1-116.e10.

2. Honor JW. 17-Hydroxyprogesterone in children, adolescents and adults. Ann Clin Biochem. 2014 Jul; 51 (4): 424-40.

Chapter 314. Hyperandrogenism

The excess of the biological action of endogenous or exogenous androgens is called hyperandrogenism and can manifest itself at different stages of development in both men and women. Hyperandrogenism is also the term used to describe the signs or clinical manifestations specifically in women with hyperandrogenemia: hirsutism, alopecia, acne, among others.

Statistics and epidemiology

The most common cause is polycystic ovarian syndrome with a prevalence of 72.1% in classic anovulatory patients.
The prevalence of idiopathic hyperandrogenism is around 15.8%.
Mild androgen excess disorders may account for about 30% of patients with clinical hyperandrogenism.

Risk groups and factors

- ✓ Use of drugs (corticosteroids, androgens, steroids, progestogens).
- ✓ Cushing's syndrome.
- ✓ Obesity.
- ✓ Neoplasms

Etiology or more frequent causes

Origin	Main causes
Adrenal	Benign and malignant tumors. Cushing's syndrome. 21-hydroxylase, 11b-hydroxylase, and 3β-hydroxysteroid

	dehydrogenase deficiency (late-onset).
Ovarian	Polycystic ovarian syndrome. Virilizing tumors.
Testicular	Tumors Testotoxicosis.
Placental	P-450 aromatase deficiency in the fetus.
Peripheral production increase	Obesity. Idiopathic hyperandrogenism.
Exogenous	Use of synthetic corticosteroids, androgens and anabolic steroids, synthetic progestogens at high doses.

Pathophysiological elements

- ✓ Excessive androgen production by the ovary or adrenal glands.
- ✓ Increased conversion of androgens (especially testosterone from steroidal precursors by certain peripheral tissues.
- ✓ Increased use by androgen-sensitive tissues.

Diagnostic criteria

Clinic	In the fetus *Male fetus:* Increase in penis size. Increased growth. *Female fetus (ambiguous genitalia):* Virilization of external genitalia to a variable degree. Growth acceleration. Development of the Wolffian ducts. In the prepubertal stage Growth increase Thickening of the voice.

	Increase in body hair. Muscle hypertrophy. Changes in body odor. Acne. Precocious pubarche. Penile growth (males). Clitoral growth (women). Seborrhea. Acceleration of bone age and premature closure of the epiphysis. In the pubertal or postpuperal stage *In women* Hirsutism Acne. Androgenic alopecia. Androgenic redistribution of body fat. Breast atrophy or breast reduction. Menstrual irregularity Infertility Increased libido. *In men:* Acne. Increased libido. Increased maturation and growth.
Paraclinical	Free testosterone levels (levels higher than 1.5 ng / mL correspond to adrenal and ovarian tumors). Measurement of LH and FSH. Prolactin levels. Cortisol measurement in morning and evening blood. Urinary cortisol. Thyroid profile. Fasting glucose and insulin. ACTH stimulation test. Quantification of serum 17-alpha-hydroxyprogesterone (very high levels suggest 21-hydroxylase deficiency). Free androgen index: *(Total testosterone (ng / mL) × 3.47 / SHBG nmol / L) ×*

	100 Request the pertinent imaging studies according to the clinical suspicion.

Treatment options

Treatment should be geared towards the specific cause of hyperandrogenism and reproductive desires.
- ✓ Oral estrogen plus progestin.
- ✓ Ethinylestradiol with antiandrogenic progestins (dienogest, drospirenone, cyproterone acetate) or neutral metabolic androgenic progestins (desogestrel, norgestimate, gestiondeno).
- ✓ Anti-androgens such as spironolactone and flutamide.
- ✓ Cosmetic treatment through temporary or permanent hair removal and acne management through topical or systemic treatment. Consider referral to dermatology.

In case of congenital adrenal hyperplasia, mineralocorticoid supplementation is used. The use of hydrocortisone infused continuously every 6 to 8 hours is recommended.

Bibliographic references

1. Shlomo Melmed, Richard J. Auchus, Allison B. Goldfine, Ronald J. Kowning, Clifford Rosen. Williams Textbook of Endocrinology 14Th edition. ELSEVIER, 2020.

2. Lavin N, editor. Manual of endocrinology and metabolism. 4th ed. Philadelphia: Wolters Kluwer / Lippincott Williams & Wilkins Health; 2009. 837 p.
3. Dorantes and Martinez. Clinical endocrinology 5th edition, Editorial El Manual Moderno 2016.

Chapter 315. Hyperhidrosis

It is a disorder that causes excessive sweating as a result of overstimulation of the cholinergic receptors of the eccrine glands. This pathology is characterized by sweating higher than what is required for the regulation of homeostatic temperature.

Statistics and epidemiology

It can affect about 3% of the population of the United States. It is common in age groups between 20 to 60 years, with no preference in the predominance for the female or male sex. It affects all races, although evidence suggests that the Japanese are the most affected ethnic group. The palmar region is the mainly affected area.

Risk factor's

- ✓ Family history of primary hyperhidrosis.
- ✓ Underlying chronic diseases
- ✓ Use of antipsychotics, dopamine agonists, or insulin.

Etiology or more frequent causes

Hyperhidrosis can be classified as primary and secondary according to its etiology and manifestation:

Primary hyperhidrosis: Unknown cause. Genetic factors are theorized to play a role in excessive neural stimulation, however this is not entirely clear.

Secondary hyperhidrosis: it is associated with drugs such as dopamine agonists, antipsychotics, insulin, alcohol, and others. It can also be the result of systemic disorders such as diabetes mellitus, hyperthyroidism, Parkinson's disease, among other neurological disorders. It can occur in lymphomas and pheochromocytomas.
Other causes are any feverish illness, alcoholism, tuberculosis.

Pathophysiological elements

Parasympathetic nervous system hyperactivity.
Excessive release of acetylcholine from the nerve ending.
Acetylcholine acts on the epidermal eccrine sweat glands in a physiological response to control core body temperature (specific during physical or psychological stress).
In hyperhidrosis, the hypothalamic negative feedback mechanism appears to be affected by the fact that the body sweats more than is required to control body temperature.
Medications or systemic disorders capable of increasing the release of acetylcholine, influence the development of hyperhidrosis.

Histopathology: The eccrine glands are of normal size and number, however, the sympathetic ganglia in these patients are larger, supporting the theory that hyperhidrosis is a disorder of excessive cholinergic stimulation.

Diagnostic criteria

Clinic	Excessive sweating frequently in various eccrine glands (palms, soles of the feet, face, head, armpits), although it can occur in a segmented or localized manner. *Diagnostic criteria for primary hyperhidrosis:* Excessive sweating for 6 months or more. Sweating affects daily activities. Age less than 25 years. Family history of hyperhidrosis. Episodes of sweating that last 7 days or more. Decrease or absence of sweating during the night. Sweating affects the soles of the feet, the palms of the hands, and the face. *Diagnostic considerations for secondary hyperhidrosis:* Use of drugs associated with secondary hyperhidrosis. Clinic associated with an underlying disorder (febrile pathology, pheochromocytoma, hyperthyroidism, Parkinson's or other). Patient over 25 years of age.
Paraclinical	Mainly, the type of hyperhidrosis that the patient presents must be established through the patient's clinic. Paraclinics should be oriented towards identifying the cause, if secondary hyperhidrosis is suspected. You can start the investigation by requesting the following paraclinics: Complete blood count. Basic metabolic panel. TSH level. Sedimentation rate. Hemoglobin A1C. Chest X-ray.

Treatment options

Treatment of hyperhidrosis depends on the type of hyperhidrosis the patient has. Treatment for secondary hyperhidrosis must be directed to the underlying cause, either discontinuation of the suspected drug or specific treatment for the disorder.

20% Aluminum Chloride Hexahydrate (Drysol): used for 3 or 4 consecutive nights. He retires in the morning. May cause skin irritation.

Topical agents such as tannic acid and potassium permanganate.

Oral anticholinergics (second line of treatment when conventional topical treatment is not well tolerated): they block cholinergic receptors, oxybutynin at 5 to 10 mg daily or topical glycopyrrolate between 0.5 to 2.0% can be used.

Iontophoresis: 2 or 3 times a week.

Botulinum toxin with or without lidocaine every 3 to 4 weeks. It can cause paralysis at the injection site, is expensive, and requires repeated treatments.

Sympathectomy (excision of the T2 and T4 nodes responsible for sweating). Lymph nodes T1 for facial sweating, T2 and T3 for palmar sweating and T4 nodes for axillary sweating can be removed. The procedure is performed thoracoscopically.

Radiofrequency ablation.

Subcutaneous liposuction.

Surgical excision of the affected area.

Follow-up peculiarities

Hyperhidrosis is not a life-threatening disorder in itself, however, it can have psychosocial impacts on patients, especially those under 25 years of age.

Current treatments are not usually definitive and hyperhidrosis is frequently recurrent. Consider follow-up and sympathectomy approach for permanent results in patients with primary hyperhidrosis with significant impact on the patient's quality of life.

Bibliographic references

1. Menzinger S, Quenan S. [Evaluation and managementofhyperhidrosis]. RevMedSuisse. 2017 Mar 29; 13 (556): 710-714.
2. Nawrocki S, Cha J. Theetiology, diagnosis, and managementofhyperhidrosis: A comprehensivereview: Etiology and clinicalwork-up. J. Am. Acad. Dermatol. 2019 Sep; 81 (3): 657-666.

Chapter 316. Hirsutism

It signifies the excessive growth of male-pattern body hair in women after puberty. Hirsutism affects androgen-dependent facial and body areas (mustache, beard, pubic hair, buttocks, and thighs). It is associated with significant emotional stress as a result of the cosmetic problem.

Statistics and epidemiology

It is the most common endocrine disorder, affects about 10% of American women, with a prevalence that can range between 10 to 50% according to the population, and the incidence is higher in dark-skinned women. In boys, it is indicative of precocious puberty.

Hyperandrogenic hirsutism represented by polycystic ovary syndrome is the most common cause, accounting for 75% of cases.

Risk groups or factors:
- ✓ Polycystic ovarian syndrome.
- ✓ Thyroid disorders.
- ✓ Pregnancy.
- ✓ Postmenopause.

Etiology

Hyperandrogenic hirsutism	Polycystic ovarian syndrome.
	Androgen-secreting tumors.
	Nonclassic congenital adrenal hyperplasia.
Non-	Use of medications (androgens, glucocorticoids,

hyperandrogenic hirsutism	estrogen antagonists, progestogens, minoxidil, cyclosporine, danazol, diazoxide, interferon, D-penicillamine, phenytoin). Endocrinopathies (Cushing's syndrome, thyroid disorders, hyperprolactinemia, acromegaly). Other causes (pregnancy, postmenopause). Idiopathic

Pathophysiological elements

It is an androgen-dependent disorder which results from the interaction between the sensitivity of the hair follicle to androgens and the amount of androgens circulating in the blood. The skin can retain testosterone in the form of dihydrotestosterone (DHT), through the enzyme 5 alpha-reductase, which has isoenzymes present in the skin and the hair follicle. In addition, both the skin and the pilosebaceous follicle have an androgen receptor.

Hirsutism can be the result of:

- ✓ Exogenous androgen intake.
- ✓ Androgen hypersecretion by the ovary or adrenal glands.
- ✓ Increased skin sensitivity to normal circulating levels of androgens (idiopathic hirsutism).

Diagnostic criteria

Clinic	Development or change of hair in terms of density and properties, especially affecting androgen-dependent areas such as facial hair, chest, areolas, white line, sacrum, inner thighs and external genitalia and buttock. *Ferriman and Gallwey system*

	They assign points from 1 to 4 according to the density of the hair that goes from the absence of the hair to the hirsutism. A score between 7 to 36 is considered normal. Other symptoms associated with hirsutism: Acne. Menstrual irregularities. Temporary recession of the hairline. Frontal alopecia.
Paraclinical	The basic evaluation should be carried out in the early follicular phase (between the 3rd and 6th day of the cycle, early morning, fasting) and after the suspension of the contraceptive, pray for 2 or 3 cycles (except in cases where neoplasms are suspected) . Total testosterone levels. Dehydroepiandrosterone sulfate. Delta 4-androstenedione. LH and FSH levels. 17-hydroxyprogesterone measurement. Steroid hormone-transporting globulin. Thyroid profile. Prolactin level. Dexamethasone suppression test (on suspicion of Cushing). ACTH stimulation test. HOMA index or a carbohydrate tolerance test.

Treatment options

Pharmacotherapy	Oral contraceptives (first line of treatment). Spironolactone Finasteride. Low dose corticosteroids (To slow down adrenal hyperandrogenism). Topical eflornithine. Electrolysis.

Non-pharmacological treatment	Shaved off. Hydrogen peroxide discoloration. Hair removal. Chemical hair removal (thioglycollates).
Surgical treatment	Surgical excision of neoplasms. Ovariectomy: indicated in women with severe hyperandrogenism in perimenopausal or menopausal women.

Bibliographic references

1. Kshetrimayum C, Sharma A, Mishra VV, Kumar S. Polycysticovariansyndrome: Environmental / occupational, lifestylefactors; anoverview. J Turk Ger GynecolAssoc. 2019 Nov 28; 20 (4): 255-263.
2. Jacobsen S, Lauszus FF. [Androgen-secretingtumoursoftheovaries]. Ugeskr. Laeg. 2019 Feb 04; 181 (6).
3. Azarchi S, Bienenfeld A, Lo Sicco K, Marchbein S, Shapiro J, Nagler AR. Androgens in women: Hormone-modulatingtherapies for skin disease. J. Am. Acad. Dermatol. 2019 Jun; 80 (6): 1509-1521.

Chapter 317. Acne

It is an inflammatory disorder of the pilosebaceous unit that can have a chronic and self-limiting course. Acne is a very common skin disorder that can present as inflammatory and non-inflammatory lesions, usually on the face, although it can appear on the upper arms, back and trunk. A rare but serious form is acne conglobata, which can occur from the same causes as common or vulgar acne and can cause deep interconnected abscesses.

Statistics and epidemiology

It can appear in adolescence and persist until the beginning of the 3rd decade of life. It is more common in men than women. Urban populations have a higher incidence of acne than rural populations. About 20% of people with acne can develop severe acne.

Asian and Afro-descendant races are more vulnerable to developing the severe manifestation of acne, while the Caucasian population more frequently develops the mild form. Childhood acne is relatively rare, affecting less than 2% of children.

Risk factors and aggravating factors
- ✓ Consumption of high glycemic index foods.
- ✓ Use of oil-based cosmetics and facial massage.
- ✓ Anxiety and anger.
- ✓ Premenstrual syndrome.
- ✓ Excessive sun exposure.

- ✓ Family history of chronic acne.
- ✓ Use of tight clothing in areas susceptible to acne development.

Etiology

Acne is caused due to the hypersensitivity of the sebaceous glands to the level of circulating androgens and aggravated by the microorganism Propionibacterium acnes, which causes an immunological reaction resulting in a chronic infectious and inflammatory process. Other associated factors:

- ✓ Use of medications (anticonvulsants, steroids, lithium).
- ✓ Endocrine disorders or changes (polycystic ovary syndrome, pregnancy).
- ✓ Excess sun exposure.
- ✓ Genetic factors affecting branched fatty acids in sebum.

Pathophysiological elements

Under the influence of androgens, sebaceous secretion increases, as 5-alpha reductase transforms testosterone into DHT, to later bind to specific receptors in the sebaceous glands, increasing sebum production.

Increased proliferation of the follicular epidermis, causing sebum retention.

Rupture of dilated follicles, releasing pro-inflammatory chemicals into the dermis, stimulating inflammation.

Staphylococcus epidermis, and *Malassezia furfur,* induce inflammation and follicular epidermal proliferation.

Histology- Shown as a dilated follicle with a keratin plug. Acne conglobata resembles hidradenitis suppurativa with large tender nodules and drained nasal passages. There may be foreign body granulomas. Acne usually shows traumatized areas with evidence of fibrosis and scarring.

Diagnostic criteria

Clinic	Acne frequently occurs on the central-facial areas of the back, upper torso, as well as the deltoid region. It is evidenced as polymorphic lesions: Grade 1: comedones. They can be open or closed. Open comedones are the result of plugging of the pilosebaceous orifice due to sebum on the surface of the skin. Closed comedones occur because sebum and keratin obstruct the pilosebaceous orifice below the skin's surface. Grade 2: inflammatory lesions similar to a small papule with erythema Grade 3: pustules. Grade 4 - Several pustules fuse together to become nodules and cysts. Soft-contoured depressed scars (boxcar scars) or ice pick scars that present as deep pits. There may also be hypertrophic or keloid scars. Seborrhea may be associated and in the presence of hyperandrogenism, hirsutism, acanthosis nigricans, menstrual irregularity and weight gain are evident.
Paraclinical	The diagnostic is fundamentally clinical. However, the following paraclinics may be ordered especially in women with a history of dysmenorrhea or hirsutism: LH and FSH levels. Testosterone levels. DHEA measurement. It may be considered a culture of the discharge in severe cases.

Treatment options

Topical therapy	Topical retinoids such as retinoic acid, adapalene, and tretinoin are used. They can be used alone or in conjunction with topical antibiotic treatments or benzoyl peroxide. The best comedolytic agent is considered retinoic acid, which can be used as a cream or gel at 0.025%, 0.05% and 0.1%. Topical clindamycin 1 to 2%. 1% nadifloxacin. Azithromycin 1% in lotion or gel. Grade 2-4 estrogen can be used. Topical benzoyl peroxide combined with adapalene at concentrations of 2.5%, 4% and 5% on a gel basis. Beta hydroxy acids like 2% salicylic acid or 10-20% chemical peel. Topical dapsone.
Systemic therapy	Doxycycline 100 mg twice a day. Minocycline in capsules of 50 to 100 mg in a single daily dose. Antibiotics such as amoxicillin, erythromycin, trimethoprim / sulfamethoxazole can be used against the excessive growth of bacteria. You can use ciprofloxacin when there is evidence of pseudomonas infection. Isotretinoin at a dose of 0.5 to 1 mg / kg body weight, following a daily or weekly pulse regimen. Oral contraceptives with 20 mcg of estrogens at low doses, in conjunction with cyproterone acetate as an antiandrogen. Spironolactone 25 mg daily (when necessary to reduce androgen production).
Other measures	Regular face washing with a balanced pH solution such as benzoyl peroxide and salicylic acid. Changing dietary measures by reducing foods with a high glycemic index. Stress management. Treat underlying endocrine causes.

Bibliographic references

1. Yan HM, Zhao HJ, Guo DY, Zhu PQ, Zhang CL, Jiang W. Gut microbiota alterations in moderate to severe acne vulgaris patients. J. Dermatol. 2018 Oct; 45 (10): 1166-1171.
2. ShlomoMelmed, Richard J. Auchus, Allison B. Goldfine, Ronald J. Kowning, Clifford Rosen. Williams Textbook of Endocrinology 14Th edition. ELSEVIER, 2020.
3. Sutaria AH, Masood S, Schlessinger J. Acne Vulgaris. [Updated 2020 Aug 8]. StatPearls Publishing; 2020.

Chapter 318. Androgenic Alopecia

It is a genetically determined disorder or pattern due to an excessive response to androgens. Androgenic alopecia is characterized by a progressive loss of terminal hair from the scalp at any time after puberty. The distribution is characteristic in both men and women, and consists of prominent hair loss in the apex and frontotemporal regions in men, while in women the frontal hairline is generally preserved with diffuse apical hair loss.

Statistics and epidemiology

It most frequently affects Caucasian populations, followed by Asian, African-descendant, and Native American populations. In men, it typically begins between 20 to 25 years of age. About 13% of premenopausal women have androgenic alopecia.

Risk groups or factors: Family history of androgenic alopecia.

Etiology or more frequent causes

Genetic predisposition and probable excessive response to androgens. The alopecic pattern constitutes a polygenic disorder with variable penetrance in which both maternal and paternal genes may be involved.

Pathophysiological elements

Increase in androgen receptors and increase in the enzyme 5-alpha reductase, which leads to a greater conversion of testosterone to dihydrotestosterone at the level of the hair follicle.
Dihydrotestosterone is accumulated in the hair follicles.
Hair follicles are sensitive to androgens and excessive activation of androgen receptors shortens the anagen phase causing follicular miniaturization resulting in shorter and thinner hair follicles unable to penetrate through the epidermis.
The pathological sample shows a reduced 5: 0 ratio of anagen hair to telogen where the norm is 12: 1.

Diagnostic criteria

Clinic	Gradual onset after puberty.
	In men:
	It begins as a bitemporal thinning of the frontal scalp first and later involves the vertex.
	The hairline can also regress in the shape of an "M".
	Norwood-Hamilton classification
	Type I: minimal bitemporal recession of the hair.
	Type II: extension of type I.
	Type III: hair loss in the area of the tonsure and slow recession of the hair.
	Type IV to VI: extension of type III.
	Type VII: more severe pattern of alopecia with confluence of bald areas, the hair is only preserved around the back and the sides of the head.
	In women:
	It is observed as the thinning of the hair between the

	frontal and the vertex of the scalp, but without affecting the frontal hairline. Unmasked by telogen effluvium 1 to 6 months after a stressor. It manifests as a wider part or a visible scalp. *Ludwig Classification* Type I: mild form of hair loss on the front and upper part of the scalp, relatively preserved frontal hairline. *Type II:* moderate. *Type III:* serious.
Paraclinical	Scalp biopsy (when the diagnosis is not clear with the clinic). Dermoscopy: evidence of miniaturized hair with brown perihilar casts useful to differentiate it from diffuse alopecia areata. It is considered useful to request paraclinics to unmask underlying causes of androgenic alopecia. Thyroid profile. Complete blood count. Total iron and ferritin binding capacity.

Treatment options

- ✓ Topical minoxidil.
- ✓ Finestaride 1 mg daily.
- ✓ Dutasteride.
- ✓ Oral antiandrogens such as spironolactone and cyproterone acetate (in women).
- ✓ Hair transplant.
- ✓ Red light or laser at 660 nm.
- ✓ Prostaglandin analogs (latanoprost and bimatoprost).

Bibliographic references

1. Sasaki GH. Review of Human Hair Follicle Biology: Dynamics of Niches and Stem Cell RegulationforPossibleTherapeuticHairStimulationforPlasticSurgeons. Aesthetic Plast Surg. 2019 Feb; 43 (1): 253-266.
2. Manabe M, Tsuboi R, Itami S, Osada SI, Amoh Y, Ito T, Inui S, Ueki R, Ohyama M, Kurata S, Kono T, Saito N, Sato A, Shimomura Y, Nakamura M, Narusawa H, Yamazaki M ., Drafting Committee for the Guidelines for the Diagnosis and Treatment of Male- and Female-Pattern Hair Loss. Guidelines for the diagnosis and treatment of male-pattern and female-pattern hair loss, 2017 version. J. Dermatol. 2018 Sep; 45 (9): 1031-1043.

Chapter 319. Clitoromegaly

It consists of an abnormal enlargement of the clitoris with a measurement of the clitoral index (width x length in mm) which exceeds 35 mm2. The causes of clitoromegaly can be acquired or congenital. It may be an obvious diagnosis in patients with ambiguous genitalia, however borderline conditions may go unnoticed.

Statistics and epidemiology

The most common hormonal cause of virilization of the external genitalia is congenital adrenal hyperplasia, whose prevalence is approximately 1 in 10,000 and its annual incidence ranges between 1 case in 5,000 to 15,000.
Polycystic ovary syndrome is a common disorder that causes clinical or biochemical hyperandrogenism and affects about 9% to 18% of women of childbearing age and may be responsible for causing signs of clitoromegaly.
Non-virilizing syndromes of genetic origin such as Fraser syndrome occur in 1 in 100,000 live births and the most common manifestation is clitoromegaly with around 36.8% occurrence.
Neurofibromatosis has an incidence of 1 in 3,000 live births, and clitoromegaly may be the first manifestation in young girls.

Risk groups or factors:
- ✓ Family background.

- ✓ Endocrine disorders.
- ✓ Exogenous administration of drugs with androgenic action (danazol, norethisterone) during pregnancy.
- ✓ Masturbation (pseudoclitoromegaly).

Etiology or more frequent causes

- ✓ Hormonal conditions
- ✓ Endocrinopathies (polycystic ovary syndrome)
- ✓ Virilizing neoplasms.
- ✓ Exposure to androgens.
- ✓ Syndromes with virilization (Turner syndrome, Antley-Bixler syndrome).
- ✓ Non-hormonal conditions
- ✓ Neurofibromatosis.
- ✓ Epidermoid cysts.
- ✓ Other tumors.
- ✓ Syndromes without virilization (Fraser syndrome, Donohue syndrome, Seckel syndrome, Beckwith-Wiedemann syndrome)
- ✓ Nevus.
- ✓ Pseudoclitoromegaly.
- ✓ Idiopathic

Pathophysiological elements

46, XY-associated disorders of sexual development

Disorder in hormone synthesis or action (AR gene, SRD5A2).

Sex chromosome disorder of sexual development (SRY gene).

Ovotesticular disorders of sexual development (SOX, RSPO, NR5A1, MAP3K1, SRY, DMRT1 genes).

Disorders of sexual development associated with 46, XX
Genetics (CYP21A2, HSD3 BETA 2, CYP11B1 genes).
Androgen excess.
Maternal or fetoplacental factors (exogenous factors such as maternal virilizing tumors or administration of hormonal drugs).
Androgen-secreting masculinizing neoplasms.

Diagnostic criteria

Clinic	Dimensions of the clitoris for the clinical diagnosis of clitoromegaly		
	Age	Long	Width
	0 to 3 years	> 12.6 mm	> 5 mm
	4 to 8 years	> 18.8 mm	> 6 mm
	9 to 12 years	> 24.2 mm	> 7 mm
	13 to 16 years	> 27.4 mm	> 8 mm
	There may be other clinical manifestations associated with the underlying cause. A complete medical history should be taken. Assess secondary sexual characteristics, hirsutism, alopecia, anthropometric measurements.		
Paraclinical	FSH and LH measurement. Testosterone level. Thyroid profile. Serum electrolytes. Measurement of 17 Hydroxyprogesterone (17-OH-P). Prolactin levels Cortisol level. HCG stimulation test. ACTH test. Karyotype. Abdominal and gynecological ultrasound (according to the clinical suspicion of neoplasms or other).		

Treatment options

Treat the underlying cause of the clitoromegaly.

Hormone replacement therapy when required (congenital adrenal hyperplasia).

Watchful waiting can be followed during hormone treatment.

Surgical procedure or clitoroplasty (controversial): clitorectomy, reduction clitoroplasty, complete excision of the corpora cavernosa, albuginea-sparing clitoroplasty, circumference reduction clitoroplasty, among others.

Bibliographic references

1. Kaefer, M., & Rink, RC (2017). TreatmentoftheEnlargedClitoris. Frontiers in pediatrics, 5, 125.https://doi.org/10.3389/fped.2017.00125.
2. Gupta, M., Saini, V., Poddar, A., Kumari, S., & Maitra, A. (2016). AcquiredClitoromegaly: A GynaecologicalProblemoranObstetricComplication ?. Journalofclinical and diagnosticresearch: JCDR, 10 (12), QD10 – QD11.https://doi.org/10.7860/JCDR/2016/23212.9072.
3. Iezzi ML, Lasorella S, Varriale G, Zagaroli L, Ambrosi M, Verrotti A. Clitoromegaly in Childhood and Adolescence: Behind One ClinicalSign, a Clinical Sea. Sex Dev. 2018; 12 (4): 163-74.https://doi.org/10.1159/000489385

Chapter 320. SHBG

The sex hormone transporter thyroglobulin (SHBG) is defined as a homodimeric transporter glycoprotein with high affinity for estrogens and androgens. The main peripheral organ responsible for the production of SHBG is the liver, although its origin has been shown to take place in the hypothalamus and pituitary, where it is closely associated with oxytocin-producing neurons.

"Free hormone" hypothesis

It is a dogma centered in endocrinology, which establishes that the biological activity of hormones is determined by their free concentrations, that is, when they are not bound to proteins.
On the contrary, in the case of estrogens and androgens, it is theorized that the concentrations of free hormones and their biological activity are determined by the presence of SHBG.

SHBG functionality

Androgens and estrogens function as key regulators of the reproductive organs, as well as other sexually dysmorphic tissues, for example, muscle, adipose tissue, and bones. In healthy adults, it is estimated that 55% of testosterone (T) in men and 17β-estradiol (E2) in women is bound to circulating SHBG, while the rest are weakly bound to proteins transporters such as albumin, and only 1 to 3% of sex hormones circulate freely. Thus:

In clinical practice, measurements of the concentrations of free sex steroids must be calculated from:
Total concentrations of sex steroids, albumin, and SHBG.
Balance dialysis.
Other methods.

SHBG clinical utility

It is useful for evaluating mild disorders of androgen metabolism.
It allows the identification of women with hirsutism who are more likely to respond to androgen therapy.
They help to discriminate subjects with excessive androgenic activity from normal individuals.
Low SHBG levels have been associated with central obesity and metabolic syndrome.
In asymptomatic men, low SHBG levels are associated with increased cardiovascular risk.
High concentrations of SHBG appear in some types of cancer, anorexia nervosa, and protein-calorie malnutrition.

SHBG reference values

Age group (years)	Reference value nmol / L	
	Man	Woman
0 to 2	24 to 56	16 to 44
3 to 9	18 to 136	18 to 136
10 to 13	17 to 123	17 to 123
14 to 17	11 to 71	11 to 71
18 to 59	7 to 49	11 to 112
> 60	20 to 63	17 to 95
Pathology related to abnormal SHBG results		
High level	**Low level**	
Liver disease. **Hyperthyroidism** **Eating Disorders.** **Testicular or pituitary disorder in**	Hypothyroidism Diabetes mellitus type 2. Cushing's syndrome. Excess use of steroid	

men. **Problem associated with the pituitary or Addison's disease in women.**	medications. Testicular cancer or adrenal cancer in men. Polycystic ovary syndrome in women.

Bibliographic references

1. Hammond GL (2011). Diverse roles for sex hormone-binding globulin in reproduction. Biology of reproduction, 85 (3), 431–441.https://doi.org/10.1095/biolreprod.111.092593
2. Laurent MR, Hammond GL, Blokland M, et al. Sex hormone-binding globulin regulation of androgen bioactivity in vivo: validation of the free hormone hypothesis. Sci Rep. 2016; 6: 35539. Published 2016 Oct 17. doi: 10.1038 / srep35539
3. Goldštajn MŠ, Toljan K, Grgić F, Jurković I, Baldani DP. Sex Hormone Binding Globulin (SHBG) as a Marker of Clinical Disorders. Coll Antropol. 2016; 40 (3): 211-218.

Chapter 321. Antiandrogens

The pharmacological group known as "Antiandrogens", is a series of drugs whose effect is put to the effect of androgens by different routes or mechanisms, among which are:

Inhibition of synthesis with analysis of LH-releasing hormone (LHRH).
Competitive antagonism.
Inhibition of 5 alpha-reductase.

LHRH analogs

They produce energetic and selective stimulation of LHRH receptors in the pituitary, causing the initial facilitation of FSH and LH release. However, when used in a sustained way, it causes desensitization in the receptors. For this reason, the LHRH analogues cause an increase in circulating testosterone during the first 2 to 4 weeks of treatment to later decrease between 90 to 95%, reaching levels of testosterone obtained in chemical castration.

LHRH analogs:

- ✓ Buserelin.
- ✓ Goserelin.
- ✓ Leuprorelin.
- ✓ Triptorelin.

Androgen antagonists

They have high affinity for the androgen receptor and can bind to it reversibly.

Steroids	
Cyproterone Acetate (ACP)	*Pharmacological action:* They also have an affinity for progesterone and glucocorticoid receptors. They inhibit secretion of pituitary gonadotropins and testicular androgens. Prevents symptoms associated with LHRH Suppresses levels of testosterone, 5 alpha-DHT and LH. Reduces adrenal production of androgens.
Non-steroidal	
Flutamide. Nilutamide. Bicalutamide	*Pharmacological action* Pure competitive antagonists with no affinity for other receptors. LH levels rise.

5 alpha-reductase inhibitors

They oppose the effects of androgens by preventing the transformation of testosterone into 5 alpha-DHT, decreasing its intracellular concentration. It mainly inhibits the type two isoenzyme of 5 alpha-reductase, which is distributed mainly in the genital skin and the urogenital tract. Due to its pharmacological action, it reduces circulating levels and the prostate concentration of 5 alpha-DHT, without modifying circulating testosterone levels.

Types of drugs

Finasteride (dose less than 1mg / day orally).
Dutasteride (dose 0.5 mg / day).
Turosteride.
4-OH-androstenedione.

Pharmacokinetic characteristics of the main antiandrogens.

Drug		Tmax hours	Metabolism	Excretion	Elimination half-life
Competitive antagonists	Cyproterone Acetate	3 to 4	Hepatic (15 and 16 beta-OH-ACP	Stool 65% Urine 35%	38 hours
	Flutamide	2	Hepatic (2-hydroxyflutamide	Urine 96% Stool 4%	4 hours.
	Bicalutamide	16	Hepatic	Urine 50% Stool 50%	7 days
	Nilutamide	1.6	Hepatic	Urine 70% Stool 30%	56 hours
5alpha-reductase inhibitors	Finasteride	6 to 8	Hepatic (CYP3A, 2 poorly active metabolites	Stool 57% Urine 39%	5 to 6 hours.
	Dutasteride	1 to 3	Hepatic, CYP3A4 and CYP3A5	Feces	3 to 5 weeks

Table 269 - 2.

Adverse reactions
- ✓ Gynecomastia (more common with flutamide).
- ✓ Mastodynia (in males).
- ✓ Breast tension (in women).

- ✓ Decreased libido
- ✓ Reduction of erection and ejaculation.
- ✓ Oligospermia
- ✓ Infertility
- ✓ Hot flushes
- ✓ Headaches
- ✓ Altered mood.
- ✓ Depression.
- ✓ Cardiovascular disorders and coagulopathies (with PCA).
- ✓ Painful increase in testicular volume (Non-steroidal antiandrogens in monotherapy).
- ✓ Methemoglobinemia (flutamide).
- ✓ Alterations in visual accommodation to darkness (nilutamide).
- ✓ Hepatic toxicity (can be severe with flutamide and less frequently with nilutamide and bicalutamide).
- ✓ Hepatomas (ACP).

Bibliographic references

1. P. Lorenzo, A. Moreno, I. Lizasoain, JCLeza, MA Moro, A.Portolés. Velazquez. Basic and Clinical Pharmacology 18th Edition. Panamerican Medical Publishing House. 2013.

Chapter 322. Hormonal Contraception

Hormonal contraception consists of using hormonal methods or treatments to prevent unwanted pregnancies. Contraceptive treatments are also used as part of other types of medical therapies, obtaining benefits in reducing the risk of endometrial and ovarian cancer, among others.

Mechanism of action fundamentals

- ✓ Inhibition of total ovulation (progestins) or partial (estrogens).
- ✓ Thickening of the cervical mucus (progestogens: make the cervical mucus viscous and thick).
- ✓ Implantation impeded by the production of decidualized endometrium with atrophic and exhausted glands (they generate an endometrial environment hostile to implantation as a result of sustained exposure).
- ✓ Effect on the uterine tubes and possible inhibition of sperm uptake (paralysis of the migration of the morula through the tube, preventing sperm transport).
- ✓ Alteration of endometrial cell structures and secretions (estrogens).

Pharmacology

Progestins	LH suppression and ovulation. In high amounts, they may inhibit folliculogenesis. Formulations: *First generation (low potency but well tolerated, heavier*

	bleeding at low doses of estrogen): Noretinodrel. Norethindrone. Norethindrone acetate. Ethinodiol diacetate. *Second generation (higher potency, less breakthrough bleeding, but more androgenic side effects):* Levonorgestrel Norgestrel. Norgestimate. *Third generation (reduction of androgenic side effects):* Desogestrel. Norgestimate. Gestodeno. *Fourth generation (antiandrogenic and antimineralocorticoid effect):* Drospirinone
Estrogen	They regulate bleeding. They inhibit FSH. They prevent the formation of the dominant follicle. Formulations: Ethinylestradiol. Mestranol Estradiol valerate.

Hormonal contraception methods

Conventional or combined pill (monophasic or constant doses with changing doses that can be biphasic and triphasic). *Sequential pill* (14 to 16 tablets with estrogen followed by 5 to 7 tablets where an estrogen and a progestogen change, followed by 7 days without administration or replaced by non-hormonal tablets with iron or vitamins). *Mini-pill.* *Parenteral contraception (*continuous, long-acting contraceptives). *Subcutaneous contraception.*

> *Medicated devices (vaginal ring, hormone-releasing contraceptive coil, others).*
> *Coital pill (*single doses of progestogens ingested 5 hours before intercourse to prevent fertilization for up to 18 hours afterwards).
> *Morning-after pill.*
> *Contraceptive skin patch (*combination of estrogen and progestin).

Progestin contraceptives

Method	Description	Side effects
Progestin implants (only)	It is a single rod containing 68 mg of etonogestrel delivered subdermally (usually in the upper limb). It can last from 3 to 5 years. *Effectiveness:* it fails in about 1 in 1000. *Non-contraceptive benefits:* Improves dysmenorrhea	Irregular or unpredictable bleeding pattern. Prolonged or frequent bleeding- Higher incidence of ovarian cysts (clinically insignificant).
Progestin-impregnated intrauterine devices	They can alter the lining of the uterus so that it is unfavorable for implantation. Releases levonorgestrel in small amounts per day. *Non-contraceptive benefits:* Treatment of	Headache. Tender breasts. Humor changes. Pelvic pain. Acne.

	menorrhagia (in uterine fibroids and adenomyosis), treatment of pain in women with endometriosis, alternative to hysterectomy in women with menorrhagia.	
Progestin-only injectable	Depot medroxyprogesterone acetate is administered via the muscle at a dose of 150 mg every 12 weeks. The pharmacologically active level is achieved within 24 hours. *Non-contraceptive benefits:* Improves menorrhagia / dysmenorrhea, improves pain in women with endometriosis, relieves symptoms of premenstrual syndrome, improves pelvic pain / dyspareunia of ovarian origin after hysterectomy.	Change in menstrual pattern. Altered mood. Weight gain. Bone loss (due to long-term use)
Mini-pills	Not used frequently	Irregularity of the menstrual

(progestin-only oral contraceptives).	today. The main indication is in women who are breastfeeding or who have contraindications for estrogen. It requires constant administration.	cycle. Stabbing or breakthrough bleeding. Amenorrhea Cycle duration reduction. Ectopic pregnancy.

Contraceptive pills

It consists of the most common form of contraception in industrialized countries. Currently available oral contraceptive tablets can be of the following types:
Estrogen-progesterone combination (most commonly prescribed).
Progesterone alone.
Pill for continuous or prolonged use.
Adverse effects:
- ✓ Hemorrhage.
- ✓ Sickness.
- ✓ Headache.
- ✓ Abdominal cramps
- ✓ Tender breasts.
- ✓ Increased vaginal discharge.
- ✓ Decreased libido

Bibliographic reference

1. Horvath S, Schreiber CA, Sonalkar S. Contraception. [Updated 2018 Jan 17]. In: Feingold KR, Anawalt B,

Boyce A, et al., Editors. Endotext. South Dartmouth (MA): MDText.com, Inc .; 2000-.
2. Finer LB, Zolna MR. Declines in unintendedpregnancy in theUnitedStates, 2008–2011. New England Journalof Medicine. 2016 Mar 3; 374 (9): 843-52.

Chapter 323. Female Infertility

It consists of a medical condition in which the woman is unable to become pregnant despite the absence of contraceptive methods. Female infertility represents psychological and physical damages in which both the patient and the couple are affected.

Statistics and epidemiology

The chances of infertility increases with age. Among women aged 15 to 34, the infertility rate ranges from 7.3 to 9.1%. In women 35 to 39 years of age, infertility rates increase up to 25%. Infertility rates in women ages 40 to 44 are 30%.

Worldwide, of women between the ages of 20 and 44 at least 2% were never able to have a live birth, while another 11% with a previous live birth were unable to have an additional birth.

Risk groups or factors:
- ✓ Sexually transmitted infections.
- ✓ Uterine neoplasms.
- ✓ Anatomical alterations.
- ✓ Prolactinomas.
- ✓ Endocrine disorders.
- ✓ Etiology or more frequent causes
- ✓ Ovulatory disorders
- ✓ Endometriosis
- ✓ Pelvic adhesions.

- ✓ Tubal blockage.
- ✓ Other tubal / uterine abnormalities.
- ✓ Hyperprolactinemia.

Pathophysiological elements

Anovulation	Hypogonadal hypogonadotropic anovulation (hypothalamic amenorrhea): decreased hypothalamic GnRH secretion
	Normogonadotropic normoestrogenic anovulation: polycystic ovary syndrome (See Chapter 268).
	Hypoestrogenic hypergonadotropic anovulation: premature ovarian failure (see Chapter 273).
	Hyperprolactinemia anovulation (pituitary adenoma).
Endometriosis	Endometrial tissue outside the uterine cavity. Infertility is associated with inflammation and increased production of cytokines, prostaglandins, macrophages, NK cells. The function of the tubes and ovaries is altered with inflammation resulting in defective follicular formation, fertilization and implantation.
	In stages III and IV, infertility is associated with pelvic adhesions or masses that alter the pelvic anatomy.
Pelvic / tubal adhesions	Intra-abdominal infectious processes are associated with infertility due to pelvic inflammatory disease. The microorganism most associated with infertility is Chlamydia trachomatis.
Uterine causes	Space-occupying lesions or reduced endometrial receptivity.

Diagnostic criteria

Clinic	The evaluation of female infertility should be indicated in women with a failed pregnancy after 12 months of

	regular sexual intercourse in the absence of contraception, or after 6 months in the case of women over 35 years of age. *Clinic history* It is essential to develop a complete medical history of the patient that emphatically meets the following characteristics: Duration of infertility. Complete obstetric and gynecological history (history of sexually transmitted infections should be included). Menstrual history. Important medical and surgical history. Sexual history (including frequency and timing of intercourse asking about probable male circumstances such as erection and ejaculation problems). Psychobiological habits: including lifestyle, tobacco habits, alcoholics, use of illicit drugs, occupation, diet and exercises. *Physical exam:* Perform a complete physical examination prioritizing the evaluation that orients toward the specific cause of infertility. Vital signs. Anthropometric measurement (BMI, weight, others). Thyroid evaluation. Breast exam (check for galactorrhea). Signs of androgen excess (inspect external genitalia and perform a dermatological study for signs of virilization). Appearance of abnormal vaginal or cervical anatomy. Pelvic tenderness or masses. Uterine enlargement or irregularity.
Paraclinical	Transvaginal ultrasound. *Evaluation of the ovarian anointing* Urine LH prediction kits. Serum progesterone level on day 21 of the cycle. Progesterone level in the mid luteal phase (should be measured 1 week before menstruation, a level higher

than 3 ng / ml is evidence of ovulation).
Ovulation determination using daily ultrasounds (more precise but invasive, not recommended).
Evaluation of the ovarian reserve
Anti-Mullerian hormone:
<0.5 ng / ml: predicts difficulty in follicular growth (more than 3 follicles).
<1.0 Ng / ml: limited egg supply (may require aggressive ovulation induction protocols).
1.0 to 3.5 ng / ml: normal values.
> 3.5 ng / ml: ample supply, may require mild induction to prevent ovarian hyperstimulation syndrome.
FSH levels:
FSH levels below 10 IU / ml indicate normal ovarian reserve.
FSH levels of 10 to 20 IU / ml indicate intermediate reserve.
Greater than 20 IU / ml indicates a poor prognosis for spontaneous ovulation.
Estradiol on cycle day 3:
Less than 80 pg / ml: normal with adequate ovarian reserve.
Greater than 80 pg / ml: low pregnancy rates.
Greater than 100 pg / ml pregnancy rate of 0%.
Tubal evaluation
Laparoscopy with chromopertubation.
Uterine cavity evaluation
Hysteroscopy
Saline infusion ultrasound.

Treatment options

Depending on the cause of the infertility, the therapeutic options may be different. Some of the most common are described below.

Lifestyle changes: measures are individualized according to the peculiar characteristics of the patient. A woman with a BMI> 27 may benefit from weight loss; however, a patient with a BMI below 17 and a history of intense exercise regimens or eating disorders may require different corrective therapies.

Clomiphene citrate (selective estrogen receptor modulator with estrogen agonist and antagonist effects): 50 mg starting dose from day 2, 3, 4, or 5 of the cycle for 5 consecutive days. Sex is started every other day for a week, starting 5 days after the last pill.

Letrozole (aromatase inhibitor): starting dose 2.5, 5 or 7.5 mg per day on days 3, 4, 5, 6, 7 of the cycle with intercourse every other day starting 5 days after finishing the treatment. It is the first line in patients with polycystic ovary syndrome.
- ✓ Gonadotropin therapy: more intensive regimen.
- ✓ Intrafallopian transfer of gametes.
- ✓ Oocyte and embryo donation.
- ✓ Controlled ovarian hyperstimulation and intrauterine insemination.
- ✓ In vitro fertilization (first-line treatment for infertility caused by bilateral tubal factor).
- ✓ Surgical hysterectomy to remove fibroids.

Bibliographic references

1. Shlomo Melmed, Richard J. Auchus, Allison B. Goldfine, Ronald J. Kowning, Clifford Rosen. Williams

Textbook of Endocrinology 14Th edition. ELSEVIER, 2020.
2. Walker MH, Tobler KJ. Female Infertility. [Updated 2020 Mar 4]. StatPearls Publishing; 2020 Jan.

Chapter 324. Ovarian and Antimullerian Reserve

Antimullerian hormone (AMH) is used in clinical practice as an endocrine marker, useful for evaluating ovarian reserve, since the serum level of this antimullerian hormone is capable of reflecting the number of follicles that have made the transition from the primordial set to the set of growth follicles and is not controlled by gonadotropins.

Biological Aspects of Anti-Mullerian Hormone and the Ovarian Reserve

It is produced exclusively by the granulosa cells of the ovarian follicles, in the early stages of follicle development. It increases until early adulthood.
Antimullerian hormone concentrations decrease slowly and progressively with age until they become undetectable 5 years prior to menopause when the reserve of primordial follicles is depleted.
Given the wide age ranges in which menopause occurs individually, there is great variability in the rate of depletion of the set of follicles and the initial size of the set of follicles.

Factors influencing AMH levels
Evaluate individually the cases where conditions are present that alter the result of AMH, measurements of the

concentration of AMH, is not a reliable indicator of ovarian reserve in certain cases.

- ✓ Biological variation.
- ✓ Clinical sample extraction conditions.
- ✓ Use of oral contraceptives (reduced levels).
- ✓ Administration of GnRH agonists in the luteal half.
- ✓ Overweight.
- ✓ Ethnicity.
- ✓ Vitamin D status.
- ✓ Polymorphisms of AMH and its receptor.
- ✓ Genetic variants in the genome.
- ✓ Smoking (associated with lower levels).

Ovarian reserve test

Its objective is to evaluate the reproductive potential of women, determined based on the quantity and quality of the remaining oocytes.

Other clinical utilities:
- ✓ Prediction of menopause.
- ✓ Evaluation of early menopause.
- ✓ Investigate causes of amenorrhea.
- ✓ Guides the diagnosis of polycystic ovary syndrome.
- ✓ Evaluation of neonates with ambiguous genitalia.
- ✓ Monitoring for some types of ovarian cancer.

Serum AMH level and relationship with fertility

Fertility	AMH level
High level	> 6.8 ng / ml
Optimal fertility	4 to 6.8 ng / ml

Satisfactory fertility	2.2 to 6.8 ng / ml
Low fertility	0.3 to 2.2 ng / ml
Very low / undetectable	0.0 to 0.3 ng / ml

The level of antimullerian hormone is strongly correlated with fertility, since it is a marker of ovarian reserve estimated as superior to other methods (FSH, LH, inhibin B and E2 on the third day of the cycle). The antimullerian hormone is highly associated with the number of antral follicles and has little variability and decreased cycle throughout the reproductive life of women.

Bibliographic references

1. Raeissi, A., Torki, A., Moradi, A., Mousavipoor, SM, & Pirani, MD (2015). Age-specific serumanti-mullerian hormone and follicle stimulating hormone concentrations in infertile Iranian women. International journal of fertility & sterility, 9 (1), 27–32.https://doi.org/10.22074/ijfs.2015.4205
2. Iwase, A., Nakamura, T., Nakahara, T., Goto, M., & Kikkawa, F. (2014). Assessmentofovarian reserve using anti-Müllerian hormone levels in benign gynecologic conditions and surgical interventions: a systematic narrative review. Reproductive biology and endocrinology: RB&E, 12, 125.https://doi.org/10.1186/1477-7827-12-125
3. Simone L. Broer, Frank JM Broekmans, Joop SE Laven, Bart CJM Fauser, Anti-Müllerian hormone: ovarian reserve testing and its potential clinical implications, Human Reproduction Update, Volume 20, Issue 5, September / October 2014, Pages 688–701, https://doi.org/10.1093/humupd/dmu020

Chapter 325. Anovulation

It consists of one of the most common gynecological disorders, which corresponds to irregular menstrual cycles, abnormal uterine bleeding, amenorrhea, and infertility. Anovulation is considered a sign of a particular underlying condition.

Statistics and epidemiology

Ovulatory disorders constitute about 30% of infertility cases.
Chronic anovulation rates range from 6% to 15% in women of childbearing age.
Some studies suggest that the higher frequency of anovulation occurs in Caucasian women than in African-descendant or Hispanic women.

Risk factor's:
- ✓ Polycystic ovarian syndrome.
- ✓ Endocrine disorders (hypothyroidism, and others).
- ✓ Stress.
- ✓ Intense exercise

Etiology or more frequent causes

Hypothalamic causes	Low concentration of gonadotropin-releasing hormone (hypogonadotropic hypogonadism). Stress. Kallmann syndrome.

	Amenorrhea related to weight or vigorous exercise. Chronic disease (AIDS, chronic liver or kidney failure).
Pituitary causes	Hyperprolactinemia. Pituitary insufficiency (hypogonadotropic hypogonadism). Brain radiation therapy. Craniopharyngioma or hypophysectomy. Sheehan syndrome.
Ovarian causes	Polycystic ovarian syndrome.
Other causes	Hypothyroidism Congenital adrenal hyperplasia.

Pathophysiological elements

In normal physiology, ovulation takes place, thanks to the presence of the hypothalamic-pituitary-ovary axis. When the hypothalamic arcuate nucleus is stimulated, it releases GnRH into the portal vessels of the pituitary stalk in a pulsatile fashion. GnRH then stimulates receptors in the anterior pituitary to produce and release both LH and FSH. In women, FSH causes ovarian follicles to mature and estrogen is produced, while LH modulates the release of androgens from theca cells of the ovaries.

This system is so sensitive that only a minimal alteration in any of its factors can cause its fluidity to be altered and trigger anovulation.

Diagnostic criteria

Clinic	*Clinic history:* Medical and surgical history. Family history associated with current symptoms. History of pubertal development.

	Detailed aspects of menstruation (including menarche, frequency, regularity, and others). Previous reproductive history. Aspects related to past and current sexual activity. Contraceptive methods. Current diet and history of weight loss. Use of medications. Psychological antecedents. Current symptoms (visual disturbances, headache, changes in the distribution and appearance of hair, deepening of the voice, breast secretions, irregular menstrual bleeding, among others). ***Physical exam*** Perform a complete organ and system physical examination to identify the cause. Evaluate symptoms of hyperandrogenism (hirsutism, acne, and others).
Paraclinical	A complete medical history and a thorough physical examination is essential to identify the underlying cause of anovulation. Paraclinical patients should be oriented according to the clinical findings and the suspected diagnostic impression. Pregnancy test (quantitative beta-HCG). It should be done in all women. FSH and LH level. Level of ovarian steroid hormones (estradiol and progesterone. TSH level. Prolactin level. Blood glucose Cortisol level with or without ACTH stimulation test. Total testosterone / free testosterone. 17-hydroxyprogesterone-CAH. Pregnenolone (17-alpha-hydroxylase deficiency. Dehydroepiandrosterone sulfate. Complete metabolic profile. Thyroid antibodies.

	C-reactive protein.
	Rheumatoid factor.
	Karyotype (usually performed in those under 30 years of age).
	Imaging studies
	Ultrasonography (transvaginal for ovaries and endometrium or abdominal for adrenals).
	Magnetic resonance imaging: pituitary and adrenal glands.
	Dual energy X-ray absorptiometry. Bone density scan.
	Nuclear thyroid scan.
	Biopsy (when endometrial hyperplasia is to be excluded).

Treatment options

Identifying the specific cause of anovulation is critical to establishing the specific diagnosis.

Dysfunctional uterine bleeding secondary to anovulation usually responds well to oral or intravenous estrogen. Parenteral therapy can be started with estrogen at 25 mg every 4 hours. When the bleeding is not very intense, an oral treatment with high-dose contraceptive pills (3 pills daily for 7 days) can be started, followed by oral continuation for 3 months.

Cases of anovulation due to hyperprolactinemia: Bromocriptine may be indicated starting at a dose of 1.25 mg with food during the night.

Medical induction. Gonadotropin-releasing hormone treatment begins in a hospital setting, this may be the appropriate treatment for women with hypothalamic causes.

Treatment with antiestrogens (clomiphene), is carried out in circumstances that allow ultrasound monitoring.

Metformin at a dose of 1500 mg / day, helps improve menstrual regularity and decreases insulin and testosterone concentrations.

Follicle-stimulating hormone injections.

Surgical induction by laparoscopic ovarian diathermy or perforation is performed by 5 to 6 diathermy or laser punctures in the ovary. The procedure must be done carefully to avoid destroying too much ovarian tissue.

Bibliographic references

1. Shlomo Melmed, Richard J. Auchus, Allison B. Goldfine, Ronald J. Kowning, Clifford Rosen. Williams Textbook of Endocrinology 14Th edition. ELSEVIER, 2020.
2. Rebar R. Evaluation of Amenorrhea, Anovulation, and Abnormal Bleeding. [Updated 2018 Jan 15]. In: Feingold KR, Anawalt B, Boyce A, et al., Editors. Endotext [Internet]. South Dartmouth (MA): MDText.com.

Chapter 326. Inducers of Ovulation

Ovulation inducers are a group of drugs belonging to the family of antiestrogens (clomiphene citrate and letrozole) and gonadotropins, which have the ability to oppose the action of estrogens and/or directly stimulate the ovary to produce eggs, through a set of mechanisms.

Ovulation inducing drugs

Antiestrogens		
Estrogen antagonists	*Mechanism of action*	*Adverse reactions*
Selective estrogen receptor modulator: Clomiphene Tamoxifen	Inhibition of estrogen synthesis by action of LHRH analogs. Blocking the binding of estradiol to its competitive antagonist receptors. Inhibiting the peripheral transformation of androgens into estrogens through aromatase inhibitors.	*Clomiphene, Tamoxifen and Letrozole:* Anti-estrogenic symptoms (hot flashes, atrophy of the genital mucosa).
Aromatase inhibitors **Letrozole**		*Clomiphene:* Coagulation disorder. Hypercalcemia Waterfalls. *Letrozole:* Lymphopenia Hypercholesterolemia Thrombocytopenia
Gonadotropins		
Description	*Mechanism of action*	*Adverse reactions*
Named for their action	Gonadotropins stimulate gametogenesis and the	Ovarian hyperstimulation

on the gonads. These are luteinizing hormone (LH), human chorionic gonadotropin (hCG), and follicle-stimulating hormone (FSH).	production of sex steroids. In women, FSH stimulates estrogen production and follicular development, while increasing ovarian receptors for FSH and improving sensitivity to it. LH acts on final follicular maturation and ovulation, while simultaneously causing luteinization of the follicle after ovulation. In addition, it stimulates the synthesis of progesterone and estradiol by the corpus luteum.	syndrome (ovarian enlargement, pain, abdominal distention). Ascites Hydrothorax Hypovolemia Increased blood velocity. Kidney dysfunction Liver dysfunction Thromboembolic phenomena. Allergic reactions. Headache Injection site reaction.
Biguanide		
Drug	Mechanism of action	Adverse reactions
Metformin	Decreases insulin levels by reducing liver gluconeogenesis. Improves the body's uptake to excrete insulin through the gastrointestinal tract and peripheral uptake. It is used in patients with polycystic ovary syndrome to improve ovulation.	Anorexy. Vomiting Taste alteration, Abdominal pain. Diarrhea. Lactic acidosis (rare).

Administration

Start with an ultrasound and blood tests before starting treatment.

Medications for ovulation induction

Drug	Dose	Cycle start day
Clomiphene citrate	50 mg x 5 days Maximum dose: 250 mg.	2 to 5
Tamoxifen	20 mg x 5 days Maximum dose 80 mg	5
Clomiphene Citrate (CC) + Tamoxifen	150 mg CC x 5 days + 40 mg tamoxifen x 5 days	3
Letrozole	2.5 mg x 5 days Maximum dose 7.5 mg	3
Metformin	500 mg per day. Holder up to 500 mg daily every week. Maximum dose: 2500 mg / day	Daily
Metformin + Letrozole	1500 mg metformin daily + 2.5 mg x 5 days	Daily for 6 to 8 weeks. Letrozole should be started according to normal protocol.
Metformin + CC	CC at doses of 50 to 250 mg per day + 850 mg daily of metformin.	The same daily for 6 to 8 weeks, starting the CC according to the normal protocol.
Gonadotropins	Initial dose 75 IU (intramuscular or subcutaneous). *Augmentation protocol:* more than 75 IU increase every 7 days in the absence of recruited follicle.	5

	Low dose escalation protocol: the initial dose is 37.5 to 75 IU plus an increase of 37.5 IU every 7 to 14 days in the absence of the recruited follicle. *Reduction protocol:* 150 IU until dominant follicle greater than 10 mm, then 112.5 IU for 5 days. 75 IU for 5 days until ovulation	

Table 276 - 2. Ovulation inducing drugs.

Bibliographic references

1. P. Lorenzo, A. Moreno, I. Lizasoain, JC Leza, MA Moro, A. Portolés. Velazquez. Basic and Clinical Pharmacology 18th Edition. Panamerican Medical Publishing House. 2013.
2. Lindheim SR, Glenn TL, Smith MC, Gagneux P. Ovulation Inductionforthe General Gynecologist. J ObstetGynaecol India. 2018; 68 (4): 242-252. doi: 10.1007 / s13224-018-1130-8

Chapter 327. Endometriosis

Endometriosis is defined as the presence of tissue with an appearance and characteristics similar to the endometrium in ectopic sites outside the uterine cavity. These sites are frequently in the pelvic peritoneum and ovaries and are characterized by being associated with chronic pelvic pain, pain during intercourse, and infertility.

Statistics and epidemiology

It affects between 5% and 10% of American women of reproductive age, in a proportion of 4 out of every 1,000 women. The prevalence rate is 20% to 50% of infertile women, and it can be found in 71% to 87% of women with chronic pelvic pain.

It is estimated that about 20 to 50% of women with endometriosis are asymptomatic according to laparoscopic studies. There is no evidence of ethnic predominance.

Risk factor's

- ✓ Family history of endometriosis.
- ✓ Early age of menarche.
- ✓ Short menstrual cycles (less than 27 days).
- ✓ Prolonged menstrual duration (more than 7 days).
- ✓ Defects in the uterus or fallopian tubes.
- ✓ Hypoxia and iron deficiency.
- ✓ Delayed motherhood.
- ✓ Inverse relationship to parity.

Etiology and pathophysiological elements

The exact cause of endometriosis is not known. Endometriosis can be inherited in a polygenic way. The main theories point to the metaplastic conversion of the coelomic epithelium and the hematogenous or lymphatic dispersion of the endometrial cells, although it can be the result of several factors.

These theories suggest the transport of viable endometrial cells by retrograde menstruation. Cells flow retrograde through the fallopian tubes to deposit in pelvic organs where they proliferate.

Factors associated with pathogenesis:
- ✓ Immune dysfunction.
- ✓ Retrograde menstruation.
- ✓ Metaplasia.
- ✓ Remnant Mullerian cells.
- ✓ Genetics.
- ✓ Dissemination and anatomical deposition.

Clinical forms:

Peritoneal endometriosis: endometriotic implants on the surface of the pelvic peritoneum and ovaries.

Endometriomas: ovarian cysts lined by endometrioid mucosa.

Rectovaginal nodule: a solid and complex mass composed of endometriotic tissue combined with adipose and fibromuscular tissue, which resides between the vagina and the rectum.

Histology: presence of endometrial epithelial or stromal cells in conjunction with chronic bleeding and inflammatory changes. Lesions can appear alone or in combination.

The inflammatory process that takes place in endometriosis can stimulate the nerve endings found in the pelvis and cause pain, as well as alter the function of the uterine tubes, reduce the receptivity of the endometrium and negatively alter the development of the oocyte and embryo.

Diagnostic criteria

Clinic	Symptoms usually appear after menarche and usually disappear after menopause. Suspect endometriosis when there is symptoms of intensely painful menstruation during adolescence, which have progressed to chronic pelvic pain. *Probable symptoms:* Dysmenorrhea Infertility Heavy or irregular bleeding. Dyspareunia Pelvic pain. Lower abdominal or back pain. Swelling. Nausea and vomiting Painful defecation, with cycles of diarrhea and constipation. Pain during exercise Dysuria Groin pain
Paraclinical	Direct visualization of lesions laparoscopically or by laparotomy (peritoneal endometriosis). Vaginal ultrasound (Endometriomas).

Treatment options

Infertility caused by endometriosis is treated by surgical removal (with or without assisted reproductive technology). Pain is treated through a combination of medical suppression of ovulation and surgery.
- ✓ GnRH agonists and antagonists.
- ✓ Oral contraceptives.
- ✓ Danazol.
- ✓ Progestins
- ✓ Aromatase inhibitor (for persistent postmenopausal endometriosis).

Currently the use of danazol is controversial due to its anabolic and androgenic effects (weight gain, muscle cramps and virilization), treatment with hormonal agents with oral contraceptives, progestogens and GNRG agonists are mainly recommended for a 6-month cycle with any of these agents to achieve pain relief.

In premenopausal women with endometriosis

The use of combined contraceptives is considered as the first line of treatment (when not contraindicated). This treatment regimen can be followed for a long time.
When relief is not achieved after 6 months of oral contraceptive treatment, a daily oral aromatase inhibitor is added to the oral contraceptive regimen:
- ✓ Anastrozole: 1 mg per day; or
- ✓ Letrozole: 2.5 mg per day.

After one year with this treatment, if pain persists or relief is not satisfactory, conservative laparoscopic surgery is considered.

Bibliographic references

1. Shlomo Melmed, Richard J. Auchus, Allison B. Goldfine, Ronald J. Kowning, Clifford Rosen. Williams Textbook of Endocrinology 14Th edition. ELSEVIER, 2020.
2. Wolf RA. Endometriosis: etiology, pathology, diagnosis, management. Comprehensive Gynecology. Philadelphia, PA: Mosby; 5th ed. 2007: chap 19.

Chapter 328. Recurring Abortions

In the United States, recurrent abortions or recurrent pregnancy loss (RPL), is defined as the loss of two or more consecutive failed pregnancies, which have been documented by ultrasound or histopathology. On the other hand, in the United Kingdom, recurrent abortions are defined as 3 or more consecutive early pregnancy losses.

It can be classified as primary RLP, when women never had a live child and as secondary RLP, when the loss of pregnancy in women in whom they had a previous live birth.

Statistics and epidemiology

It occurs in only 2% of pregnant women. About 50% of women with recurrent abortions do not have a clearly defined cause. Congenital uterine anomalies are present in about 12.6% of patients with recurrent abortions.

Etiology and / or risk factors

Genetics	Aneuploidy Balanced, reciprocal, and fetal robertsonian translocations.
Anatomical	Congenital anomalies of the Müllerian tract. Uterine abnormalities: Septate uterus. Unicornuate uterus. Bicornuate uterus. Didelphos.

	Arched.
	Septate uterus.
	Fibroids
	Polyps.
	Asherman's syndrome.
Endocrine	Mellitus diabetes.
	Thyroid dysfunction
	Hyperprolactinemia.
Antiphospholipid antibody syndrome	It causes an increased risk of thrombosis and placental insufficiency.
Environmental factors	Smoking (affects trophoblastic function).
	Obesity.
	Alcohol consumption (3 to 5 drinks a week).
	Cocaine use.
	Caffeine consumption (more than 3 cups a day).
Immunological	Hereditary thrombophilias

Pathophysiological elements

Recurrent abortions correspond to a multifactorial condition, in which various factors (genetic, anatomical, endocrine, environmental, immunological, antiphospholipid antibody syndrome) may be responsible.

FOXD1 mutations have been closely involved in recurrent abortions, because it is a molecule involved in embryonic implantation, through the regulation of endometrial and placental ennes.

Diagnostic criteria

Clinic	The diagnosis is fundamentally clinical and is established based on the loss of 2 or more consecutive

	pregnancies. The medical history is essential to establish the diagnosis and should gather details pertinent to the syndrome: Details associated with previous pregnancies. Gestational age of the previous pregnancy. Method of treating anterior loss (dilation, curettage). Medical history (thyroid problems, diabetes or other). Surgical history. Menstrual pattern Description of psychobiological habits (smoking, alcoholism, drug use, exposure to environmental pollutants). Family background. The physical examination must be complete and detailed, including a pelvic exam.
Paraclinical	Once the diagnosis based on the loss of d Thyroid profile. Blood glucose Prolactin level. Karyotype evaluation. Evaluation of uterine abnormalities: Pelvic ultrasound. Sonohysterography with saline infusion. Hysteroscopy Hysterosalpingogram. Magnetic resonance. Measurement of anticardiolipin antibodies, lupus anticoagulant and anti-beta 2 glycoprotein. Microarray analysis of 24 chromosomes (genetic evaluation of the product of conception).

Treatment options

Treatment is aimed at treating the specific underlying cause. Consider indicating emotional support for anxious partners, regardless of the cause.

Refer your patients with chromosomal abnormalities for genetic counseling. Inform your patients about the possibility of developing fetal chromosomal abnormalities in subsequent pregnancies.

In hypothyroidism, start hormone replacement therapy.

Administer metformin in patients with type 2 diabetic and polycystic ovary syndrome, and treatment relevant to the patient's metabolic status.

Some congenital and acquired uterine anomalies responsible for recurrent miscarriage can sometimes be treated surgically by hysteroscopic resection of the septum, myomectomy, adhesion lysis, and single bicornuate repair.

Patients with antiphospholipid antibody syndrome can be treated with aspirin and low molecular weight heparin.

TNF inhibitors and granulocyte colony stimulating factor may be beneficial in some cases of recurrent miscarriage.

Bibliographic references

1. Practice Committee of American Society for Reproductive Medicine. Definitions of infertility and recurrent pregnancy loss: a committee opinion. Fertile. Steril. 2013 Jan; 99 (1): 63.
2. Shlomo Melmed, Richard J. Auchus, Allison B. Goldfine, Ronald J. Kowning, Clifford Rosen. Williams Textbook of Endocrinology 14Th edition. ELSEVIER, 2020.

Chapter 329. Artificial Insemination

Artificial insemination is an assisted conception technique, which involves the deposition of a semen sample, previously processed in the upper uterine cavity in such a way that it overcomes the natural barriers for the ascent of sperm through the female reproductive tract. It can be used either donor semen or homologous semen.

Methods

- ✓ In vitro fertilization.
- ✓ Intracytoplasmic sperm injection.
- ✓ Sub-zonal insemination.
- ✓ Intrauterine insemination.

Clinical utility and indications

It is considered a non-invasive and profitable first-line therapy indicated for selected patients with functionally normal uterine tubes, but with infertility of the couple associated with other causes such as:

Female causes	Male causes
Anti-sperm antibodies.	Mild to moderately altered male factor:
Ovulatory disorders.	
Infertility of unexplained cause.	Oligospermia
Coital dysfunction.	Asthenospermia.
Altered cervical factor:	Teratospermia.
Cervical stenosis	Difficulty for sperm penetration into the uterine cavity.

	Retrograde ejaculation Coital dysfunction.

Limited use:
- ✓ Endometriosis (may be indicated in certain cases).
- ✓ Severe male factor infertility.
- ✓ Infertility associated with tubal factor.
- ✓ Ovarian dysfunction (currently it can be indicated in these cases).
- ✓ Maternal age over 35 years.

Contraindications
- ✓ Severely affected male factor.
- ✓ Severe tubal disorder.
- ✓ Baseline FSH (cycle day 2 to 5) > 15 IU / L.
- ✓ Presence of any absolute contraindication to pregnancy due to medical or psychiatric reasons.
- ✓ Active genital infection.
- ✓ Severe pelvic endometriosis.
- ✓ Women over 40 years old.

Requirements for the procedure
- ✓ Women over 18 years of age.
- ✓ Good general health.
- ✓ Consent of both parties.
- ✓ At least one normal, patent fallopian tube.
- ✓ Ovulatory cycle (induced with ovulation inducers or spontaneous).

Process

Ovulation stimulation is recommended, since higher success rates have been recorded in induced ovulation than in natural ovulation. Gonadotropins and recombinant human follicle-stimulating hormone are used with greater success (see Chapter 276).

Ultrasound or serological follow-ups should be performed to ensure ovulation and identify the most appropriate time for fertilization.

The semen sample must be delivered on the day of insemination and less than one hour after being collected.

After a sperm capacitation procedure (selection and recovery of the sperm with better morphology and mobility), the sample is placed in a flexible catheter, which will be introduced into the uterus.

A modified application technique consists of the slow release of sperm for 3 hours.

After having practiced insemination, supplementation of the luteal phase with progesterone is indicated for 15 days.

After 16 days, blood and urine HCG should be measured.

Adverse effects

Symptoms associated with the introduction of the catheter through the cervix:
Crampy pain.
Scanty bleeding
Multiple pregnancy.
Ovarian hyperstimulation syndrome.

Ectopic pregnancy
Psychological disorders:
Anxiety and depression.
Perinatal risks (in elderly women).

Cancellation criteria

- ✓ Premature ovulation
- ✓ Sperm sample less than 3 million / ml
- ✓ GCh administration failure.
- ✓ Inadequate follicular development (less than 1mm day).
- ✓ Follicular growth failure.

Bibliographic references

1. Zhang, A., Ma, X., Zhang, L., Zhang, X., & Wang, W. (2019). Pregnancy and off spring outcomes after artificial insemination with donor sperm: A retrospective analysis of 1805 treatment cycles performed in Northwest China. Medicine, 98 (16), e14975.https://doi.org/10.1097/MD.0000000000014975
2. Farquhar, C., & Marjoribanks, J. (2018). Assisted reproductive technology: an overview of Cochrane Reviews. The Cochrane data base of systematic reviews, 8 (8), CD010537. https://doi.org/10.1002/14651858.CD010537.pub5

Chapter 330. In Vitro Fertilization

About 10 to 20% of couples have trouble conceiving. In vitro fertilization (IVF) is an assisted reproductive technique used to treat infertility.

This technique involves ovarian stimulation using gonadotropic hormones followed by the retrieval of oocytes under anesthesia for subsequent fertilization by sperm in the laboratory to, in this way, develop embryos in culture before being transferred to the uterus.

Since 1978, there have been about 5 million births conceived through IVF. This technique can also be combined with intracytoplasmic sperm injection (ICSI), which consists of a technique to fertilize the oocyte in the laboratory, through the direct injection of a single sperm into the cytoplasm of the oocyte.

Indications

Damage or blockage of the fallopian tubes.
Uterine fibroids.
Endometriosis
Ovulation disorders
Previous removal of the fallopian tubes.
Genetic disorders
Preservation of fertility before medical treatment (cancer or other cause).
Male infertility associated with a deficiency in the production or function of sperm.
Polycystic ovarian syndrome.
Infertility with no apparent cause.
Previous failed attempts at artificial insemination.
Single Women.

Summary of the procedure

Controlled ovarian stimulation (GnRH analog and human chorionic gonadotropin)
Follicular aspiration or follicular capture (guided by olaparoscopic transvaginal ultrasound, performed about 34 to 36 hours after hCG administration) and collection of the seminal sample (ICSI is recommended for couples with male infertility).
Classification of oocytes and fertilization (the fertilization of the oocytes must be confirmed by observing two pronuclei found in the zygote about 17 hours, after fertilization, embryos with high implantation potential are selected).
Transfer (often waiting up to 72 hours after fertilization to transfer the embryos to the uterus, through a catheter from the cervix to the fundus of the uterus or into the fallopian tubes so that they are later carried to the uterus through the peristaltic action of tubes).

Adverse outcomes

The direct association between IVF and some gestational adverse effects is difficult to determine, because IVF is frequently used by elderly women and / or with underlying comorbidities that increase the risk of obstetric complications.

Outcome	Description
Hypertensive disorder of pregnancy	Includes gestational hypertension, pre-eclampsia, and eclampsia.
Gestational diabetes	The incidence of GDM among IVF / ICSI-assisted pregnancies was about 43% higher compared to unassisted pregnancies.
Preterm delivery (before week 37).	An increased risk of preterm delivery has been evaluated in children conceived after IVF, however, the transfer of frozen / thawed embryos could reduce this risk by more closely simulating the hormonal levels found in an unassisted pregnancy, thus avoiding Thus the potential impacts of elevated estradiol and VEGF levels on placentation.
Low birth weight	Less than 2500 g Higher risk found in IVF / ICSI assisted pregnancies.
Congenital defects and imprinting disorders.	Congenital cardiovascular defects. Musculoskeletal. Urogenital. The congenital defect rate ranges from 8%. The imprinting disorders are associated with conditions such as Beckwith-Wiedemann syndrome, Angelman syndrome, Prader-Willi syndrome. However, its incidence is rare. Epidemiological studies are lacking.
Neurodevelopmental disorders	The manipulation of the hormonal and physical environment of the embryo can cause disorders in the development of the brain, for example: Cerebral palsy. Autism and autism spectrum disorder.

Other adverse effects
- ✓ Spontaneous abortion.
- ✓ Ectopic pregnancy.

- ✓ Cancer.
- ✓ Low weight for gestational age.
- ✓ Multiple pregnancies
- ✓ Ovarian hyperstimulation syndrome.

Bibliographic references

1. Sullivan-Pyke, CS, Senapati, S., Mainigi, MA, & Barnhart, KT (2017). In Vitro fertilization and adverse obstetric and perinatal outcomes. Seminars in perinatology, 41 (6), 345–353. https://doi.org/10.1053/j.semperi.2017.07.001
2. Casper, R., Haas, J., Hsieh, TB, Bassil, R., & Mehta, C. (2017). Recent advances in in vitro fertilization. F1000Research, 6, 1616. https://doi.org/10.12688/f1000research.11701.1

Chapter 331. Pregnancy Hormonal Adjustments

Pregnancy constitutes a dynamic state that includes multiple and varied adaptations in the physiology of women, which are necessary to ensure the ideal environment and the continuous supply of essential metabolites required for fetal growth and development to take place satisfactorily.

In the endocrine system, pregnancy has a profound impact on women, beginning early with the production of hCG from the trophoblast, which occurs at the time of implantation.

Pituitary gland

- ✓ The anterior pituitary gland enlarges approximately 36% due to the increase in the number and size of the lactotrophs, while the posterior pituitary decreases in size during pregnancy.
- ✓ Improves the synthesis and release of prolactin due to the marked increase in estrogens during pregnancy.
- ✓ Increase in serum prolactin (around 207 ng / ml with a range between 35 to 600 ng / ml).
- ✓ The levels of growth hormone (GH) in the maternal serum do not change during pregnancy. However, the immunoreactive source during pregnancy is modified due to placental hormone production.
- ✓ The corpus luteum of pregnancy secretes relaxin, while estrogens stimulate the release of GH in early gestational stages.
- ✓ The pituitary GH (Gh1 or hGH-N) is reduced after the 25th week of gestation and after the 4th month of pregnancy. Meanwhile, placental syncytiotrophoblasts release a variant of

- GH known as GH2 or hGH-V in a non-pulsatile pattern.
- ✓ In the first half of pregnancy, an improvement in the GH response occurs, although this is reduced in the second half.
- ✓ Insulin-like growth factor 1 (IGF1) increases in the second half of pregnancy (5 times higher than in non-pregnant women).
- ✓ The synthesis and secretion of the pituitary gonadotropin-releasing hormone (GnRH) is reduced during pregnancy, although placental production of this is increased. This indicates a marked reduction in gonadotropin immunoreactivity from the 10th week of pregnancy.
- ✓ Decrease in serum levels of luteinizing hormone (LH) and follicle stimulating hormone (FSH).
- ✓ Decreased thyrotropin or hTSH, during the first trimester of pregnancy.
- ✓ Maternal adrenocorticotropic hormone (ACTH or corticotropin) levels increase during pregnancy, reaching four times its concentrations compared to the non-pregnant state. This occurs between the 7th and 10th week of gestation. There is a gradual increase between weeks 33 to 37. The values decrease up to 50% shortly before delivery to rise again during the stress of delivery up to 15 times.
- ✓ Biologically active CRH is produced and released by the placenta, to a lesser extent by the fetal and decidual membranes. Glucocorticoids stimulate the expression of placental CRH.
- ✓ The CRH and ACTH ratio is altered during pregnancy.
- ✓ Arginine vasopressin (AVP) concentrations are similar between pregnant and non-pregnant women.
- ✓ Oxytocin levels progressively increase in maternal blood. Its increase parallels the increase in the serum level of estradiol and progesterone. During cervical dilation and vaginal distention during labor, oxytocin levels are further increased, stimulating the contraction of the smooth muscles of the uterus.

Thyroid gland

The thyroid increases in size by approximately 18%.

Thyroid growth is associated with an increase in the size of the follicles with greater amounts of colloid and a greater volume of blood.

Increased uptake of iodine by the maternal thyroid gland.

Increased estrogen concentrations in pregnancy promote greater sialylation of TBG and increased hepatic synthesis of thyroxine transporter globulin (TBG). This results in a twofold increase in TBG, and in increased levels of thyroxine and triiodothyronine in the maternal circulation throughout pregnancy.

No significant changes in thyroxine-binding prealbumin occur, although albumin levels are reduced as a result of increased vascular volume.

Criteria for the hypothyroidism detection approach in pregnant women

Family history of thyroid disease.
Personal history of thyroid disease.
Previous radiation to the head or neck.
Morbid obesity.
More than 30 years old.

Parathyroid glands

Maternal total serum calcium levels are reduced during pregnancy.

In parallel with the increase in GFR, the rate of urian calcium excretion increases.

It is theorized that parathyroid hormone (PTH) levels increase during pregnancy. Although measurements of intact PTH through immunometric assays indicate the normal parameter associated with non-pregnant women.

Concentrations of the protein associated with PTH increase during pregnancy.

The level of 25-hydroxyvitamin D is not modified by pregnancy, however, the increase in vitamin D binding globulin driven by estrogen causes an increase in the concentration of 1,25 dihydroxyvitamin D (1,25 (OH) 2D).

Increases the free and biologically active fraction of 1,25 (OH) 2D.

Pancreas

Increased estrogen and progesterone cause hyperplasia and hypertrophy in the beta cells of the islets of Langerhans.

Fetal glucose requirements increase glucose delivery through the placenta by facilitated diffusion. This can lead to maternal hypoglycemia.

Although insulin levels are normal, postprandial insulin hypersecretion can occur.

Due to increased insulin synthesis and secretion, increased glycogen storage occurs, as well as reduced hepatic glucose production.

As pregnancy progresses, hPL levels increase as well as glucocorticoid levels, leading to insulin resistance during the last half of pregnancy.

In late pregnancy, glucose intake results in higher and sustained levels of insulin and glucose, as well as a greater degree of glucagon suppression.

Kidney glands

Increased hepatic production of cortisol transporter globulin.

Decreased metabolic clearance of cortisol.

Plasma cortisol increased up to 3 times in the 26th week of pregnancy.

High concentrations of progesterone cause an antiglucocorticoid effect, preventing the development of stigma caused by excess glucocorticoids.

Increased levels of androstenedione and testosterone.

Adrenal levels of dehydroepiandrosterone (DHEA) and dehydroepiandrosterone sulfate (DHEAS) doubled, although your maternal serum DHEAS concentration decreases 1/3 or even half of the level outside of pregnancy, as a result of the increase of the -hydroxylation and placental utilization of 16-hydroxyhydroepiandrosterone sulfate, to form estrogens.

The levels of catecholamines in the 24-hour urine, epinephrine and serum norepinephrine are similar to those found in non-pregnant women.

Bibliographic references

1. Shlomo Melmed, Richard J. Auchus, Allison B. Goldfine, Ronald J. Kowning, Clifford Rosen. Williams Textbook of Endocrinology 14Th edition. ELSEVIER, 2020.
2. Tal R, Taylor HS, Burney RO, et al. Endocrinology of Pregnancy. [Updated 2015 Dec 7]. In: Feingold KR, Anawalt B, Boyce A, et al., Editors. Endotext [Internet]. South Dartmouth (MA): MDText.com, Inc .; 2000-.

Chapter 332. Female Sexual Dysfunction

It consists of disorders of female sexual interest or arousal, as well as female orgasmic disorder and painful disorders with genitopelvic penetration. All disorders to be considered as female sexual dysfunctions must include symptoms of distress and have occurred for at least a 6-month period.

Statistics and epidemiology

It is estimated that female sexual dysfunction has an incidence of 10% when anxiety is considered as a diagnostic criterion.
The incidence is at least 75% in menopausal women when only symptoms are considered as diagnostic criteria.
The age peak of highest incidence ranges between 51 and 59 years.
Female sexual dysfunction can occur in women of all ages.

Risk factor's
- ✓ Social stress
- ✓ History of psychiatric disorders.
- ✓ History of physical or sexual abuse.
- ✓ Endocrine diseases.
- ✓ Estrogen therapy.

Etiology and pathophysiological elements

Neurotransmitters play a critical role in proper female sexual function, requiring a delicate balance of dopamine for desire and a high level of epinephrine, norepinephrine, and serotonin to stimulate arousal and orgasm.

Any disorder that interferes with the function of these neurotransmitters can be responsible for female sexual dysfunction. Hormonal deficiencies can also be responsible for the pathophysiology of this dysfunction.

The etiologies can include organic disorders such as hormonal, neurological and vascular problems, however, psychosocial factors are also involved, such as, for example, interpersonal problems in the relationship, social stress, mood, history of physical or sexual abuse and psychiatric history .

Diagnostic criteria

Clinic	Clinic history
	To establish the diagnosis, a complete sexual history is essential, including a description of the event, specifically indicating whether the patient has difficulty in sexual desire, arousal, orgasm, or presents sexual pain or a combination thereof, as well as the appearance of symptoms. (gradual or abrupt).
	Sexual interest disorder or sexual arousal
	Difference between desire level at baseline before the patient identified the problem.
	Female sexual pain or penetrating disorder
	Describe nature, severity of pain, location, and time course.
	Ask about sexual practices or positions that cause or

	lessen pain. Female orgasmic disorder Ask about previous orgasmic experience. (same partner, particular environment or other condition). *Physical exam* Examine the thyroid (thyroid disease can contribute to female sexual dysfunction). Pelvic exam: Look for signs that suggest the cause. It is more useful in women who report sexual pain. Findings may include atrophy or tender areas associated with the complaint. Genital Exam: Perform bimanual exam prior to speculum inspection. Probable Findings: Pain in the levator and perineal muscles of the body (vaginismus). Rectovaginal nodule (endometriosis). Pain in the anterior wall in relation to the bladder, can be synonymous with painful bladder syndrome or interstitial cystitis. Vaginal dryness Common gynecological conditions: leiomyomas, adnexal masses, cervical cancer, vulvar dermatosis, pelvic organ prolapse, endometriosis, vaginismus, adenomyosis, vulvodynia.
Paraclinical	Paraclinics are often not necessary to establish the diagnosis. Prioritize medical history and clinical manifestations for diagnosis. You can indicate the paraclinics that you consider useful based on the clinical etiological suspicion, they may be useful: Estrogen levels. Blood glucose Nieles of FSH. Thyroid tests. Androgen levels. *Imaging tests* Consider its use in patients with sexual pain and pain

	associated with cervical, bladder, adnexal, or uterine masses identified on clinical examination. Transvaginal ultrasound is the most indicated for these patients. A laparoscopy may be indicated when adenomyosis, endometriosis, or adhesive disease is suspected.

Treatment options

Treatment options are guided by the underlying cause and the context of the patient. Consider referring your patient to psychiatry, sex therapist, physical therapy, among others.

Sexual desire or arousal disorder:

Adjust the prescriptions for medications associated with female sexual dysfunction that your patient is taking.
Flibanserin: indicated for premenopausal women with low sexual desire. It is required to be administered overnight on a daily basis (prohibit alcohol consumption during treatment due to risk of syncope and hypotension).
Bremelanotide: indicated for acquired generalized hypoactive sexual desire disorder in premenopausal women. It is administered subcutaneously 45 minutes before sexual intercourse.
Supplemental androgens (controversial).

Genitopelvic pain or penetration disorder

Topical estrogen: indicated in women with perimenopausal or postmenopausal atrophy. It is available in a continuous-release cream, tablet, or ring form.

Topical prasterone: applied every night as a vaginal suppository.

Ospemifene - Approved to treat dyspareunia by reversing genital atrophy.

Non-estrogenic lubricants and moisturizers.

Pelvic Floor Physiotherapy - Indicated to help with painful muscle contractions of the vaginal muscles.

Vestibulectomy indicated for women with vulvodynia.

Female orgasmic disorder
Adjustment of antidepressant therapy.
Sildenafil (controversial in women).

Follow-up peculiarities:
Currently there are no formal guidelines for the follow-up interval in patients with female sexual dysfunction, however, it is recommended to evaluate the progress of the treatment every 3 to 6 months and in case of improvement, the follow-up begins annually. According to the underlying cause, the follow-up visit intervals should be adjusted according to the patient.

Bibliographic references

1. American Psychiatric Association. Diagnostic and Statistical Manual of Mental Disorders. FifthEdition. Washington, DC: American Psychiatric Publishing; 2013.
2. American College of Obstetricians and GynecologistsCommitteeonPracticeBulletins-Gynecology. ACOG PracticeBulletin No. 119: Female

sexual dysfunction. ObstetGynecol. 2011 Apr. 117 (4): 996-1007.
3. Al-Abbadey M, Liossi C, Curran N, Schoth DE, Graham CA. Treatment of Female Sexual Pain Disorders: A Systematic Review. J Sex Marital Ther. 2016. 42 (2): 99-142.

Chapter 333. Fibrocystic Condition of the Breast

It is considered the most common benign pathology of the breast. It is also known as fibrocystic breast disease, which is a condition diagnosed in around women around the world. These are benign epithelial breast lesions. Due to their high incidence and benign behavior, the term "disease" is often not designated to refer to this condition.

Fibrocystic changes in the breast correspond to a general term that includes mastalgia, breast cysts, and benign tumors.

Statistics and epidemiology

According to the literature, the incidence ranges from 30 to 60% and up to 50 to 60% of all women. It is most common among women 30 to 50 years of age.

The most common form is fibroadenomas and they represent between 70 to 95% of all benign breast diseases.

Etiology and pathophysiological elements

The etiology of this condition has been strongly associated with a history of estrogen and progestin therapies for more than 8 years. The pathophysiological elements of the fibrocystic breast condition are determined by the predominance of estrogens and the deficiency of progesterone causing a hyperproliferation of the connective tissue or fibrosis, followed by the facultative epithelial proliferation.

Because the breast tissue is affected by the levels of estrogen and progesterone, the states of hyperestrogenism and anovulation are associated with the development of benign breast conditions.

Types of benign breast diseases:
- ✓ Hyperplasia
- ✓ Cysts (fibrous hyperplastic, adenosis, papillomatosis).
- ✓ Fibroadenomas.
- ✓ Sclerosing adenosis.
- ✓ Mastitis.

Histopathology

- ✓ Extracellular matrix of collagen.
- ✓ Peri-canalicular stromal cell patterns.
- ✓ Florid epithelial hyperplasia.
- ✓ Involution of fibroadenomas in menopause (the dense collagen stroma and the atrophic glands are affected).
- ✓ Cystic changes derived from the lobular unit of the terminal duct, caused by the expansion of the efferent ducts of the lobular unit of the terminal duct.
- ✓ Cyst formation occurs as a result of fluid accumulation.
- ✓ Flat lining with myoepithelial layer.

Diagnostic criteria

Clinic	*Cysts*
	Benign cysts are mobile within the glandular breast tissue.
	The thoracic wall and skin have a rubbery texture.
	Breast discomfort and tenderness absent or mild (except in inflammatory cysts).
	Most patients have multiple cysts.
	Frequent location in the upper outer quadrant of the breast.
	The texture is usually from firm to multiple subcentimetric cysts.
	Fibroadenomas
	Fibroadenomas are oval in shape and present in variable sizes and well-defined margins. They are mobile and often multiple.
Paraclinical	Any woman with a clinical finding of a discrete palpable mass requires a triple test consisting of a complete physical examination, imaging studies, and excisional biopsy.
	Women over 35
	Mammogram with ultrasound examination
	Complex cysts (both liquid and solid matter), require a biopsy.
	Solid lesions: require an x-ray or ultrasound guided core biopsy.
	Women in their 30s
	Clinical surveillance.
	Follow-up exam in 2 to 3 months.
	Mammography and ultrasound when nodularity, asymmetric thickening or changes in the lump are evidenced in follow-up visits.

Treatment options

The fibrocystic breast condition is a benign situation, however, it can present painful symptoms. The treatment is oriented individually according to the patient, consider watchful waiting in asymptomatic patients with low risk of breast cancer.
Lifestyle changes (avoiding foods or drinks with high caffeine content, wearing a supportive bra).
Dose modification of the hormone replacement therapy regimen.
Metformin.
Aspirin or ibuprofen in patients with mastalgia. Evening primrose oil is justified as supportive measures in case pain persists despite treatment. It can be used for 3 to 6 months under observation of the effects.
Tamoxifen, bromocriptine or danazol are considerable options when, despite regular measures for 6 months, the pain is intense and persistent.
Aspiration of fluid from cysts for symptomatic relief (FNAB). Cyst fluid appears macroscopically stained with blood; any unusual appearance requires cytological evaluation.
Surgery: it is indicated for cysts with a persistently solid intracystic appearance on ultrasound despite frequent PAAF or when these present atypical cellularity on cytological evaluation.

Follow-up peculiarities

Proliferative type lesions have a higher risk of malignancy in both breasts. When the increase in pleomorphic calcifications is evidenced by mammographic studies, start a follow-up regimen at 6-month intervals.

Bibliographic references

1. Schünemann HJ, Lerda D, Quinn C, Follmann M, Alonso-Coello P, Rossi PG, Lebeau A, Nyström L, Broeders M, Ioannidou-Mouzaka L, Duffy SW, Borisch B, Fitzpatrick P, Hofvind S, Castells X, et to the. EuropeanCommissionInitiativeonBreastCancer (ECIBC) ContributorGroup. BreastCancer Screening and Diagnosis: A SynopsisoftheEuropeanBreastGuidelines. Ann. Intern. Med. 2020 Jan 07; 172 (1): 46-56.
2. Mitchell, Kumar, Abbas, Aster. Compendium of Robins and Cotran Structural And Functional Pathology. 9th Edition. Editorial Elsevier. 2017.
3. ShlomoMelmed, Richard J. Auchus, Allison B. Goldfine, Ronald J. Kowning, Clifford Rosen. Williams Textbook of Endocrinology 14Th edition. ELSEVIER, 2020.

Chapter 334. Functional Tumors of the Ovaries

These are those neoplasms developed in the ovaries, which secrete one or more hormones and which can manifest clinically in the patient. Functional tumors of the ovary can include various responsible histological categories and which produce a variety of hormonal effects. They are usually symptomatic once they are large.

Statistics and epidemiology

The age of incidence depends on the type of tumor. Stromal and sex cord tumors account for 7% of malignant neoplasms of the ovaries. Leydig cell tumors represent less than 0.5% of all ovarian tumors. Stromal and sex cord tumors of the ovary (TECS) account for about 70% of ovarian tumors. TECS are the tumors that most frequently have functional behavior. Germ cell tumors account for 15-20% of ovarian tumors.

Etiology or pathophysiological elements

Ovarian tumors can be classified according to their histological origin into 3 groups:

Histological classification of ovarian tumors	Type	Description	Clinical presentation
Tumors derived from the superficial epithelium (Müllerian) or ovarian epithelial tumors (non-functional).		Associated with malignancy	Not functional
Germ cell-derived tumors.	Mature cystic teratoma of the ovary (benign)	Associated with paraneoplastic syndromes. Unilocular cysts containing hair and sebaceous material. Karyotype 46, XX	It can behave as a carcinoid tumor or as a thyroid hormone-secreting neoplasm. May cause thyrotoxicosis.
	Dysgerminoma (usually non-functional).	Composed of large vesicular cells with clear cytoplasm. They express Oct3, Oct4 and Nanog	Ambiguous genitalia. Elevated chorionic gonadotropin levels (some).
Stromal origin and sex cord tumors (TECS).	Granulosa cell tumors (most common).	They can produce female or male hormones. Cellular elements similar to the granular layer of the ovarian follicle.	Virilizing effect in women. Endocrine activity analogous to normal follicular cells. Isosexual peripheral precocious puberty.

				Clitoromegaly, acne, hirsutism, deep voice (when it occurs in postmenarchic girls). Lower abdominal pain, increased abdominal girth. In the adult variant, menstrual cycle alterations occur in women of childbearing age. Gynecological bleeding (in postmenospause)
		Tecota and fibrothecomas.	Often unilateral. Cellular elements similar to those of the internal theca of Graff's follicle (lipid content, benign behavior).	They occur around menopause frequently. Associated with polycystic ovary syndrome. Producers of estrogen. They can cause isosexual peripheral precocious puberty (in girls). Associated with

			irregular uterine bleeding in adult women of childbearing age.
	Sertoli-Leydig cell tumors.	Also known as androblastomas or arerenoblastomas. Unilateral tumors of moderate size. Cell component includes Sertoli and Leydig cells in variable proportions and different degrees of differentiation.	Common virilizing ovarian tumors in women ages 13 to 40. Androgen secretors. Oligomenorrhea, followed by frank amenorrhea. Hoarsely. Hirsutism Acne, frontotemporal alopecia. Clitoromegaly
	Lipid cell tumors (Leydig cell tumor and hilar cell tumor).	Also known as a Grawitz tumor. Contains cellular debris from the adrenal cortex. Large neoplasms (> 8cm).	It can produce testosterone, estrogens, androstenedione, cortisol, erythropoietin, and progesterone.

Table 257 - 1. Functional ovarian tumors.

Diagnostic criteria

The clinical manifestations of functioning ovarian tumors depend on the age of presentation and the type of precursor cell of the neoplasia. The clinical manifestations were described according to the tumor in Table 257-1.

Clinical manifestations:

Paraneoplastic syndrome (most common of ovarian functioning tumors): tumor hypercalcemia.
Thyrotoxicosis
Chorionic gonadotropin syndrome.
Early puberty.
Female virilization.

Paraclinical:

Thyroid function tests.
Chorionic gonadotropin level.
ACTH levels (frequently greater than 200 pg / mL).
Androgen and estrogen levels.
Transvaginal ultrasound.
Tumor markers.

Treatment options

According to the characteristics of the tumor and its functionality, an expectant follow-up can be followed.
The usual therapeutic options consist of surgery (oophorectomy or cystectomy), although depending on the

malignancy, radiation therapy or chemotherapy may be required.

Bibliographic references

1. Mitchell, Kumar, Abbas, Aster. Compendium of Robins and Cotran Structural And Functional Pathology. 9th Edition. Editorial Elsevier. 2017.
2. Cruz Hernández Jeddú, Yanes Quesada Marelis, Hernández García Pilar, Isla Valdés Ariana, Turcios Tristá Silvia Elena. Functional tumors of the ovary. Rev Cubana Endocrinol. 2007 Dec
3. Roth, LM, Billings, SD Hormonally functional ovarian neoplasms. Endocr Pathol 11, 1–17 (2000). https://doi.org/10.1385/EP:11:1:1.

Chapter 335. Climacteric Syndrome

The climacteric syndrome corresponds to the transition period between the fertile or reproductive stage to the menopausal stage, as well as an undetermined fraction of the postmenopause. This transition period is characterized by a set of particular clinical manifestations associated both physical and psychological.

Statistics and epidemiology

Menopause occurs around 50 years of age, the median age of onset of perimenopause is 47.5 years. Hot flashes are the most frequent and striking symptoms. More than four fifths of women experiencing postmenopause experience hot flashes in the first 3 months after ovarian function cessation.

Etiology and pathophysiological aspects

The climacteric syndrome is a physiological process of ovarian aging, probably determined by genes, although the associated regulatory mechanisms have not been fully elucidated. Among the modifying factors of the age of onset, prolonged smoking and the use of medications capable of causing ovarian damage such as cyclophosphamide, medorethamine, among others, stand out.

The physiological and psychological aspects take place in response to the gradual degradation of ovarian function and the reduction of estrogen production.

Etiological classification: Natural- Surgical- Estrogen withdrawal (due to GnRH agonists).

Diagnostic criteria

Clinic	Irregular menstruation frequency followed by amenorrhea. Vasomotor instability (hot flashes and sweats): hot flashes are a subjective sensation of intense heat in the upper part of the body that lasts for about 30 seconds to 5 minutes followed by palpitations, headache, weakness, among others. Urogenital atrophy (pain during intercourse). Fatigue. Headache Dizziness Numbness. Pain in the extremities Attention problem. Nervousness. Anxiety. Insomnia. Humor changes. Depression.
Paraclinical	Quantification of FSH (greater than 25 mIU / ml). Estradiol level (less than 20 pg / mL). Estrone level (37 pg / ml). Antimullerian hormone Cervical cytology (regular screening every 2 to 3 years up to 65 years).

Treatment options

Estrogenic hormone therapy: indicated for hysterectomized women

- ✓ Standard dose of oral conjugated estrogen 0.625 mg / day.
- ✓ Standard dose of micronized estradiol 17β: 1 mg / day.

Combined estrogen-progestational hormone therapy: daily administration of estrogen by adding the progestogen for a few days a month (7 to 14 days).

Topical hormonal treatment:
- ✓ Hormonal vaginal cream (Conjugated estrogens 0.625 mg / g of excipient): 0.5 to 2 g per day.
- ✓ Eggs, vaginal capsules: estriol, ovules at a dose of 0.5 to 3.5 mg per day.

Antidepressants:
- ✓ Paroxetine at a dose of 12.5 to 25 mg per day.
- ✓ Fluoxetine at a dose of 20 mg daily.
- ✓ Veralipride (dopamine antagonist): dose of 100 mg / day for 20 days.

Non-hormonal lubricants.

Bibliographic references

1. Shlomo Melmed, Richard J. Auchus, Allison B. Goldfine, Ronald J. Kowning, Clifford Rosen. Williams Textbook of Endocrinology 14Th edition. ELSEVIER, 2020.
2. Dorantes and Martinez. Clinical endocrinology 5th edition, Editorial El Manual Moderno 2016.

Chapter 336. Premature Ovarian Failure

Also known as premature ovarian failure, or premature menopause, it consists of the early depletion of the ovarian follicles before the age of 40. These patients are characterized by normal puberty and a variable period of regular menstrual cycles, followed by episodes of oligomenorrhea or amenorrhea in conjunction with urogenital atrophy and hot flashes.

Statistics and epidemiology

At least 1% of women enter menopause before the age of 40.

Risk groups or factors:
- ✓ Family history of premature ovarian failure.
- ✓ Family or personal history of autoimmune disorders.
- ✓ Chemotherapy.
- ✓ Radiotherapy.

Etiology and pathophysiological elements

Premature ovarian failure occurs as a result of early depletion of ovarian follicles, this can occur as a result of a small amount of ovarian reserve (or the number of primordial follicles in a woman at the time of gametogenesis) or as a result of accelerated destruction of the oocyte complement: In most cases, the cause is unknown, although some disorders are associated with premature ovarian failure.

Causes of premature ovarian failure.

Genetic disorders
Gonadal dysgenesis with mosaic X chromosome defects.
Premutation of the FMR1 gene, a variant of Fragile X syndrome.
Blepharophimosis-ptosis-epicanthosis reversus syndrome (FOXL2 mutation).
Galactosemia (GALT mutation).
Autoimmune disorders
Autoimmune poliendocrine syndrome.
Others:
Sudden destruction of follicles
Chemotherapy.
Radiotherapy.
Infections (mumps oophoritis).

Diagnostic criteria

Premature ovarian failure can be diagnosed in patients with the following characteristics:
Woman under 40 years of age.
Amenorrhea, oligomenorrhea or menstrual irregularity.
Hot flushes.
Menopausal serum FSH levels (40 IU / L), at least 2 times

Other probable clinical manifestations:
- ✓ Infertility or subfertility.
- ✓ Vaginal dryness
- ✓ Sleep disturbances
- ✓ Pigmentation changes in the skin.
- ✓ Vitiligo (autoimmune).

- ✓ Hair loss (autoimmune alopecic pattern).
- ✓ Goiter
- ✓ Fatigue.
- ✓ Anxiety or depression
- ✓ Signs of virilization.

The risk of abnormal karyotypes increases when premature ovarian failure begins at an earlier age. Indicate chromosome analysis in patients with premature ovarian failure younger than 30 years.

Paraclinical:
- ✓ Thyroid stimulating hormone.
- ✓ FMR1 gene premutation carrier state test.
- ✓ Follicle-stimulating hormone (establishes a diagnosis of premature ovarian failure).
- ✓ Karyotype (in women under 30 years of age or sexual infantilism).

Treatment options

The treatment of premature ovarian failure is oriented according to the specific cause. However, the main treatment is hormonal therapy, using combined estrogen and progestin or a low-dose oral contraceptive. Androgen replacement is controversial.

Follow-up peculiarities

Early menopause is associated with an increased risk of cardiovascular mortality, as well as stroke, bone fractures, and cancer. These patients present a decrease in the quality of life and a reduction in life expectancy. It is recommended to start a comprehensive follow-up plan emphasizing the reduction of risks associated with premature menopause.

Bibliographic references

1. Shlomo Melmed, Richard J. Auchus, Allison B. Goldfine, Ronald J. Kowning, Clifford Rosen. Williams Textbook of Endocrinology 14Th edition. ELSEVIER, 2020.
2. Torrealday S, Kodaman P, Pal L. Premature Ovarian Insufficiency - anupdateonrecentadvances in understanding and management. F1000Res. 2017; 6: 2069. Published 2017 Nov 29. doi: 10.12688 / f1000research.11948.1.

Chapter 337. Female Hormone Replacement

Hormone replacement therapy in women, allows to replace hormonal losses during the transition to the menopausal stage, among others. With the increase in life expectancy, women can spend about a third of their lives in the menopausal period, and sometimes have physically and mentally intolerable symptoms, where clinical counseling is a useful option.

Indications

Problems associated with menopause
Treatment of menopausal vasomotor symptoms.
Treatment of genitourinary syndrome of menopause (vaginal and vulvar atrophy).
Prevention of osteoporosis.
Primary or secondary amenorrhea.
Dysfunctional uterine bleeding.
Endometrial hyperplasia.
Assisted reproductive technology treatment.

Estrogen and progesterone preparations

Hormone	Preparation
Oral estrogen	Conjugated estrogen.
	Ethinyl-estradiol.
	Esterified estrogens.
	17 beta-estradiol.
Transdermal estrogen	17 beta-estradiol patch.
	17-beta estradiol gel.
	17-beta estradiol emulsion.

	17-beta estradiol spray.
Vaginal estrogen	17beta-estradiol cream. Conjugated estrogen cream. 17 beta-estradiol ring. 17 beta-estradiol tablets.
Oral progestogen	Drosperinone. Micronized progesterone. Medroxyprogesterone acetate. Norethindrone acetate. Megestrol acetate.
Transdermal progestogen	Norethindrone acetate. Levonorgostar.
Progestin (intrauterine system)	Levonorgostar IUS

Tibolone

It is a progestogen with selective tissue estrogenic activity. Suppresses vasomotor problems and improves mood, as well as libido. The recommended dose is 2.5 mg / day. It is considered the therapy of choice for women with a history of endometriosis or who have had unwanted effects with conventional therapy.

Transfer of menopausal replacement therapy to tibolone

Mastalgia or breast tension.
Humor changes.
Sexual appetite disorders.
Increase in breast density with the need for a repeat mammogram or when it cannot be read properly.
Irregular bleeding without histopathological finding.

Contraindications of female hormone replacement therapy

Breast carcinoma: history, current, or suspected.
Invasive breast carcinoma.
Premalignant changes of the breast (lobular neoplasia, atypical ductal hyperplasia).
In situ ductal carcinoma (intraductal carcinoma).
Untreated estrogen-dependent carcinoma.
Endometrial carcinoma.
Endometrial stromal sarcoma.
Estrogen-dependent malignant carcinoma (suspected or known).
Unfounded genital bleeding (as a sign of endometrial carcinoma).
Active liver disease.
Idiopathic thromboembolic disease (previous or current).
Pulmonary embolism
Phlebothrombosis.
Active or recent arterial thromboembolism.
Coronary thrombosis.
Angina pectoris.
Known intolerance to a certain component of the preparation.

Adverse effects of female hormone replacement therapy

Risk of venous thromboembolism.
Risk of cardiovascular accident.
Coronary heart disease.
Breast cancer
Gynecological cancer.

Bibliographic references

1. Agarwal, S., Alzahrani, FA, & Ahmed, A. (2018). Hormone Replacement Therapy: Would it be Possible to

Replicate a Functional Ovary ?. International journal of molecular sciences, 19 (10), 3160.https://doi.org/10.3390/ijms19103160
2. Fait T. (2019). Menopause hormone therapy: latest developments and clinical practice. Drugs in context, 8, 212551.https://doi.org/10.7573/dic.212551

Chapter 338. Transgender Teen

At the beginning of puberty, gender dysphoria appears to arise or worsen, implying the high probability of transgender identity in adulthood. These patients require a thorough evaluation by a qualified mental health specialist so that the specialist can identify the diagnosis of gender dysphoria and determine the coexistence of other mental health problems. Studies show the existence of an association between the autism spectrum and gender dysphoria in adolescents, which is why referral to a mental health specialist is essential.

Endocrine Society Guidelines for Puberty Induction in Transgender Adolescents

Induction of female puberty
Induction of female puberty by oral 17 beta-estradiol, increasing doses every 6 months.
5 μg / kg / day
10 μg / kg / day
15 μg / kg / day
20 μg / kg / day
Adult dose: 2 to 6 mg / day.
In postpubertal trans adolescents, the estradiol dose may increase faster: 1 mg per day for 6 months or 2 mg / day.
Induction of female puberty by transdermal 17 beta-estradiol (the dose increases every 6 months and a new patch is placed every 3 to 5 days.
06.25 to 12.05 μg / 24h
25 μg / 24 h
37.5 μg / 24 h
Adult dosage: 50 to 200 μg / 24 h.

Induction of male puberty
Induction of male puberty by testosterone esters, dose increase every 6 months (subcutaneous or intramuscular route).   25 mg / m2 every 2 weeks (alternative: half this dose weekly or double every 4 weeks).   50 mg / m2 every 2 weeks.   75 mg / m2 every 2 weeks   *Adult dosage:* 100 to 200 mg every 2 weeks.   In postpubertal male transgender adolescents, the dose may increase faster: 75 mg every 2 weeks for 6 months.   125 mg every 2 weeks.

Endocrine Society Guidelines for Reference Protocol, Physical Examination, Follow-up, and Monitoring During Pubertal Suppression with GnRH Agonist

Every 3 to 6 months
Anthropometry, blood pressure, Tanner stages.
Every 6 to 12 months
LH and FSH.   E2 / T   25 (OH) D.
Every 1 or 2 years
DMO using DXA   Bone age by left hand radiography.

Endocrine Society guidelines for the initial evaluation, follow-up and monitoring of paraclinics of transgender youth during puberty induction

Every 3 to 6 months
Anthropometric: Weight.

Height. Sitting height. Tanner stadiums. Blood pressure.
Every 6 to 12 months
Transgender males: Hemoglobin / hematocrit. Lipids Testosterone. 25-hydroxyvitamin D. Transgender women: Prolactin Estradiol 25 (OH) D
Every 1 to 2 years
BMD by dual energy X-ray absorptiometry (DXA). Bone age on left hand X-ray (provided clinically indicated)

Potential Adverse Effects of Puberty Blockers in Transgender Youth

Currently there are few long-term studies on potential adverse effects, however, the following effects have been observed:
- ✓ Decrease in BMD.
- ✓ Infertility
- ✓ Cognitive disorders.

Bibliographic references

1. Shlomo Melmed, Richard J. Auchus, Allison B. Goldfine, Ronald J. Kowning, Clifford Rosen. Williams

Textbook of Endocrinology 14Th edition. ELSEVIER, 2020.
2. Kaltiala-Heino, R., Bergman, H., Työläjärvi, M., & Frisén, L. (2018). Gender dysphoria in adolescence: current perspectives. Adolescent health, medicine and therapeutics, 9, 31–41.https://doi.org/10.2147/AHMT.S135432

Chapter 339. Transgender Woman

According to the definitions of the 2017 guidelines of the Endocrine Society, it is defined as "transgender woman", also known as "trans woman" and "male-to-famale" (Man to woman), those individuals who were assigned to the male sex at birth but who, on the contrary, identify and live as women.

Prevalence

It is estimated that around 0.5 to 1.3% of men assigned at birth live as transgender.
About 1 in 2,800 men assigned at birth live as a transgender woman.

Initial evaluation

- ✓ Complete medical history.
- ✓ History of the duration and severity of gender dysphoria.
- ✓ Careful review of chronic medical problems (especially those that can be exacerbated by hormone therapy).
- ✓ Serve as a liaison between mental health providers and surgeons.
- ✓ Evaluate psychiatric history, emphasizing depressive history and suicide risk. Indicate antidepressant treatment or urgent referral to mental health if deemed necessary.

Endocrine Society Recommendations for Hormone Administration

Estrogens	
Oral estradiol	2.0 to 6.0 mg / day
Transdermal	
Estradiol transdermal patch (new patch every 3 to 5 days)	0.025-0.2 mg / day
Parenteral	
Valerato **or** **Estradiol cypionate**	5 to 30 mg intramuscular every 2 weeks 2 to 10 mg intramuscularly every week
Antiandrogens	
Spironolactone	100 to 300 mg / day.
Cyproterone Acetate	25 to 50 mg / day.
GnRH agonist	3.75 mg SQ (SC) monthly 11.25 mg SQ (SC) 3 months

Endocrine Society Recommendations for Physical Examination and Follow-up

Perform follow-up evaluation every 3 months for the first year. Subsequently, the consultations will be held once or twice a year to monitor signs of feminization and assess the development of adverse reactions.
Measure testosterone and serum estradiol levels every 3 months: Serum testosterone should be below 50 ng / dL.   Serum estradiol should not exceed the maximum range of 100 to 200 pg / ml.
If spironolactone is administered, serum electrolytes, especially potassium, should be measured every 3 months during the first year, followed by an annual assessment of serum potassium levels.
Perform routine cancer screening following protocol as a non-transgender person, on all tissues present.

> Consider having bone mineral density tests at the beginning of the evaluation. In low-risk people, screen for osteoporosis at age 60.

Risks associated with transfemale hormonal administration
- ✓ Venous thrombosis and pulmonary embolism.
- ✓ Myocardial infarction and cerebrovascular accidents.
- ✓ Hypertriglyceridaemia.
- ✓ Hyperprolactinemia.
- ✓ Osteoporosis.
- ✓ Breast cancer
- ✓ Liver dysfunction

Bibliographic references

1. Hembree WC, Cohen-Kettenis PT, Gooren L, et al. Endocrine treatment of people with gender dysphoria / gender inconsistencies: a clinical practice guideline from the Endocrine Society. J Clin Endocrinol Metab. 2017; 102: 3869-3903.
2. Shlomo Melmed, Richard J. Auchus, Allison B. Goldfine, Ronald J. Kowning, Clifford Rosen. Williams Textbook of Endocrinology 14Th edition. ELSEVIER, 2020.

Chapter 340. Transgender Man

The definition outlined in the Endocrine Society's 2017 guidelines, on transgender man also known as "trans man," "female-to-male," or "transgender man," refers to people who have been assigned as female at birth, however, they identify and live as male.

Prevalence

It is estimated that around 0.4 to 1.2% of women identify as transgender male.

Initial evaluation

As in the case of the transgender woman, any initial encounter with a transgender adult should include the full development of the patient's medical history and pertinent family medical history in search of underlying medical conditions that may be aggravated by hormonal administration.

An evaluation associated with the individual's social and family support structure should be carried out, especially if the current social environment does not coincide with the stated gender role.

The doctor must carry out an appropriate evaluation of depressive signs and identify the risk of suicide, given the high risk of autolysis in transgender people. Consider referral to mental health provider when deemed necessary.

Endocrine Society Recommendations for Hormone Administration

Testosterone	
Parenteral testosterone	
Testosterone enanthate or cypionate	100 to 200 mg SQ (intramuscular route) every 2 weeks or SQ (subcutaneous route) half a week.
Testosterone undecanoate	1000 mg every 12 weeks
Transdermal testosterone	
1.6% Testosterone Gel	50 to 100 mg / day.
Testosterone transdermal patch	2.5 to 7.5 mg / day.

Endocrine Society Recommendations for Follow-Up Visits, Physical Examination, and Monitoring

Evaluate your patient every 3 months during the first year, then a consultation is made 1 or 2 times a year to monitor signs of virilization and the appearance of adverse reactions.
Measure serum testosterone levels every 3 months until levels are in the normal male range: Testosterone Enanthate / Cypionate Injections: Testosterone should be measured midway through the administration between injections. ***Target level***: 400 to 700 ng / dl to 400ng / dL. The maximum and minimum levels of testosterone must be measured, supervising that they remain in the normal male range. ***Parenteral Testosterone Undecanoate:*** Testosterone is measured before injection. When the level is less than 400 ng / dl, the dose interval should be adjusted. ***Transdermal testosterone:*** Testosterone level is measured no earlier than 1 week of daily application (minimum 2 hours after application).

Hematocrit or hemoglobin should be measured at the beginning of the study and the measurement repeated at 3-month intervals during the first year. Subsequently, the measurement is carried out 1 or 2 times a year. Regular follow-up checks should include measurement of weight, blood pressure, and lipids.
Osteoporosis screening should be performed when testosterone administration is interrupted or there is a risk of bone loss.
In case of presence of cervical tissue, the controls indicated by the American College of Obstetricians and Gynecologists should be carried out.
Subareolar and periareolar breast exams are performed annually for mastectomy. In the absence of mastectomy, a mammogram should be indicated as recommended by the American Cancer Society.

Potential risk associated with transmasculin hormonal administration

- ✓ Erythrocytosis
- ✓ Hyperlipidemia
- ✓ Cancer of the cervix and uterus.

Bibliographic references

1. Shlomo Melmed, Richard J. Auchus, Allison B. Goldfine, Ronald J. Kowning, Clifford Rosen. Williams Textbook of Endocrinology 14Th edition. ELSEVIER, 2020.
2. Note NM, den Heijer M, Gooren LJ. Evaluation and Treatment of Gender-Dysphoric / Gender Incongruent Adults. [Updated 2019 Jul 21]. In: Feingold KR, Anawalt B, Boyce A, et al., Editors. Endotext [Internet]. South Dartmouth (MA): MDText.com, Inc .; 2000-.

Chapter 341. Andrology

It is the branch of medicine and science, which is responsible for the reproductive function of man according to physiological and pathological conditions. Andrology deals with male reproductive health. Andrology ranges from genetic studies to male pubertal changes and includes the study of sterility and assisted reproductive techniques to alterations of the prostate, contraception and sexual function.

Male reproductive system

The male reproductive system is made up of a set of organs that act in a coordinated way, in order to produce functional sperm to be transported to the female reproductive tract. Sperm is a haploid cell which is produced in the testes. Spermatozoa undergo maturation changes through their transit through the epididymis to the ejaculatory ducts found in the prostate.

Components of the male reproductive system:

Component	Description
Testicles	In charge of spermatogenesis
Scrotum	Houses and protects the testes, while maintaining optimal testicular temperature for spermatogenesis.
Epididymis	It consists of a single tubule, very folded and connected to the testicle by a set of efferent ducts. Its function is to bring testicular sperm to its full functional maturation.
Different	Its primary function in conjunction with the ejaculatory

conductor	duct, is to transport mature sperm, as well as secretions from the seminal vesicle to the prostatic urethra.
Seminal vesicles	It is located immediately above the prostate gland. The secretions of the seminal vesicles are rich in prostaglandins and fructose and form about 70% of the ejaculate volume.
Prostate	It produces secretions rich in zinc, citric acid, choline and several proteins such as acid phosphatase, seminin, prostate antigen and plasminogen activator, whose role is presumed relevant for sperm function during ejaculation.
Penis	It is responsible for depositing male germ cells in the female genital tract during intercourse. It consists of two corpora cavernosa and a corpus spongiosum.

Endocrine and nervous control of the male reproductive system

In order for the male reproductive system to function properly, a comprehensive hormone-dependent balance must be maintained.

The pituitary is responsible for producing follicle-stimulating and luteinizing gonadotropins, regulated by hypothalamic control. The initiation of spermatogenesis requires FSH, while the luteinizing hormone stimulates the production of androgens in testicular Leydig cells.

The testes need testosterone concentrations to remain high to maintain spermatogenesis, for their part, accessory organs are dependent on androgens to carry out their own secretory function.

In addition, the male reproductive organs are under the neural control of the sympathetic and parasympathetic nervous system, through which the erectile function of the penis can be carried out through parasympathetic control and the ejaculatory function through sympathetic control.

Each of the pathologies at any of the indicated levels that interferes with the functioning of the male reproductive system is evaluated by andrology, which in turn encompasses branches such as urology, anatomy, genetics, and biochemistry.

Bibliographic references

1. Rupert P. Amann, Ph.D., John K. Amory, MD, Janice L. Bailey, Ph.D., William J. Bremner MD, Ph.D. et al. The American Society of Andrology. HandbookofAndrology. 2nd Edition. Allen Press, 2010.
2. Mario Brassesco. Spanish Fertility Society. Andrology Manual. 2011 EdikaMed, SLISBN: 978-84-7877.
3. Barak S, Baker HWG. Clinical Management of Male Infertility. [Updated 2016 Feb 5]. In: Feingold KR, Anawalt B, Boyce A, et al., Editors. Endotext [Internet]. South Dartmouth (MA): MDText.com, Inc .; 2000-.

Chapter 342. The Testicles

They are male sex glands, which have both endocrine and exocrine functions. The adult testes are paired ovoid organs that are found outside the abdominal cavity within the scrotum and hanging from the inguinal canal through the spermatic cord, which is made up of a neurovascular pedicle, cremasteric muscle, and vas deferens.

Embryology

For the formation of the testes they comprise 3 main types of cells:

Germ cells	They originate in the wall of the yolk sac and migrate between the fifth and sixth weeks of gestation towards the genital ridges.
Support cells	They derive from the coelomic epithelium of the genital ridges
Stromal or interstitial cells	They derive from the mesenchyme of the genital ridges

Both the adrenal glands, the gonads, the kidney, and the reproductive system are derived from the urogenital ridges which are located in the coelomic cavity of the embryo.

The early bipotential gonad is programmed to become a testis around the 6th to 7th week of gestation, due to the action of the specific region of the sex of the Y chromosome, which is located on the short arm of this chromosome.

Anatomy

The testicles are milky white ovoid structures whose consistency is resistant and elastic. The left testicle hangs lower in the scrotum than the right in 60% of men.

- ✓ *Dimensions:* They are about 4 to 5 cm long and 3 cm thick (each).
- ✓ Average volume 18.6 ± 4.8 ml. (ranges between 15 to 30 ml)

They are located in the scrotum (structure that confers protection, maintaining a temperature 2°C lower than abdominal temperature).

Each testicle is wrapped in 3 layers:
- ✓ Outer or vaginal layer: made up of mesothelial cells.
- ✓ Middle layer or albuginea: formed by fibroelastic connective tissue and smooth muscle cells.
- ✓ Inner or vascular layer: formed by networks of blood vessels.

Blood supply	Testicular arteries, branches of the internal spermatic arteries.
Innervation	Sympathetic and parasympathetic innervation.
Venous drainage	Pammpiniform plexus, which fuses into the testicular (internal spermatic) vein. The right testicular vein drains into the inferior vena cava, while the left testicular vein drains at right angles to the left renal vein.

Histology

The seminiferous tubules are about 0.2 mm in diameter, they are lined by an epithelium that contains Sertoli cells (elements of nutrition and support) and germ or spermatogenic cells. The germ cells are forming a large mass and are the precursors of sperm.

The epithelium rests on a thin basal lamina that is covered by a specialized area of fibrous tissue which has fibroblasts, connective tissue fibers and cells similar to smooth muscle, which can modify the diameter of the seminiferous tubule by contracting to facilitate transport of sperm.

Cells	Description
Sertoli cells	Tall, their bases rest on the basement membrane, the outline is irregular, the nucleus is ovoid and pale. *Features:* They provide an essential medium for the differentiation of germ cells. Participates in the movement of germ cells from the base of the tubule to the light. It is responsible for engulfing damaged germ cells and residual bodies. They secrete protein with a high affinity for androgens to maintain adequate testosterone levels.
Spermatogenic cells	They comprise a stratified layer of epithelium, they have between 4 to 8 cells in height with different degrees of differentiation. They can be classified according to their differentiation into: Spermatogonia (multiplying by mitotic division). Primary spermatocytes. Secondary spermatocytes (which divide by meiosis). Spermatids. Sperm.
Leydig cells	They are found in compact groups in the interstitium, between the seminiferous tubules. It is a large cell, with a vacuolated cytoplasm, a nucleus with thick chromatin granules and a precise nucleolus.

Spermatogenesis

It consists of the process by which stem cells, or spermatogonia, differentiate into mature spermatozoa, through 3 functionally distinct phases:
Mitotic or proliferative phase: in which most of the spermatogonia undergo mitosis to be able to renew the set of stem cells, while a small part is committed to greater differentiation and, in this way, to produce spermatocytes.
Meiotic phase: spermatocytes undergo successive meiotic divisions to produce spermatid cells which are haploid germ cells.
Spermiogenesis: Finally, the immature, round spermatid cells go on to differentiate into mature sperm.
The mature spermatozoa are released into the lumen of the seminiferous tubule and transported to the rete testis, the vas deferens and later to the epididymis by peristaltic contractions and flow of intratubular fluid.

Spermatozoon: most are composed of an oval-shaped head, which contains condensed chromatin and nucleoproteins. They also have an acrosomic cap which covers about 2 anterior thirds of the head. They have a short neck, which contains centrioles essential for the union of the tail and the division of the zygote after fertilization. They also contain a long tail known as a flagellum, which allows normal and progressive forward mobility.

Bibliographic references

1. Shlomo Melmed, Richard J. Auchus, Allison B. Goldfine, Ronald J. Kowning, Clifford Rosen. Williams Textbook of Endocrinology 14Th edition. ELSEVIER, 2020.
2. Dorantes and Martinez. Clinical endocrinology 5th edition, Editorial El Manual Moderno 2016.

Chapter 343. Anabolic Steroids

Also known as androgenic steroids, it is a set of synthetic derivatives of testosterone. Androgens exert their effects in various parts of the body, including the muscles, bones, hair follicles, liver, kidneys, reproductive tissues, the central nervous system, hematopoietic and immune systems. Its effects are often associated with masculinization and anabolic effects, especially in the formation of skeletal muscle and bone proteins.

Types of anabolic steroids

Alkylated derivatives (obtained by substitutions in position 17 alpha)	Oxandrolone. Oxymetholone. Fluoxymesterone Danazol
Testosterone esters (Obtained by esterification in position 17beta)	Testosterone Cypionate. Testosterone enanthate. Testosterone heptylate. Testosterone propionate. Nandrolone Decanoate Nandrolone Phenpropionate Dromostanolone.

Indications of anabolic steroids

FDA approved indications
Primary hypogonadism.
Delayed puberty
Hypogonadotropic hypogonadism
Gonadotropin and luteinizing hormone-releasing hormone deficiency.
Hypothalamic-pituitary axis dysfunction (various tumors, lesions, and radiation).

Primary testicular failure:
Cryptorchidism.
Orchitis
Testicular torsion.
Missing testicle syndrome.
Previous history of orchiectomy.
Klinefelter syndrome.
Chemotherapeutic agents.
Toxic damage from alcohol and heavy metal consumption.
Most common indications in Spain
Endometriosis
Benign breast disease.
Menorrhagia Precocious puberty.
Hereditary angioneurotic edema.
Protein metabolism disorders associated with severe malnutrition.
Impotence, male climacteric.
Postmenopausal and senile osteoporosis.
Lactation suppression.

Pharmacological actions

Growth and development of male sexual organs and maintenance of secondary sexual characteristics.

In skeletal muscle, they regulate the transcription of target genes that regulate the accumulation of DNA in skeletal muscle to allow muscle growth.

Positive regulation and increase in the amount of androgen receptors (contributes to increased muscle size and strength).

Brain stimulating effect through effects on neurotransmitters, stimulation of the growth hormone-insulin-like growth factor-1 axis and glucocorticoid antagonism.

Nitrogen retention in muscles increasing muscle size and alleviating joint pain by promoting collagen synthesis and enhanced bone mineralization (Nandrolone Decanoate and Nandrolone Fenpropionate).

Anti-estrogenic properties (dromostanolone)

Administration of anabolic steroids

Drug	Dose
Testosterone Cypionate	50 to 400 mg intramuscularly 1 to 4 times a month.
Testosterone undecanoate	750 mg (initial dose), then 750 mg 4 weeks after the first dose and another 750 mg thereafter (10-week intervals between doses). Or 10 to 25 mg / day
Enanthate	200 mg every 10 to 14 days.
Propionate	10 to 25 mg 2 to 3 times a week
Fluoxymesterone	5 to 40 mg daily

Adverse effects

Cardiovascular	Hypertension. Cardiomyopathy Coronary heart disease.
Metabolic and endocrine	HDL cholesterol reduction. Hypokalemia Hyperlipidemia Hypertriglyceridaemia. Increased thyroid stimulating hormone. Increased estradiol. Hot flushes. Weight gain.
Genitourinary	Increased prostate specific antigen. Testicular atrophy.

	Benign prostatic hypertrophy. Spermatogenesis suppression. Mastalgia. Hypogonadism Prostatitis. Hematuria Dysuria Impotence. Pelvic pain. Urinary infection.
Gastrointestinal	Irritation of the mouth. Gingivitis. Increased bilirubinemia. Decreased appetite. Dysgeusia. Gastroesophageal reflux disease. Gastrointestinal bleeding.
Dermatological	Skin blisters. Acne vulgaris. Crusty skin Nasal excoriation Acne. Pruritus. Contact dermatitis.
Neuromuscular and skeletal	Myalgia. Premature epiphyseal closure. Pain in extremities. Tendon rupture Abnormal bone growth Hemarthrosis.
Neuropsychiatric	Emotional lability. Depression. Nervousness. Body ache. Insomnia Aggressive behavior and violence. Anosmia. Mood disorders.

Others	Nandrolone causes hirsutism and a deep voice in women with long periods.

Bibliographic references

1. P. Lorenzo, A. Moreno, I. Lizasoain, JC Leza, MA Moro, A. Portolés. Velazquez. Basic and Clinical Pharmacology 18th Edition. Panamerican Medical Publishing House. 2013.
2. Lusetti M, Licata M, Silingardi E, Bonsignore A, Palmiere C. Appearance / Image- and Performance-EnhancingDrugUsers: A ForensicApproach. Am J ForensicMedPathol. 2018 Dec; 39 (4): 325-329.

Chapter 344. Ambiguous Genitalia

Ambiguous genitalia are defined as genitalia whose external appearance in the newborn does not resemble those of a boy or a girl, but has an intermediate appearance between the two sexes. This definition could also include phenotypic appearance not corresponding to genetic sex, with a discordance between genital appearance and karyotype. However, these types of cases are discovered at puberty.

Statistics and epidemiology

Congenital adrenal hyperplasia is the most common cause of virilization in 46XX people. The most common deficit is that of the enzyme 21-hydroxylase in 90-95% of cases of congenital adrenal hyperplasia.

Etiology or more frequent causes

Ovary	Congenital adrenal hyperplasia. Placental aromatase deficiency. Maternal virilization syndrome.
Tests	Androgen insensitivity. Leydig cell hypoplasia. 5 alpha-reductase deficiency. Testosterone biosynthesis deficiency.
Dysgenetic gonads	Denys-Drash and Frasier syndrome. Gonadal dysgenesis. Smith-Lemli-Optz syndrome. Camptomelic dwarfism.

Pathophysiological elements

Enzyme deficiencies:
Of glandular origin (testis and adrenal):   46 XY / 17β-hydroxysteroid dehydrogenase (17β-HSD3) deficiency.   46 XY / 3β-hydroxysteroid dehydrogenase deficiency.   46XY / StAR deficiency.   Of peripheral origin: 46 XY / 5 alpha reductase deficiency 2.
Developmental abnormalities of the gonads
Klinefelter syndrome.   Turner syndrome.   Pure or mixed gonadal dysgenesis.   Leydig cell hypoplasia type 1 and 2.   46, XX or 46, XX / XY or 46, XY / Ovo-testis (formerly called true hermaphroditism).
Androgen receptor abnormalities
Complete androgen insensitivity syndrome.   Androgen insensitivity syndrome.
Maternal androgen excess (rare)
Virilized by maternal tumor.   Virilized by exogenous androgens.

Diagnostic criteria

Clinic	***Apparently male:*** Bilaterally non-palpable testicles in a full-term newborn. Hypospadias and undescended testicles. Penoscrotal hypospadias. Associated hypospadias and separation of the scrotal sacs (bifid scrotum). ***Apparently feminine:***

	Hypertrophy of the clitoris in any degree. Inguinal hernia with gonadal content. Lip fusion. Palpable gonads.
Paraclinical	Serum electrolytes. Glucose level (cortisol deficiency can manifest as hypoglycemic disorders due to congenital adrenal hyperplasia). Karyotype. Hormonal study: especially measurements of gonadotropins, androgens and andron precursors, adrenal steroids and Müller inhibitors. Ultrasound or MRI (evaluation of the development of internal organs). Massively parallel sequencing or full exome / genome sequencing.

Treatment options

Treatment must be planned by a multidisciplinary team consisting of a neonatologist, pediatric endocrinologist, psychologist, and pediatric surgeon.

A 46XX neonate with ambiguous genitalia is usually adjudicated female, especially in congenital adrenal hyperplasia. Surgical reconstruction is proposed for the female sex.

Surgical treatment is performed based on the civil sex awarded. Removal of non-ovarian gonads is considered due to the risk of malignancy of dysgenetic gonads.

In the case of male choice, reconstruction requires a minimum size of the corpora cavernosa, descent into the male gonadal inguinal sac or duct (removal when they cannot be preserved) and correction of hypospadias. In the absence of gonads, testicular prostheses are placed for aesthetic purposes.

Hormone therapy will be started between 11 to 12 years of bone age in girls and between 12 to 13 years of bone age in boys. Treatment is continued into adulthood.

Follow-up peculiarities

The sex assignment diagnosis must be followed in conjunction with the parents' choice of parenting, functional aspects, karyotype, among other elements. From a functional and surgical point of view, gender reassignment due to an incorrect diagnosis causes a very negative psychological situation, which is why some literatures choose to delay the surgical procedure until adolescence.

Bibliographic references

1. Krishnan S, Meyer J, Khattab A. AmbiguousGenitalia in theNewborn. [Updated 2019 Dec 2]. In: Feingold KR, Anawalt B, Boyce A, et al., Editors. Endotext [Internet]. South Dartmouth (MA): MDText.com, Inc .; 2000-.
2. Pelayo Baeza FJ, Carabaño Aguado I, Sanz Santaeufemia FJ, La Orden Izquierdo E. Ambiguous genitalia. RevPediatr Aten Primaria. 2011 Sep; 13 (51): 419-33.
3. Acimi S. (2019). WhatTermtoChoose: AmbiguousGenitaliaor Disorders of Sex Development (DSD) ?. Frontiers in pediatrics, 7, 316.https://doi.org/10.3389/fped.2019.00316

Chapter 345. Prepubertal Male Hypogonadism

This is the reduction in the production of sperm or testosterone, although on occasion, a reduction in the response to testosterone can occur and as a result, delayed puberty or reproductive failure occurs in prepubertal patients.

Statistics and epidemiology

The most common causes are the primary type. Klinefelter syndrome is the most common sexual disorder, approximately 10% of patients diagnosed with this syndrome are identified at puberty.
Cryptorchidism occurs in 3% of term infants and up to 33% of preterm infants. In other statistics, about 26 to 36% of male pediatric cancer survivors have hypogonadism after treatment.

Risk groups or factors:
- ✓ Head injury.
- ✓ History of cancer treatment (chemotherapeutics).
- ✓ Parotitis.
- ✓ Cryptorchidism.

Etiology and pathophysiological elements

Primary hypogonadism		Secondary hypogonadism	
Congenital	Acquired	Congenital	Acquired
Klinefelter syndrome. Cryptorchidism.	Cancer treatment. Testicular	Kallmann syndrome Idiopathic	Damage disease of the pituitary gland.

| Noonan syndrome. Congenital adrenal hyperplasia. | damage. Orchitis secondary to mumps. | hypogonadotropic hypogonadism. Panhypophyseal insufficiency. | Head trauma Alcohol or drug abuse |

Prepubertal hypogonadism can occur as a result of a disorder that interferes with the development of testosterone and / or sperm, or a peripheral insensitivity to testosterone. Sometimes both circumstances can coexist. A testicular disorder alters the production of testosterone or is capable of damaging the seminiferous tubules, on the other hand, congenital or acquired disorders that affect the hypothalamus or pituitary function, cause gonadotropin deficiency and consequently failure to stimulate the testicles.

Before puberty, gonadotropin and steroid levels are at low levels according to age, however, this represents a diagnostic difficulty for the hypogonadotropic state in this age group.

Diagnostic criteria

| **Clinic** | Inadequate differentiation of the internal Wolffian ducts and external genitalia (when androgen deficiency occurs during the first trimester of gestation). Ambiguous external genitalia or normal-appearing female external genitalia. Microfalo and partial cryptorchidism (deficiency during the second and third trimesters of gestation). Alteration of secondary sexual development: high voice, |

	absence of body hair, little pubic hair, poor muscle development, gynecomastia (delayed puberty).
Paraclinical	Blood glucose level. Testosterone determination. LH and FSH levels. Karyotype (when genetic causes are suspected). Human chorionic gonadotropin (hCG) stimulation test.

Treatment options

Treatment is established according to the specific cause. Therapy often consists of surgery and replacement therapy.
Cryptorchidism is corrected by surgery early.
Secondary hypogonadism requires androgen replacement therapy starting at a low dose and increasing progressively.
In Kallmann syndrome, treatment is performed with hCG to correct cryptorchidism and establish fertility. Puberty can be induced by administration of injectable or gel testosterone.
Prader-Willi syndrome patients benefit from human growth hormone replacement therapy.

Follow-up peculiarities

The follow-up should be carried out in the long term, in conjunction with a multidisciplinary team that evaluates future risk factors associated with testicular cancer, fertility disorders or other.

Bibliographic references

1. Shlomo Melmed, Richard J. Auchus, Allison B. Goldfine, Ronald J. Kowning, Clifford Rosen. Williams Textbook of Endocrinology 14Th edition. ELSEVIER, 2020
2. Brito VN, Berger K, Mendonca BB. Male hypogonadism: childhood diagnosis and future therapies. Pediatric Health. 2010 Oct; 4 (5): 539-55.

Chapter 346. Micropenis

Also known as microcephalus, it is defined as a length of the stretched penis less than 2.5 standard deviations (SD), below the mean for age. The term micropenis can also be associated with a normal form, while the term microcephalus is used to describe associated hypospadias.

Statistics and epidemiology

The incidence of micropenis is estimated to range from 1.5 out of 10,000 newborn boys. A high prevalence of micropenis has been reported in populations with intensive use of pesticides. The most common cause is abnormal hypothalamic or pituitary function.

Etiology or more frequent causes

Insufficient testosterone secretion
Hypogonadotropic hypogonadism Kallmann syndrome. Laurence-Moon syndrome. Prader-Willi syndrome. In conjunction with another pituitary defect. Rud syndrome. Bardet-Biedl syndrome.
Primary hypogonadism Robinow syndrome. Trisomy 21. Noonan syndrome Klinefelter syndrome and poly-X Gonadal dysgenesis (incomplete form). Testosterone steroidogenesis.

Anorchia. Luteinizing hormone receptor defect.
Testosterone activation defects
Growth hormone / IGF-1 deficiency. Fetal hydantoin syndrome. 5-alpha reductase deficiency (incomplete form). Androgen receptor defect (incomplete form).
Developmental abnormalities
Agenesis of the penis. Cloacal exstrophy.
Idiopathic
In conjunction with another congenital malformation

Pathophysiological elements

Fetal production of testosterone and its conversion to dihydrotestosterone (DHT) in peripheral tissues is essential for the male apparatus to develop normally. Also, intact peripheral androgen receptors are essential for normal development. Any alteration in these elements can cause micropenis:

- ✓ Hypothalamic-pituitary-gonadal axis.
- ✓ Defect of the action of peripheral androgens.
- ✓ Isolated deficiency of growth hormone.
- ✓ Primary structural anomaly.
- ✓ Genetic syndrome.

Diagnostic criteria.

Clinic	The physical examination should be thorough looking for dysmorphic features. An abnormal growth rate after the first 6 to 12 months of life may indicate a pituitary deficiency.

	Measurement must be done carefully. Traditional methods use a ruler or gauge to measure penis length. This should be done with the penis fully stretched, not flaccid. Hold the glans penis with your thumb. Measurement starts from the pubic ramus extending to the distal tip of the glans on the dorsal side. The foreskin should be retracted during measurement while the suprapubic fat pad is pressed inward. Another approach involves the use of a syringe adapted to measure the length of the penis. The diagnosis of micropenis is fundamentally clinical, when the measurement of the length of the penis is at -2.5 SD, below the normal expected for the age.
Paraclinical	Paraclinical tests are indicated to establish the underlying cause of the micropenis. Measurement of serum gonadotropins. Testosterone level before or after hCG stimulation test (administer hCG intramuscularly, doses of 1000 IU for 3 days or 1500 U every 2 days for 12 days): testosterone levels below 300 ng / dL may indicate gonadal dysgenesis. DHT level. Testosterone precursors. Pituitary hormones (when necessary). Measurement of inhibin B and AMH. Pelvic ultrasound: when it is required to visualize internal genitalia. Magnetic resonance: suspicion of structural defects of the midline. Genetic testing.

Treatment options

Intramuscular testosterone therapy at doses of 25 to 50 mg. Testosterone cypionate or enanthate can be given once every 3-4 weeks for 3 months.

Topical Testosterone Therapy (5% Testosterone Ceme), used for 30 days.

5-a dihydrotestosterone topical gel: daily dose of 0.2 to 0.3 mg / kg for 3 or 4 months.

Recombinant human LH and FSH.

Surgical treatment: When the micropenis does not reach the expected length despite the administration of medical treatment, penile reconstruction may be considered.

Follow-up peculiarities

Treatment is often aimed at achieving aesthetic and functional results acceptable to the patient. However, general dissatisfaction of patients with their genital appearance is common. Follow-up visits are geared towards the specific cause of the micropenis.

Bibliographic references

1. Hatipoğlu, N., & Kurtoğlu, S. (2013). Micropenis: etiology, diagnosis and treatmentapproaches. Journalofclinicalresearch in pediatric endocrinology, 5 (4), 217–223.https://doi.org/10.4274/Jcrpe.1135.
2. Bonomi M, Vezzoli V, Krausz C, et al. Characteristics of a nation wide cohort of patients presenting with isolated hypogonadotropic hypogonadism (IHH). Eur J Endocrinol. 2018 Jan. 178 (1): 23-32

Chapter 347. Cryptorchidism

Cryptorchidism, or undescended testicle, is a congenital anomaly, which consists of the absence of at least one testicle in the scrotum. It is the most common congenital defect in the male external genitalia. Although it can occur in both testicles, it frequently affects the right testicle.

Statistics and epidemiology

At least 3% of full-term male newborns have cryptorchidism. The prevalence of cryptorchidism in preterm infants is 30%. Heritability among first degree relatives is estimated to range from 0.5 to 1%. About 7% of siblings of children with cryptorchidism may have this abnormality.

Risk groups or factors
- ✓ Smaller placental weight.
- ✓ Premature babies before testicular descent.
- ✓ Smaller babies for gestational age.
- ✓ Maternal obesity.
- ✓ Maternal diabetes.
- ✓ Pesticides
- ✓ Chemical endocrine disruptors.
- ✓ Preeclampsia.
- ✓ In vitro fertilization.
- ✓ Alcohol consumption during pregnancy.
- ✓ Syndrome associated with congenital malformations (Noonan, Down, Prader-Willi syndrome).

✓ Family history of cryptorchidism in a first-degree relative.

Etiology

In most cases of cryptorchidism, the etiological aspects are unknown, however, in some cases of cryptorchidism, the cause may be due to a combination of hormonal, environmental, genetic and anatomic factors.

Anatomical etiology
Inguinal canal abnormalities.
Persistent vaginal process and inguinal hernia.
Anomaly of the testicle, epididymis and vas deferens.
Inadequate governmental attachment
Hormonal
Deficient INSL3 production or insensitivity of the INSL3 receptor.
Deficient GnRH and / or gonadotropin production. GnRH or LH receptor insensitivity.
Poor androgen production or receptor insensitivity to androgens.
Poor CGRP production or receptor insensitivity.
Poor AMH production or insensitivity to the AMH receptor.
Genetic
Mutations of the 5 alpha reductase gene.
HOXA10 gene mutations.
Higher incidence of a polymorphic allele of steroidogenic factor 1 (SF-1), with reduced transcription activity. SF-1, affects the expression of LGR8 and INSL3.
Heterozygous mutations of the Lgr8 and Insl3 genes on chromosome 19.
Mutations in the androgen receptor on the X chromosome, increases the repeat length of GAG or GGN.

Pathophysiological elements

In the pathophysiology of the undescended testes, the increase in temperature stands out mainly. For spermatogenesis to take place effectively, the testicular temperature must be 2 to 7 °C below body temperature. The unique anatomical features of the scrotum for thermoregulation provide the optimal environment for spermatogenesis to take place. However, a reduction in the recto-scrotal temperature gradient by only 1 to 2°C is capable of suppressing spermatogenesis.

Transient hormonal deficiencies are likely to cause a lack of testicular descent and cause alterations in the development of spermatogenic tissue.

Classification
- ✓ Congenital and acquired.
- ✓ Palpable and not palpable.
- ✓ Unilateral or bilateral.

Diagnostic criteria

Clinic	*Medical record:* You must collect data associated with pregnancy, medication used, exposure to toxins, birth weight, positions of the testicles at birth, among other details. *Physical exam:* carefully examine the patient in a supine and standing position (in older children) in a warm environment. Palpation is mandatory to determine testicular aspects (palpable or not, retractable, sliding or others). Examine gonadal size, turgor, and abnormalities. Rule out hernias or hydrocele. About 70% of cryptorchidism is palpable, so imaging

	studies are not usually necessary in most cases. When the diagnosis is not made in childhood, infertility can be a reason for consultation in the adult with cryptorchidism.
Paraclinical	*Imaging studies:* Ultrasound: evaluates the size of the inguinal testicles. It is less reliable for testicles located in the abdomen. CT scan and MRI: useful when the testicles are not palpable in both scrotums. Young children may require general anesthesia. Venography and angiography: it is not useful in children, it is difficult to perform and has high complication rates. Karyotype: it can be useful to exclude the diagnosis of primary dysgenetic hypogonadism. Gonadotropin levels. Anti-Mullerian hormone levels.

Treatment options

Hormonal therapies should not be used to induce testicular descent.

The American Pediatric Association recommends hormonal therapy for cases of undescended testicles that are associated with Prader-Willi syndrome, because surgery is more risky for this group of patients due to the high risk of respiratory compromise.

Human chorionic gonadotropin is used frequently through a series of injections and recurrent evaluations.

Surgical treatment is the first treatment option for children with congenital cryptorchidism between 6 and 18 months of age. Fertility improves when orchiopexy is performed early.

When the testicles are not palpable, an exploratory laparoscopy may be indicated and if they are found during the procedure, the following options can be performed:
Laparoscopic orchiopexy with preservation of vessels.
Fowler Stevens laparoscopic orchiopexy in one or two stages.

Follow-up peculiarities

These patients may have fertility problems, especially if diagnosed in adulthood.
On the other hand, the risk of testicular cancer if the orchiopexy is performed before puberty is between 2 to 3 times higher than in the general population, while the risk can rise between 5 to 6 times when the orchiopexy is performed after puberty. It is recommended to teach your patients the technique to perform testicular self-examination and to establish follow-up investigations.

Bibliographic references

1. Niedzielski, JK, Oszukowska, E., & Słowikowska-Hilczer, J. (2016). Undescendedtestis - currenttrends and guidelines: a reviewoftheliterature. Archives of medical science: AMS, 12 (3), 667–677.https://doi.org/10.5114/aoms.2016.59940
2. Shlomo Melmed, Richard J. Auchus, Allison B. Goldfine, Ronald J. Kowning, Clifford Rosen. Williams Text book of Endocrinology 14Th edition. ELSEVIER, 2020.

3. Braga LH, Lorenzo AJ, Romao RLP. Canadian Urological Association-Pediatric Urologists of Canada (CUA-PUC) guidelineforthe diagnosis, management, and followupofcryptorchidism. Can UrolAssoc J. 2017 Jul; 11 (7): E251-E260

Chapter 348. Kallmann Syndrome

It is a congenital form of hypogonadotropic hypogonadism which manifests itself with olfactory disorders such as hypo or anosmia.

The decrease in gonadal function of this syndrome is caused as a result of the failure in the differentiation or migration of neurons during embryological development, which arise in the olfactory mucosa, to establish themselves in the hypothalamus that acts as neurons of the releasing hormone gonadotropin (GnRH).

The decrease in GnRH levels results in a decrease in the amount of sex steroids, leading to a lack of sexual maturity and the absence of secondary sexual characteristics.

Statistics and epidemiology

The prevalence of Kallmann syndrome (KS) is around 1 case per house in 8,000 to 10,000 men.

There is a marked male predominance with a male: female ratio of 4: 1 to 5: 1.

Between 30-40% of cases occur as a result of a known mutation of genes involved in the migration of GnRH neurons from the olfactory plate to the hypothalamus.

Etiology and elements of pathophysiology

The cause of this syndrome is a genetic alteration that results in a defect in the hypothalamic GnRH neurons or in their differentiation and migration to the hypothalamus in the course of embryonic development. Mutations have been reported in approximately 40 different genes. The most common genetic defects are related to KS, the ANOS1 and FGFR1 genes

Associated genetic mutations:

FGFR1 / KAL2, TAC3R and PROK2: leptin genes (LEP) and its receptor (LEPR).
PROKR2.
KISS1R: encodes the kisspeptin 1 / metastin receptor (an important neuropeptide-stimulating GnRH.
TAC3: encodes neurokinin B.
*GNRH1 (*on rare occasions).

Diagnostic criteria

Clinic	Delayed or absent puberty.
	Symptoms associated with hypogonadism.
	Hyposmia or anosmia.
	Clinic associated with heart disease: fatigue, cyanosis, dyspnea, palpitations, syncope.
	Colour blindness.
	Hearing impairment
	Paraplegia.
	Epilepsy.
	Sterility.
	Osteoporosis, skeletal abnormalities.

	In men:
	Erectile dysfunction.
	Decreased libido
	Decreased muscle strength.
	Reduction of aggressiveness and impulse.
	In women:
	Amenorrhea
	Dyspareunia
	Physical exam
	Eunucoid body proportion.
	Arm extension greater than height by more than 5 cm.
	Distance between the symphysis and the floor less than 5 cm greater than the distance between the crown and the symphysis.
	Legs disproportionately long in relation to the arms (men).
	Micropenis or small penis, unpigmented and non-rough scrotum, small or absent testicles, cryptorchidism.
	Pubic hair, arms, thoracic and facial hair absent.
	Predominance of fat on the face, chest and hips.
	Gynecomastia
Paraclinical	Pregnancy test.
	Thyroid profile.
	IGF-1 measurement.
	LH and FSH levels.
	Serum testosterone level (decreased less than 100 ng / dl in adults).
	Low serum estradiol level.
	Ferritin level (normal in SK).
	Magnetic resonance imaging of the brain (75% have abnormal olfactory systems).
	Bone densitometry.

Treatment options

Kallmann syndrome can often be treated by hormone replacement therapy, by administering steroids such as testosterone or estrogen-progestin supplementation. All complications associated with Kallmann syndrome should be identified and specific treatment indicated and specialist referrals should be indicated if required.

Follow-up peculiarities
Kallmann syndrome has a good prognosis with the administration of adequate treatment. By itself, it is not associated with a reduction in life expectancy, although it may be associated with heart disorders and osteoporosis. It is recommended to plan regular follow-up visits according to the conditions present in the patient to evaluate the effectiveness of the treatment and the appearance of complications related to Kallmann's syndrome.

Bibliographic references

1. Shlomo Melmed, Richard J. Auchus, Allison B. Goldfine, Ronald J. Kowning, Clifford Rosen. Williams Textbook of Endocrinology 14Th edition. ELSEVIER, 2020.
2. Boehm U, Bouloux PM, Dattani MT, de Roux N, Dodé C, Dunkel L, Dwyer AA, Giacobini P, Hardelin JP, Juul A, Maghnie M, Pitteloud N, Prevot V, Raivio T, Tena-Sempere M, Quinton R , Young J. Expert consensus document: European Consensus Statement on congenital hypogonadotropic hypogonadism - pathogenesis, diagnosis and treatment. Nat Rev Endocrinol. 2015 Sep; 11 (9): 547-64

Chapter 349. Klinefelter Syndrome

It consists of a common sex chromosomal abnormality which is responsible for causing primary hypogonadism. It is characterized by very small and firm testes, in conjunction with azoospermia and infertility, as well as varying degrees of androgen deficiency and signs of eunucoidism and increased gonadotropin concentrations.

Statistics and epidemiology

About 1 case occurs for every 500 to 700 neonates and prenatals.
The prevalence among adults is 1 case in 2,500.
It is estimated that 75% of men with Klinefelter syndrome will never be diagnosed.
The risk of children with Klinefelter syndrome increases with increasing maternal and paternal age.

Risk groups or factors:

- ✓ Advanced maternal and paternal age.
- ✓ Etiology or more frequent causes
- ✓ A disease of genetic origin in which different disorders have been described:
- ✓ Mosaic karyotypes such as: 46, XY / 47, XXY.
- ✓ Aneuploidies such as 48, XXXY and 49, XXXXY.
- ✓ Karyotype 47, XXY (represents more than 90% of cases).

The extra X chromosome is acquired randomly and is often due to meiotic nondisjunction or postzygotic nondisjunction. The phenotype is more serious in relation to the amount of X chromosomes added.

Pathophysiological elements

The mechanisms underlying primary testicular failure and the phenocytic variety of neurocognitive and physical characteristics are not well characterized. It has been shown that the added X chromosome can cause hyalinization of the testes, as well as the fibrosis that causes primary gonadal failure, which evolves during adolescence and adulthood. As early as dysfunction manifests itself, the clinical manifestations will be more evident, finding characteristic features of hypogonadism in the neonate.

The additional amount of the SHOX gene located in the pseudoautosomal region of the X chromosome, causes characteristic features such as long limbs, elevated stature, and a reduction in the ratio between the upper and lower segments.

Diagnostic criteria:

Clinic	Micropenis, hypospadias, cryptorchidism, small testes (newborns).
	Developmental delay.
	Tall statue.
	Clinodactyly.
	Hypertelorism
	Gynecomastia
	Elbow dysplasia.
	High arched palate.
	Hypotonia
	Language or learning delay.
	Reading disabilities.

	Behavior problems In adults, the most relevant clinical characteristic is very small testes with at least 4 ml of volume and less than 2.5 cm in length. Infertility Eunucoidism. IQ reduced from 10 to 15 points, but without reaching a degree of intellectual disability.
Paraclinical	The diagnosis is established by karyotype analysis. Non-invasive prenatal free DNA testing. Elevated gonadotropin level. Reduced serum testosterone level. Elevated estradiol Increase in SHBG concentrations.

Treatment options

Treatment consists of correcting the androgen deficiency.

Infants with a micropenis may receive testosterone (topical to the penis or systemic).

Older children require early intervention with speech and reading therapy especially if there is dyslexia or speech delay.

During puberty, the administration of testosterone is necessary for the proper development of secondary sexual traits, muscle mass and strength, maximum bone mass, among others.

Adults should receive testosterone replacement therapy, additionally advanced reproductive technology can be used.

Gynecomastia can be treated by medical treatment such as tamoxifen or by surgery depending on the time of onset and the degree of gynecomastia.

Follow-up peculiarities

The Klinefelter syndrome has a risk of developing other associated disorders such as type 2 diabetes mellitus, dyslipidemias, cardiovascular disease and long-term thromboembolism. Regular screening and control exams are recommended.

Bibliographic references

1. Shlomo Melmed, Richard J. Auchus, Allison B. Goldfine, Ronald J. Kowning, Clifford Rosen. Williams Textbook of Endocrinology 14Th edition. ELSEVIER, 2020.

Chapter 350. Noonan Syndrome

Formerly known as male Turner syndrome, it consists of an autosomal dominant or occasional sporadic hereditary disease, whose phenotypic manifestations are heterogeneous.

Statistics and epidemiology

It affects about 1 case per 1000 to 2500 live births, both men and women, without ethnic preferences.

Risk groups or factors: Associated with advanced paternal age.

Etiology or more frequent causes

It is an autosomal dominant pleomorphic disease, that is, the parents present the Noonan syndrome mutation with a 50% probability of transmitting it to their offspring. It can also occur as a sporadic or de novo mutation.

Half of men with Noonan syndrome have alterations in the non-receptor gene for protein tyrosine phosphatase type 11 (PTPN11). Another mutation that can occur in the SOS1, RAF1 or KRAS genes.

Pathophysiological elements

Men with Noonan syndrome present hypogonadism, the main characteristic of which is androgen deficiency and impaired sperm production with increased gonadotropin concentrations.

Diagnostic criteria

Clinic	*Prenatal stage:*
	Increased nuchal translucency in the uterus.
	Polyhydramnios for kidney disorders.
	Congenital heart disease.
	Mild limb shortening.
	Fetal macrosomia.
	Postnatal stage, childhood and adults.
	Macrocephaly
	Cryptorchidism.
	Eyes wide open.
	Short stature.
	Pulmonary stenosis.
	Infertility (more common in men).
	Hypertrophic cardiomyopathy.
	Difficulty feeding and growth retardation (infants).
	Squint.
	Hearing loss.
	Intellectual and developmental delay.
	Unusual facial features (hypertelorism, downward slanting eyes, low set ears or thick jelices, high nasal bridge, ptosis, micrognathia, triangular shaped face, high palate, dental malocclusion, low hairline).
	Short, webbed neck.
	Shield-shaped chest.
	Pectus excavatum or carinatum.
	Scoliosis
	Ulna worth.
	Joint laxity.
	Hepatosplenomegaly.
	Intellectual disability.
Paraclinical	The diagnosis is mainly clinical. Molecular genetic

	testing can be done to confirm the diagnosis. Once the diagnosis of Noonan has been established, paraclinics should be indicated to evaluate the complications associated with it: Cardiac evaluation: echocardiography and electrocardiograph. Audiological and ophthalmological evaluation. Renal ultrasound. Coagulation profile. Development evaluation. Chest and back images.

Treatment options

The treatment of Noonan syndrome consists of symptomatic improvement and multidisciplinary supportive care. According to the organs and systems affected by the syndrome, specific treatment may be necessary:
Orchiopexy is indicated in patients with cryptorchidism in 1-year-old boys to reduce the risk of testicular cancer during adulthood.
A cardiac evaluation should be obtained every 5 years with echocardiography and electrocardiogram.
Growth hormone therapy may be indicated for short stature.

Follow-up peculiarities

The follow-up will be carried out in conjunction with an interdisciplinary team based on the patient's pathologies. The prognosis depends on the severity of the phenotype. There may be high mortality and morbidity according to the severity of the heart defect.

Bibliographic references

1. Shlomo Melmed, Richard J. Auchus, Allison B. Goldfine, Ronald J. Kowning, Clifford Rosen. Williams Textbook of Endocrinology 14Th edition. ELSEVIER, 2020.

Chapter 351. Functional Testicular Tumors

Functional tumors of the testes are defined as neoplasms that originate within the testes, capable of secreting hormones. Germ cell neoplasms are usually hormone or enzyme producers, and these secretions can be used as biomarkers for tumor diagnosis and monitoring.

Statistics and epidemiology

Germ cell tumors correspond to 95% of cases and are usually malignant.
They can occur at any age, although more than 90% have a maximum prevalence between 25 to 40 years of age.
Seminomas account for about a third of all malignant germ cell tumors of the testes and is one of the most treatable cancers.
The survival rate for seminomas is 98% to 99% in the early stage.
It affects Caucasians 5 times more than Afro-descendants.

Risk groups or factors:

- ✓ History of cryptorchidism.
- ✓ Testicular dysgenesis syndrome.
- ✓ Family history of germ cell tumors.
- ✓ Exposure to pesticides.

Etiology and pathogenesis

Most neoplasms originate from a focus of intratubular germ cell neoplasia, which appears intrauterine, although it remains silent until puberty. These cells maintain the expression of the transcription factors known as OCT3 / 4 and NANOG, which are associated with totipotentiality. They are also keeping sharing some genetic alterations.

Classification of the most common testicular tumors

Germ cell tumors	
Seminomatous tumors	Seminomas.
	Spermatocytic seminomas.
Non-seminomatous tumors	Embryonal carcinoma.
	Yolk sac tumor (endodermal sinus).
	Choriocarcinoma
Teratoma	
Sex cord and stromal tumors	
Leydig cell tumors.	
Sertoli tumors	

Seminomas

Macroscopic: homogeneous, lobed, greyish-white masses with no evidence of areas of hemorrhage or necrosis. The albuginea tunic is intact.

Microscopic: polyhedral seminoma cells, abundant cytoplasm, large nucleus, fibrous stroma with variable density. Irregular lobes, presence of lymphocytic infiltrate, diffuse positivity for c-KIT, OCT4 and PLAP. They may contain syncytiotrophoblastic cells.

Spermatocytic seminoma

Macroscopic: soft, grayish cut surface with occasional mucoid cysts.

Microscopic: mixture of three cell populations including small cells similar to secondary spermatocytes, medium cells with rounded nuclei and cytoplasmic eosinophilia, and scattered giant cells.

Embryonal carcinoma

Macroscopic: corresponds to poorly delimited masses of small size, whitish-greyish with hemorrhagic presence or punctate necrosis. It spreads through the tunica albuginea and can involve the cord and epididymis.

Microscopic: primitive epithelial cells with poorly defined margins. They grow forming irregular sheets with tubules, alveoli and papillary structures. Mitosis and large cells are common. They express OCT3 / 4, PLAP, CD30, and cytokeratin, but not c-KIT.

Yolk sac tumor (endodermal sinus tumor)

Macroscopic: It appears as a homogeneous, mucinous, infiltrating tumor with a yellowish-white color.

Microscopic: neoplastic cells arranged in a web in a reticular or network fashion, and solid areas and papillae can be found. Schiller-Duval bodies can be identified, and their cells can be associated with eosinophilic hyaline globules, containing immunoreactive alpha 1-antitrypsin.

Choriocarcinoma

Macroscopic: Small lesion, it can appear as a hemorrhagic mass up to an inconspicuous lesion replaced by a fibrous scar.
Microscopic: Polygonal and uniform cytotrophoblastic cells which grow in cords and sheets mixed with multinucleated syncytiotrophoblastic cells. They demonstrate hCG.

Teratoma

Macroscopic: Large neoplasms between 5 and 10 cm with a heterogeneous appearance. It contains foci of necrosis and hemorrhage that suggest choriocarcinoma, embryonal carcinoma, or both.

Microscopic: differentiated elements mesodermal, ectodermal and endodermal, which are arranged irregularly. These elements can be mature or immature with features similar to embryonic or fetal tissue.

Diagnostic criteria

Clinic	Non-painful testicular enlargement. Subfertility or impaired spermatogenesis. There may be testicular pain, although it is rare. Single firm or hard palpable mass in the scrotum. There may be hydrocele. In the case of metastatic disease, retroperitoneal and anterior mediastinal lymphadenopathy is evident.

Paraclinical	Testicular ultrasound: relatively homogeneous hypoechoic intratesticular mass. It can become less homogeneous due to hemorrhage and necrosis as it increases in size. An initial chest X-ray may be ordered and in case of abnormal findings, a CT scan is ordered. *Biomarkers:* AFP: increased in endodermal sinus tumors, it can be found to a lesser extent in other germ cell tumors. hCG: typically elevated in choriocarcinomas, although seminomas may be less intense. Lactate dehydrogenase: it is nonspecific, although it contributes an ADI of the tumor burden.

Treatment options

Radical orchiectomy: used more frequently as the first therapeutic option with a high success rate.

Low-dose radiation therapy.

Chemotherapy presents persistence or relapse in a large number of cases, so it is not considered as the treatment of choice, however, in the postoperative management of disseminated tumors, systemic combination chemotherapy and cytotoxic drugs (etoposide, bleomycin, others).

Follow-up peculiarities

The highest rates of relapse occur in the first 2 years after initial treatment, although late relapses have been observed, therefore, lifelong follow-up of the patient through regular consultations is recommended. Follow-up should be carried out with post-surgical oncological management and controls and appropriate andrological follow-up.

Bibliographic references

1. Rajpert-De Meyts E, Skakkebaek NE, Toppari J. Testicular CancerPathogenesis, Diagnosis and EndocrineAspects. [Updated 2018 Jan 7]. In: Feingold KR, Anawalt B, Boyce A, et al., Editors. Endotext [Internet]. South Dartmouth (MA): MDText.com, Inc .; 2000.
2. Stephenson A, Eggener SE, Bass EB, Chelnick DM, Daneshmand S, Feldman D, Gilligan T, Karam JA, Leibovich B, Liauw SL, Masterson TA, Meeks JJ, Pierorazio PM, Sharma R, Sheinfeld J. Diagnosis and Treatment ofEarlyStage Testicular Cancer : AUA Guideline. J. Urol. 2019 Aug; 202 (2): 272-281.

Chapter 352. Male Infertility

We speak of infertility when a couple is unable to produce a pregnancy after 6 months or a year of regular sexual intercourse (2 to 3 days), without protection. Infertility in men can be the result of deficiencies in the formation, transport or concentration of sperm.

Statistics and epidemiology

About 30% of the causes of infertility in a couple correspond to male causes and another 30% occur due to infertility in both men and women. It is estimated that 10 to 15% of couples are infertile.

Male infertility rates vary greatly between regions. The highest fertility rates are in Finland, while the lowest in Great Britain.

Risk groups or factors:

- ✓ History of radiotherapy.
- ✓ History of chemotherapy.
- ✓ Testicular trauma.
- ✓ Mellitus diabetes.
- ✓ Multiple sclerosis.
- ✓ Use of alpha-agonist drugs.
- ✓ Smoking
- ✓ Consumption of marijuana.

Etiology or more frequent causes

Pre-testicular causes
Idiopathic hypogonadotropic hypogonadism.
Prader-Willi syndrome.
Laurence-Moon-Biedl syndrome.
Prolactinoma.
Isolated LH deficiency.
Isolated FSH deficiency.
Thalassemia
Cushing's disease.

Primary testicular causes of infertility
Klinefelter syndrome.
Sex inversion syndrome (XX man).
XYY man.
Noonan syndrome.
Mixed gonadal dysgenesis (45, X / 46, XY).
Androgen receptor dysfunction.
Y chromosome microdeletion syndrome.
Missing testicle syndrome or bilateral anorchia.
Down's Syndrome.
Myotonic dystrophy.
Varicocele.
Non-chromosomal testicular failure.
Cryptorchidism.
Trauma.
Chemotherapy.
Sertoli cell syndrome only.
Orchitis
Radiotherapy.

Post-testicular causes of infertility
Congenital blockage of the ductal system.
Cystic fibrosis.
Acquired obstruction of the ductal system.
Anti sperm antibodies.
Defects in the cilia.
Obstruction of the ejaculatory duct.
Ejaculatory disorders (retrograde ejaculation or anejaculation).

Pathophysiological elements

According to the cause, the pathophysiological mechanisms can be diverse, however, the mechanisms can involve alterations in the formation, concentration and transport of spermatozoa.

- ✓ Insufficiency of the primary seminiferous tubule.
- ✓ Sperm autoimmunity.
- ✓ Obstructive azoospermia.
- ✓ Gonadotropin deficiency.
- ✓ Disorder of sexual function.
- ✓ Reversible effects of toxins.
- ✓ Oligospermia
- ✓ Asthenospermia and teratozoospermia.
- ✓ Normospermia with functional defects.

Diagnostic criteria

Clinic	*Medical record* It must contain complete information on the medical and urological history, describing the duration of previous infertility or fertility, the time of puberty, underlying chronic disorders, among others. *Physical exam* Make a thorough inspection of the penis, testicles and secondary sexual characteristics, as well as body habit. You can use the Prader orchidometer or ultrasound to estimate testicular volume. Probable Findings: Signs of testicular atrophy. Swelling with pain (orchitis).

	Non-painful testicular enlargement (neoplasms, tuberculosis, tertiary syphilis). Enlarged and indurated epididymis with cystic component suggests ductal obstruction. Tenderness in the epididymis suggests epididymitis. Varicocele. Gynecomastia The evaluation of the penis focuses on the permeability and location of the ureteral meatus, ruling out the presence of meatus stenosis. The rectal examination is geared toward examining the prostate and evaluating prostate cysts, indurations, or masses.
Paraclinical	Semen analysis (semen volume, sperm concentration, morphology, motility, sperm antibodies). Antisperm antibody test. FSH and LH levels Testosterone levels. Prolactin levels. *Imaging tests* Transrectal ultrasound (suspected azoospermia or severe oligospermia, useful to evaluate ejaculatory duct obstruction). Scrotal ultrasound evaluates the anatomy of the testicle, the spermatic cord and the epididymis. It is used to properly assess testicular volume and testicular or paratesticular masses and rule out varicocele). Vasography (evaluates ductal patency). *Other studies* Postcoital testing. Sperm function test. Testicular biopsy.

Treatment options

The specific cause of infertility may require different treatment options. It is essential to find the underlying cause of infertility and guide treatment accordingly. There are a limited number of treatments available to improve conception in men.

Lifestyle modification (stress relief therapy, smoking cessation, reducing environmental exposure and harmful conditions, dietary supplements and vitamins).
Epididymal and vascular surgery (obstruction of the male genital tract). Vasovasostomy or vasoepididymostomy.
Imipramine or alpha-sympathomimetics such as pseudoephedrine can be helpful in retrograde ejaculation.
Preparation of semen for insemination.
Varicocelectomy.
Varicocele embolization.
Electroejaculation.
Assisted reproduction techniques.

Follow-up peculiarities

The follow-up is done according to the cause. Follow-up consultations are recommended in conjunction with an endocrinologist.

Bibliographic references

1. Barak S, Baker HWG. Clinical Management of Male Infertility. [Updated 2016 Feb 5]. In: Feingold KR, Anawalt B, Boyce A, et al., Editors. Endotext [Internet]. South Dartmouth (MA): MDText.com, Inc .; 2000-.

2. Shlomo Melmed, Richard J. Auchus, Allison B. Goldfine, Ronald J. Kowning, Clifford Rosen. Williams Text book of Endocrinology 14Th edition. ELSEVIER, 2020

Chapter 353. Spermatogram

It is an essential laboratory test to evaluate fertility for the study of male genital disorders, as well as other pathologies associated with infertility such as those caused by exposure to chemicals, medications and other environmental factors, among others.

Collection instructions

Recommendations of the World Health Organization and the European Society for Embryology and Human Reproduction:

- ✓ The seminal sample should be collected with a period of sexual abstinence between 2 to 7 days.
- ✓ The sample should be deposited in a clean, sterile wide-mouthed container, which allows all seminal fluid to be deposited in the container. In case of loss of a drop of semen, the procedure should be repeated with the same previous abstinence period. You should inform your patient that the first drop of semen contains about 50% of the total sperm.
- ✓ The container must be hermetically covered and marked with the patient's name.
- ✓ Transport the container to body temperature and deliver to the laboratory within one hour after the sample has been collected. The sample must be collected in the patient's home or laboratory, providing an environment of security and privacy.
- ✓ When the patient rejects self-stimulation, he can use special condoms (without spermicides) to collect a sample through intercourse. The patient should not wash the genital organs with surgical soaps that could alter the semen on the day of collection.

Results analysis

The spermiogram provides information on physical factors related to the glands and information on the cells related to the testicle, among others.

Semen volume

The normal volume for 2 days of abstinence is 2 cc minimum.

A lower value suggests hypospermia associated with low testosterone.

When, despite an orgasm, there is no external seminal fluid, it is called aspermia and is common among diabetics or in patients with spinal cord injury. If this happens, a urine sample is requested from the patient after sexual intercourse, if sperm are evidenced, it is a retrograde ejaculation.

Seminal pH

Normal reference value is equal to or greater than 7.2

The acid pH causes sperm death, the volume is usually less than 2cc. It can be confirmed by a fructose titration in the semen.

Elevated pH (greater than 8.0) suggests inflammatory processes or related chronic infections.

Mucolysis

The increased viscosity of the seminal fluid is associated with inflammatory processes of the glands, which prevents the free movement of sperm, causing asthenozoospermia.

Colour
It is usually described as grayish-white.
Yellowish color: prostatitis.
Purulent white: acute infection.
Brown: presence of blood or hemospermia, it may be due to an occasional rupture of a blood vessel in the ureteral or bladder. If it persists, the presence of neoplasms should be ruled out.

Odor
Sui generis related to the smell of sodium hypochlorite.

Cellular aspects of semen

Sperm count	<20 million / cc or less than 40 million in total count: oligozoospermia. Absence of sperm: azoospermia. Associated with secretory disorder or testicular damage due to inflammation, infection, varicocele or other. It can also occur as a result of congenital or acquired disorders.
Mobility	*Grade a:* mobile and fast with rectilinear mobility. *Grade b:* slow spermatozoa with non-rectilinear movement. *Grade c:* there is no sperm displacement, but there is flagellar mobility. *Grade d:* immobile sperm.
Morphology	Morphological alterations are classified according to head, neck, flagellum and combined location. Currently, up to 70% and 30% of normal sperm morphology is accepted as a normal morphological irregularity. Failure to comply with the percentage of normality is

	called teratozoospermia and can be the result of sexually transmitted diseases, drugs, environmental, toxic, among others.
Vitality	The eosin test allows to identify the amount of live or dead sperm.
Other cells	Other cells such as lymphocytes, viruses (HIV, hepatitis B), bacteria, and fungi can be identified.

Bibliographic references

1. Vásquez, F., Soler, C., Camps, P., Valverde, A., & García-Molina, A. (2016). Spermiogram and sperm head morphometry assessed by multivariate cluster analysis results during adolescence (12-18 years) and the effect of varicocele. Asian journal of andrology, 18 (6), 824–830.https://doi.org/10.4103/1008-682X.186873.
2. Fernando Vasquez R., Daniel Vasquez Echeverri. Spermogram and its clinical utility. Uninorte Health. Barranquilla (Col.) 2007; 23 (2): 220-230.

Chapter 354. Oligospermia

These are the concentrations of sperm found in the semen less than 15 million / mL or less than 39 million in the total concentration of the semen volume, it is described as the sperm density below the fifth percentile in fertile men. Clinically it is perceived as a decrease in the probability of getting a pregnancy.

Statistics and epidemiology

Infertility can affect 1 in 20 men. Infertility caused by male factor represents around 50% of infertility problems in couples.
It is estimated that more than 90% of male factor infertility is characterized by a low amount of sperm in the semen or by the production of poor quality of these.
Untreated oligospermia can worsen with age, progressing to azoospermia by up to 12.8% depending on the underlying cause.

Risk groups or factors:
- ✓ Genital infection
- ✓ Testicular surgery.
- ✓ Use of drugs of abuse.
- ✓ Obesity or being overweight.
- ✓ Smoking
- ✓ HIV infection.

Etiology and pathophysiological elements

	Idiopathic spermatogenic insufficiency	Idiopathic
Primary testicular failure	Testicular damage	Infection (orchitis) Vascular (torsion) Varicocele Surgery (orchiectomy, orchidopexy, pelvic or inguinoscrotal).
	Medications and toxins	Chemotherapeutic agents. Salazopyrin (sulfasalazine) Anti metabolic agents.
	Chromosomal disorders	Numerical or structural Translocation or investments Yq microdeletions
	Genetic	Single gene defect (myotonic dystrophy).
Mixed (primary and secondary)	Non-reproductive disease	Acute or chronic disease Liver or kidney failure Hepatitis. HIV Starvation. Iron overload (thalassemia
	Acute febrile illness	Transient disease.
Secondary testicular failure	Partial GNRH deficiency	Hypogonadotropic hypogonadism. Kallmann syndrome. Other
	Partial gonadotropin deficiency	Suppression mediated by sex steroids. Sex steroid secreting neoplasm. Adrenal Leydig cells. Use of androgenic steroids (abuse).
	Hypothalamic-pituitary	Prolactinoma. Macroadenoma (ACTH-secreting,

disorders	acromegaly, non-functioning adenoma). Trauma Infiltrative disease. Iron overload (hemochromatosis, transfusions in chronic anemia).

Diagnostic criteria

Clinic	Specifically, oligospermia does not present additional clinical manifestations to fertility problems. However, according to the cause, severity and age of onset, clinical manifestations associated with it can be observed and are valuable in identifying the cause. ***Clinic history*** Gather reproductive history such as age of puberty, previous fertility attempts, history of genital infections, mumps, surgeries, among others. Ask about the medications or drugs the patient is taking. ***Clinical presentation*** Severe prepubertal hypogonadotropic hypogonadism may have poor signs of virilization, micropenis, small testes (less than 4 ml). In androgen abuse, excessive androgenic action can occur characterized by excess muscle, acne, and small, soft testicles.
Paraclinical	Testosterone tests. Serum LH and FSH level. Semen analysis (spermogram). *Sperm count:* Normal:> 15 million / ml Oligospermia 5 to 14 million / ml Moderate oligospermia 1 to 5 million / ml Severe oligospermia <1 million / ml

Treatment options

Treatment options should focus on resolving the specific cause of oligospermia.

Modification of lifestyle and nutrition: adequate nutrition should be started, especially in obese patients, the diet should be oriented towards weight loss and the appropriate intake of nutrients. Instruct your patients to stop smoking and other harmful habits such as the use of drugs of abuse.

In the case of a varicocele, a varicocelectomy should be considered. Although its effectiveness on fertility is controversial.

- ✓ Vitamins E, C, B6, antioxidants and other supplements can improve sperm production.
- ✓ Clomiphene or aromatase inhibitors.
- ✓ Testosterone treatment.
- ✓ Assisted reproduction treatment for fertility (in vitro fertilization, artificial insemination, IVF-ICSI).

Bibliographic references

1. Robert I. McLachlan, Approach to the Patient With Oligozoospermia, The Journal of Clinical Endocrinology & Metabolism, Volume 98, Issue 3, 1 March 2013, Pages 873–880, https://doi.org/10.1210/jc.2012-3650
2. Kirby EW, Wiener LE, Rajanahally S, Crowell K, Coward RM. Undergoing varicocele repair before assisted reproduction improves pregnancy rate and live

birthrate in azoospermic and oligospermic men with a varicocele: a systematic review and meta-analysis. Fertile Steril. 2016; 106 (6): 1338-1343.

Chapter 355. Erectile Dysfunction

It was previously known as male impotence or erectile dysfunction. It is defined as the inability to achieve or maintain an erection. It also includes the inability to stiffen the penis sufficiently so that it can produce a satisfactory sexual intercourse.

The DSM-5, to define erectile dysfunction requires that an inability to achieve or maintain an erection occurs in 75 to 100% of sexual encounters, for a period of 6 months or more.

Statistics and epidemiology

About 52% of men between the ages of 40 to 70 have been affected by erectile dysfunction to some degree. The prevalence among men 20 to 39 years of age is estimated to be approximately 5.1%. Among men aged 40 to 59, the prevalence is approximately 14.8%.

Men with chronic diseases (kidney disease ends, debates, hypertension and cardiovascular disease), have a significantly higher prevalence than healthy men.

The incidence ranges from 12.4 cases per 1000 people per man for men between 40 to 49 years, and 29.8 cases per 1000 men per year in men between 50 to 59 years of age. For men 60 to 69 years of age the incidence is 46.4 per 1000.

Risk groups or factors:
- ✓ Advanced age.

- ✓ Mellitus diabetes.
- ✓ Arterial hypertension.
- ✓ Smoking
- ✓ Depression.
- ✓ Use of medications.
- ✓ Dyslipidemias.
- ✓ Cardiovascular diseases.

Etiology and pathophysiological elements

Category of dysfunction	Most common disorder	Pathophysiology
Neurogenic	Alzheimer disease. Spinal cord injury. Cerebrovascular accident Diabetic neuropathy. Pelvic injury	Neural innervation interrupted. Failed to initiate nitric oxide (NO) release
Hormonal	Androgen deficiency. Chronic opioid use. Mellitus diabetes Hyperprolactinemia.	Loss of libido Inadequate release of NO. Morphological changes in the penis (atrophy).
Psychogenic	Depression Psychological stress. Interpersonal problems. Anxiety.	Inadequate release of NO. Activation of the sympathetic nervous system. Decreased or loss of libido.
Systemic diseases	Aging. Mellitus diabetes. Generalized atherosclerotic disease. Chronic kidney disease	Multifactorial. Alteration of neuronal and vascular function.

Vasculogenic (arterial and cavernous)	Arterial hypertension. Obesity. Hyperlipidemia Atherosclerosis Trauma or pelvic fracture. Smoking Peyronie's disease.	Inadequate arterial irrigation. Occlusion alteration of the vein of the penis.
Drug induced	Antihypertensives. Alcohol abuse. Antidepressants Antiandrogens	Central nervous system suppression. Alcoholic neuropathy. Decreased libido Vascular insufficiency.

Table 292. Etiology and pathophysiology of erectile dysfunction. Source. Shindel AW, Brandt WO, Bochinski D, et al. Medical and Surgical Therapy of Erectile Dysfunction. [Updated 2018 Jul 10]. In: Feingold KR, Anawalt B, Boyce A, et al., Editors. Endotext.

Diagnostic criteria

Clinic	*Clinic history* Determine the psychosexual history (nature of the dysfunction, ejaculatory characteristics, sexual desire, others, depression, stress, anxiety about sexual performance, among others). Determine risk factors (underlying chronic disorders, previous surgeries, use of medications, use of drugs, alcohol, smoking, among others). Ask about the factors that may cause interaction with the therapy of choice for dysfunction (current use of nitrates, alpha-adrenergic blockers, vasodilators, among others). *Physical exam* Examine for signs of androgen deficiency (loss of body hair, small testicular volume, eunucoid proportions, gynecomastia. Evaluate neurologic deficit for traumatic injury,

	neurologic, or vascular disorder by examining genital and perineal sensation. Measure blood pressure and variations against postural changes in blood pressure. Examine femoral and foot pulses, as well as lower extremity ischemia. The penis should be examined to rule out deformities and Peyronie's disease.
Paraclinical	The basic paraclinical evaluation to be performed in all patients with erectile dysfunction, consists of: Fasting blood glucose. Plasma lipids. Total and free testosterone level in the blood. Indicate the pertinent paraclinics based on the clinical findings identified during the physical examination and collection of the medical history. Additional paraclinics are indicated based on the clinical suspicion of the patient.

Treatment options

Lifestyle modification to improve general health and reduce cardiometabolic risk.
Psychosexual counseling.
Selective phosphodiesterase 5 inhibitors (contraindicated in men who use nitrates regularly or severe heart disease):
Sildenafil at an initial dose of 50 mg, 100 mg or the maximum tolerated dose can be used in case of ineffectiveness at the initial dose, provided there is no evidence of adverse effects (1 to 2 hours before sexual intercourse)

Vardenafil: starting dose of 10 mg and can be increased to 20 mg or maximum tolerated dose. It can be reduced to 5mg depending on the effect of the drug (1 or 2 hours before sexual intercourse).

Avanafil: starting dose from 20 to 100 mg and can be adjusted up to 200 mg (30 minutes before intercourse).

Vacuum devices to induce erection (second line of treatment)

Intraureteral therapy: alprostadil at an initial dose of 250 to 500 μg. It should be applied in the office to assess changes in blood pressure or if ureteral hemorrhage occurs secondary to misapplication.

Intracavernous injection of vasoactive agents.

Penile prosthesis (third line of treatment).

Testosterone replacement in androgen-deficient men.

Follow-up peculiarities:

Follow-up should be established based on the underlying cause and the patient's risk of the treatment of choice.

Bibliographic references

1. Shlomo Melmed, Richard J. Auchus, Allison B. Goldfine, Ronald J. Kowning, Clifford Rosen. Williams Text book of Endocrinology 14Th edition. ELSEVIER, 2020.
2. Shindel AW, Brandt WO, Bochinski D, et al. Medical and Surgical Therapy of Erectile Dysfunction. [Updated 2018 Jul 10]. In: Feingold KR, Anawalt B, Boyce A, et al., Editors. Endotext.

Chapter 356. Orchiectomy

Orchiectomy consists of a surgical procedure by which the testicle is removed. It can be a unilateral orchiectomy when you want to remove a single testicle or a bilateral orchiectomy for simultaneous removal of both testicles.

Indications for orchiectomy
- ✓ Antiandrogen therapy in advanced or metastatic prostate cancer.
- ✓ Testicular torsion with complete testicular necrosis.
- ✓ Testicular infarction or destruction after trauma.
- ✓ Testicular abscess secondary to infection, for example, epididymitis.
- ✓ Testicular cancer.
- ✓ Breast cancer in men.

Types of approach

Process	Description
Scrotal approach	
Subcapsular orchiectomy	Riba technique. It is indicated in advanced prostatic carcinoma and avoids the sensation of an empty scrotum after orchiectomy. Once the incision has been made in the skin and in the tunica vaginalis parietalis, an incision is made in the tunica albuginea starting from the upper pole towards the lower pole. Protruding testicular tissue is detached from the tunica

	albuginea until the parenchyma only attaches to the hilum. The testicular tissue should be dissected and removed, keeping the hilar vessels secure with forceps.
Orchidoepididymectomy	It is indicated for testicular torsion or for infections. Once the skin incision is made, the testicle is mobilized together with the intact tunica vaginalis parietalis. The spermatic cord is opened and the vas deferens and testicular vessels are dissected separately between overholt forceps and suture ligatures. A careful cautery is performed to prevent bleeding.
Inguinal approach	
Radical orchiectomy	The incision is made starting 2 cm above the pubic tubercle extending about 5 to 7 cm in parallel with the inguinal ligament so as to expose the external inguinal ring. The incision can be extended to the upper part of the scrotum, especially for large tumors. Subcutaneous fat, Camper fascia and finally Scarpa fascia are then excised while carefully holding the found blood vessels. Identify and mobilize the ilioinguinal nerve, being careful not to resect it during the procedure. The spermatic cord is dissected and the pubic tubercle is exposed. The testicle is removed from the scrotum by pulling the cord near the pubic tubercle and applying upward pressure on the scrotum below the testicle.

Before the procedure, the option of placing an aesthetic prosthesis in place should be discussed with the patient, as well as the possibility of performing a biopsy on the presumed healthy contralateral testicle. The scrotum and lower abdomen must be completely shaved. During the procedure, one or both testicles can be extracted according to the peculiarities of the patient.

Bibliographic references

1. Hashim H., Abrams P. (2008) Radical Orchidectomy (Orchiectomy). In: Hashim H., Abrams P., Dmochowski R. (eds) TheHandbookof Office UrologicalProcedures. Springer, London.https://doi.org/10.1007/978-1-84628-706-0_8.

Chapter 357. Chemical Castration

It consists of a reversible and temporary medical procedure in which hormonal substances are used to achieve inhibition of libido and control of sexual impulses. It is a method used to suppress the violent sexual urges of sexual offenders, especially pedophiles or pedophiles. However, it is a controversial procedure.

Medications used in chemical castration

Various drugs with antiandrogen effect are used to suppress or reduce testosterone levels and consequently the sexual drive.
- ✓ Estrogenic derivatives.
- ✓ Steroidal and non-steroidal antiandrogens.
- ✓ LHRH analogs.
- ✓ LHRH antagonists.

The most widely used drugs are medroxyprogesterone acetate (MPA) or cyproterone acetate (CPA).

However, according to animal studies, it is presumed that CPA could induce the development of carcinoma in liver cells, therefore, it has not been approved in the United States, with MPA being the most widely used in that country.

For its part, MPA is not used in the European continent, due to the side effects caused by the drug, among which andropause, severe mood instability causing clinical depression, insomnia, diabetes, feminization, migraines, bone demineralization among others, so in Europe, CPA is mainly used.

GnRH agonists have been used more recently to drastically reduce testosterone levels in the blood, as well as attenuation of self-reported inappropriate sexual behavior.

Expected effects of chemical castration
- ✓ Decrease in testosterone levels.
- ✓ Decrease in the rates of recidivism in sexual crimes (especially paraphilic).
- ✓ Reduction of sexual interest.
- ✓ Decreased sexual performance.

Adverse effects
- ✓ Andropause.
- ✓ Severe mood instability.
- ✓ Clinical depression
- ✓ Feminization.
- ✓ Migraines
- ✓ Bone demineralization.
- ✓ Weight gain.

Countries where chemical castration is currently practiced
- ✓ Canada.
- ✓ Argentina.
- ✓ Spain.
- ✓ United States (some states).
- ✓ Korea.

Currently, chemical castration does not have enough evidence-based medicine studies to confirm the effects of the technique in a sufficient population to consider it effective. Its application is a controversy both in terms of effectiveness and ethical conflicts due to its secondary effects.

Bibliographic references

1. Douglas, T., Bonte, P., Focquaert, F., Devolder, K., & Sterckx, S. (2013). Coercion, incarceration, and chemical castration: an argument from autonomy. Journal of bioethical inquiry, 10 (3), 393–405.https://doi.org/10.1007/s11673-013-9465-4.
2. Sandra Mayerly Méndez Bejarano. Chemical castration, the last option in pedophile and pedophile patients, considering their autonomy and dignity. El Bosque University • Colombian Journal of Bioethics. Vol. 14 No 02 • July-December 2019.
3. Lee, JY, & Cho, KS (2013). Chemical castration for sexual offenders: physicians' views. Journal of Korean medical science, 28 (2), 171–172. https://doi.org/10.3346/jkms.2013.28.2.171

Chapter 358. Adult Gynecomastia

The term known as "gynecomastia" is derived from the Greek "gyne" (female) and "masto" (breasts) and corresponds to benign enlargement of the male breast, which frequently occurs bilaterally. Clinically it is defined by the appearance of a firm or rubbery mass which can extend concentrically from the nipples.

Statistics and epidemiology

About 60-90% of babies have transient gynecomastia as a result of elevated estrogen levels during pregnancy. The peak of gynecomastia during puberty can vary from 4 to 69%.
Children between the ages of 10 and 12 may have pubertal gynecomastia, and it disappears by 18 months. Persistence is estimated to be rare in 17-year-old males.
The third peak of gynecomastia appears in men over 65 years between 24 to 65%.

Risk groups or factors:
- ✓ Family history of gynecomastia.
- ✓ Chronic kidney disease
- ✓ Liver disease.
- ✓ Thyroid disorders.
- ✓ Use of drugs of abuse.
- ✓ Use of medications.

Etiology and pathophysiological elements

Physiological gynecomastia	Newborns (due to stimulation of maternal estradiol and progesterone). Puberty (an imbalance between estradiol and testosterone. It disappears around 2 or 3 years later). Older adults (increased peripheral aromatase activity secondary to increased body fat, increased LH, and decreased testosterone)
Pathological gynecomastia	Increased estrogen Tumors: Leydig cell tumor. Sertoli cell tumor. Adrenal tumor Granulosa tumor. Gonadal or extra gonadal germ cell tumor. Non-tumor: Higher aromatase activity. Displacement of estrogen from sex hormone-binding globulin. Decreased resistance to testosterone and androgens: Klinefelter syndrome. 17-oxosteroid reductase deficiency. Kallmann syndrome. Kennedy disease. Other diseases End-stage kidney disease. Liver disease. Thyrotoxicosis Spinal cord disorders. Drugs or drugs Marijuana Ketoconazole. Ranitidine. Cimetidine.

	Spironolactone Ethanol Metronidazole. Others.

Histopathology

The typical features of gynecomastia include proliferation of the stroma and ducts, as well as loose stroma, in acute cases, while dense stroma with few ducts appears in chronic cases.

Diagnostic criteria

Clinic	***Clinic history*** Onset and duration of gynecomastia. Associated additional symptoms. Investigate problems with specific systems (adrenal, prostate, lungs, liver, kidneys, testicles, thyroid). Family, genetic, medical or recreational drug history. ***Physical exam*** On head and neck examination look for abnormal masses. Carefully evaluate the thyroid. The breast examination should describe the nature of the tissue, especially skin changes, nipple discharge, tenderness, asymmetry, atrophy, or enlargement. Differentiate from pseudogynecomastia (circumferential fat in the subareolar area). Examine for presence of feminizing traits. *Classification* *Grade I*: small enlargement, no excess skin. *Grade IIa:* moderate enlargement, without excess skin. *Grade IIb:* moderate enlargement with extra skin. *Grade III:* marked enlargement with extra skin
Paraclinical	Based on clinical findings and medical history, orient

	paraclinicians for the specific cause. Serum testosterone levels. LH and FSH levels. Estradiol Thyroid function tests. Kidney function tests Liver function tests. Karyotype. Testicular ultrasound. Mammogram or ultrasound. Abdominal computed tomography.

Treatment options

The main goal of treatment is to resolve the specific underlying cause. Medical treatment aimed at reducing gynecomastia is not very effective when it lasts for a long time. Drugs such as clomiphene, danazol and tamoxifen are used frequently in acute cases with variable success.
Grade I or IIa patients: liposuction and surgical excision may be indicated in chronic cases.
Grade IIb patients: open surgical excision is indicated. Resection of the skin is possible if there is a large ptosis.

Follow-up peculiarities

Although gynecomastia is not life-threatening, it does cause significant emotional distress. Consider performing specific follow-up in cases where there is a high risk of other complications associated with the underlying cause, for example, in Klinefelter syndrome, screening for male breast cancer should be performed.

Bibliographic references

1. Brown JD. Critique of "Risk of Gynecomastia with Users of Proton Pump Inhibitors". Pharmacotherapy. 2019 Jul; 39 (7): 791.
2. Rasko YM, Rosen C, Ngaage LM, Al Fadil S, Elegbede A, Ihenatu C, Nam AJ, Slezak S. Surgical Management of Gynecomastia: A Review of the Current Insurance Coverage Criteria. Plast. Reconstr. Surg. 2019 May; 143 (5): 1361-1368.

Chapter 359. Andropause

Also known as late-onset hypogonadism, defined as a clinical and biochemical syndrome related to advanced age in men, and which is characterized by the deficiency of serum levels of testosterone, which is below the expected level in a healthy adult man. Andropause corresponds to the normal aging process of man, in which there is a decrease in the functional capacity of Leydig cells, as well as a slight reduction in testicular volume, among others. However, it is a controversial term today.

Statistics and epidemiology

An elderly man is considered to be over 65 years old. It is estimated that by 2030 the elderly population of the United States will be about 22%. With aging, testosterone levels decrease by 1% per year.
The level of testosterone is reduced in aging in patients with chronic pathologies.

Risk groups or factors:

It is an expected process of aging. However, testosterone reductions are more significant in subjects with chronic pathologies:
- ✓ Obesity.
- ✓ Diabetes mellitus type 2.
- ✓ Emotional stress
- ✓ Polypharmacy.

Etiology and trigger mechanisms

After the age of 30 or 40, a slow, almost imperceptible decrease in the frequency of pulsatile GnRH stimuli begins at the hypothalamic level. As age advances, the defect in GnRH production becomes more and more marked, causing hypogonadotropic hypogonadism. It is likely that this condition is associated with the increase in body fat that accompanies the aging process, especially the increase in visceral fat.

In addition, during aging, alterations in the testicular microcirculation begin to develop and degenerative changes appear in the Leydig cells, together with a reduction in the sensitivity to LH in them. This results in a decrease in testosterone production.

The etiopathogenic mechanisms therefore involve hypothalamic and testicular defects, associated with biological aging, which leads to a reduction in circulating testosterone and the development of andropause symptoms.

Diagnostic criteria

Clinic	Be sure to collect a complete medical history that allows you to identify other pathologies or risk factors not associated with andropause. Reduced testosterone in the elderly man is associated with: Changes in body composition. Anemia. Depression.

	Fatigue or decreased energy. Reduction of muscle strength. Decrease in bone mineral density. Decreased libido and morning erections. Erectile dysfunction.
Paraclinical	Two different measurements of free testosterone (below 8 nmol / L or below 300 ng / dl). LH level (elevated)

Treatment options

Lifestyle changes, especially in obese or overweight patients. Encourage your patients to reduce body fat through dietary changes and physical exercise. Consider referral to nutritionist.

Testosterone replacement therapy. Different preparations can be indicated according to the individual characteristics of the patient:

Testosterone enanthate or cypionate intramuscularly every 2 or 3 hours.

It may indicate testosterone gel, when required to maintain constant appropriate values. However, the price is higher.

The oral presentation of testosterone has an alkyl radical at carbon 17, which gives it a hepatotoxic potential, this administration is not recommended.

Follow-up peculiarities:

For treatment monitoring, it is recommended to establish follow-up visits 3 to 6 months after the start of testosterone treatment. In the consultation, you should ask about the patient's experience with the drug, both its effectiveness and the appearance of adverse effects. If the patient does not report symptomatic improvement, it is recommended to suspend the drug.

Check hemoglobin levels, hematocrit, prostate antigen, and rectal exam periodically during treatment.

Bibliographic references

1. Dorantes and Martínez. Clinical endocrinology 5th edition, Editorial El Manual Moderno 2016.
2. Parminder Singh. Andropause: Current concepts. Indian J Endocrinol Metab. 2013 Dec; 17 (Suppl 3): S621-S629.
3. Shlomo Melmed, Richard J. Auchus, Allison B. Goldfine, Ronald J. Kowning, Clifford Rosen. Williams Textbook of Endocrinology 14Th edition. ELSEVIER, 2020.

Chapter 360. Male Hormone Replacement

Maintaining proper physical and emotional well-being in men requires the presence of the sex hormone known as testosterone, an essential hormone for men. However, in male hypogonadism, an endocrine condition characterized by testosterone deficiency, it is associated with the potential to cause psychosocial complaints and multiple morbidities. Testosterone is a hormone necessary for differentiation, growth, development, and maintenance of the male phenotype.

Indications

The FDA approves the use of testosterone as replacement therapy in men with symptoms of hypogonadism and low levels of testosterone.

Symptoms suggestive of hypogonadism

Decreased spontaneous erections.
Decrease in nocturnal tumescence of the penis.
Reduction of beard growth.
Decreased libido
Reduction of the testicles.

Initial laboratory tests

They should include 2 measurements of serum testosterone during the morning (8 to 10 am), if both results indicate reduced levels (total testosterone <300ng / dL or free testosterone <5 to 9 ng / dL), complementary studies are carried out to identify secondary hypogonadism (See chapter 231).

For low normal testosterone results and positive cynical symptoms, tests to assess free or bioavailable testosterone are indicated:

- ✓ Sex hormone transporter globulin.
- ✓ Albumin.

Administration of male hormone replacement therapy

Objective: normalization of total testosterone levels combined with improvement of signs and symptoms.

General recommendations

Avoid 17-alpha-alkylated androgens and methylated oral formulations due to risk of hepatotoxicity.
Initial treatment should consist of short-acting formulations for rapid discontinuation in case of adverse effects.
It is recommended to prescribe commercially manufactured testosterone products avoiding the use of compound testosterone, however, if these preparations are prescribed, do additional monitoring and dose adjustment to ensure that therapeutic levels are appropriate.
Perform regular hematologic evaluations:
Before treatment (including Hemoglobin / Hematocrit)
At 3, 6 and 12 months after starting treatment and then annually.
When you need to make dose adjustments or change the preparation.

Formulations considerations

Transdermal gels and muscle injections are the main options.
Forms of administration:
Oral.

Oral.

Transdermal (granule, solution, gel, patch).

Intramuscular

Oral testosterone tablets and capsules should not be used for the treatment of testosterone deficiencies due to probable adverse hepatic effects and reduced therapeutic efficacy.

Oral formulations should not be swallowed or chewed.

The administration of a testosterone gel should be applied to the shoulder, upper part of the arms or the abdomen. It should not be applied to the scrotum.

The nasal testosterone gel is administered three times a day.

The recommended testosterone patch application site is on the back, abdomen, thigh, or upper arm.

The subcutaneous testosterone granules are placed every 3 to 6 months in the subdermal fat of the buttocks, thigh, or abdominal wall.

Intramuscular injections of testosterone (with testosterone cypionate or testosterone enanthate) should be administered in recommended doses of 50 to 100 mg per week, or 100 to 200 mg every two weeks.

An extra-long-acting form of intramuscular injection (testosterone undecanoate) is currently approved, which can be administered at a dose of 750 mg followed by another dose 4 weeks after the initial administration and subsequent doses every 10 weeks.

Adverse effects associated with the formulations

Testosterone presentation	Adverse effect
Buccal tablets	Irritation of the gums and oral mucosa.
Testosterone gels	Transfer to children or women who come into contact with the gel.
Patches	Skin reactions
Injectables	Fluctuations in mood, libido and energy.
All	They increase cardiovascular risk. Erythrocytosis (increased risk of venous thromboembolism). Increased PSA levels (prostate cancer should be ruled

	out before starting therapy, as it can aggravate the disease process).

Contraindications

Elevated PSA> 4 ng / ml.
Undiagnosed palpable prostate nodule.
History of breast cancer.
Prostate cancer.
Myocardial infarction or stroke (in the last 6 months).
Uncontrollable heart failure.
Untreated obstructive sleep apnea.
Men planning fertility.
Hematocrit greater than 48%.
Increase in PSA level greater than 3vng / ml in high-risk patients (African-American, first-degree family history of prostate cancer).

Follow-up strategies

One month after starting treatment, the morning testosterone level should be assessed.

After one year of treatment, the morning testosterone level should be requested for the next 3-6 months, as well as other studies such as LFT, PSA, lipid profile, DRE, estradiol, hemoglobin, hematocrit, blood pressure.

Annually after one year, the lipid profile, DRE, estradiol, PSA, Hgb and Hct, and blood pressure are measured again.

Bibliographic references

1. Park, HJ, Ahn, ST, & Moon, DG (2019). Evolution of Guidelines for Testosterone Replacement Therapy.

Journal of clinical medicine, 8 (3), 410.https://doi.org/10.3390/jcm8030410
2. Zitzmann M. Hormoners atz therapie des Mannes [Hormone Replacement Therapy in Males]. Dtsch Med Wochenschr. 2018 Sep; 143 (19): 1405-1416. German. doi: 10.1055 / s-0043-118752. Epub 2018 Sep 19. PMID: 30231287.
3. Sizar O, Pico J. Androgen replacement. [Updated May 24, 2020]. In: StatPearls [Internet]. Treasure Island (FL): Stat Pearls Publishing; 2020 January-. Available in:https://www.ncbi.nlm.nih.gov/books/NBK534853/
4. Osterberg, EC, Bernie, AM, & Ramasamy, R. (2014). Risks of testosterone replacement therapy in men. Indian journal of urology: IJU: journal of the Urological Society of India, 30 (1), 2–7.https://doi.org/10.4103/0970-1591.124197

Key Topics in Endocrinology

Abstracts

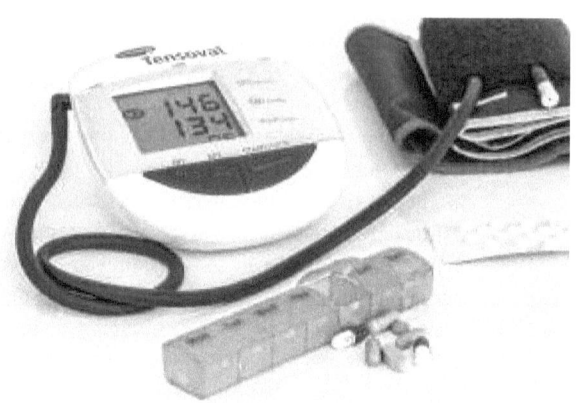

1885

I. Suspicious clinical symptoms and signs of endocrine disease

Because the endocrine glands are inaccessible on routine physical examination (with the exception of the thyroid gland and gonads), the physician must take a thorough and complete medical history, and appropriately ask about endocrine signs and symptoms by apparatus and systems. , family and personal history, evolution of puberty, menarche, sexual development and maturation, skin alterations, neurological manifestations, among others, in order to guide the physical examination in the most enriching way to identify and diagnose endocrine pathologies.

Sign / symptom	Definition / Description	Probable diagnoses
Alteration of body weight		
Thinness	Body weight below the estimated average for your sex, height and age in the community in which you reside.	Idiopathic, malnutrition, eating pattern disorders (anorexia nervosa, etc.), hyperthyroidism, use of slimming drugs, chronic infections, psychiatric disorders, malignant neoplasms, pheochromocytoma, diabetes with glycosuria, Addison's disease, Hypercalcemia.
Slimming	Individual with a previous weight greater than the current one.	
Malnutrition	Consequence of a diet deficient in calories, protein and nutrients for a prolonged period.	
Weight gain (overweight, obesity, morbid obesity)	Adipose tissue gain. Weight gain as a result of an excessive increase in body fat storage. It exceeds	Overfeeding, sedentary lifestyle. Cushing syndrome (central obesity pattern)

	20% of desirable weight, while morbid obesity is considered when it has exceeded 40% of body weight.	Acromegaly. Hypothyroidism Diabetes mellitus type 2. Metabolic syndrome. Cyclic or indeterminate edema. Genetic predisposition, Hypogonadotropic hypogonadism. Lipomastia
Central or android obesity	Subcutaneous fatty deposit predominantly in the abdominal region.	
Gynecoid obesity	Gluteofemoral subcutaneous adipose deposit. Typically female obesity pattern.	
Growth disturbances		
Dwarfism	Growth defect consisting of a delay in height. It corresponds to a height lower than 40% of the mean for age and sex in the subject's population group. When the reduction in height is 20%, it is called a subject of small stature.	Craniopharyngioma. Chronic infections Down's Syndrome. Celiac Disease. Infant hypothyroidism. Rickets. Turner syndrome.
Giantism	Height growth that exceeds normal height. In adults, gigantism is estimated when the height is greater than 203 cm, while in children it is 3 standard deviations above the normal height for their sex and age.	Acromegaly. Hypogonadism Hyperthyroidism
Skin and adnexal changes		
Thick skin	Manifestation of rough, hard and thick skin.	Giantism. Acromegaly. Hypothyroidism
Thin skin	Evidence of thin, hot and humid skin with sweating and easy dermographism.	Hyperthyroidism
Purple stretch marks	They especially appear in the anterolateral and lower abdomen, buttocks, breasts,	Adrenocortical syndromes with increased plasma cortisol (Cushing's

	and upper arms and thighs.	syndrome).
Acne	Common open comedones among healthy young men and women during pubertal.	Physiological Corticosadrenal hyperfunction Androgen-producing ovarian tumor. Polycystic ovarian syndrome.
Alopecia	Significant hair loss caused by physical, chemical or genetic predisposition reasons.	Malnutrition, genetics, ringworm of the scalp, burns, mechanical or chemical injuries, trichotillomania, discoid lupus, tumors, X-linked ichthyosis, hypoparathyroidism, hypopituitarism, hypothyroidism.
Telogen effluvium	Rapid hair loss throughout the scalp, often reversible resulting from disturbances in the normal hair cycle.	Systemic diseases that cause alopecia, pregnancy, intense emotional stress, sudden weight loss.
Androgenic alopecia	Condition that combines genetic predisposition and action of androgenic hormones. It can occur in men and women.	Genetic predisposition.
Hypertrichosis	Exaggerated increase in normal hair in women in areas where they exist according to the female pattern (legs and forearms)	Genetic predisposition.
Hirsutism	Male pattern of hair growth in women. It is generally triggered by excessive androgen production.	Cushing's disease, polycystic ovary disease, 21-hydroxylase deficiencies, 3 beta hydroxysteroid dehydrogenase isomerase, 11 beta-hydroxylase, adrenal tumors, use of drugs (diazoxide, minoxidil,

		phenytoin, glucocorticoids), other conditions associated with hyperandrogenism.
	Mood disturbance	
Asthenia	Feeling of tiredness or exhaustion prior to doing any strenuous activity.	It can be associated with almost any pathology. When accompanied by changes in body weight, it can be associated with Addison's syndrome and hyperthyroidism (decreased body weight), Cushing's syndrome, and hypothyroidism (weight gain).
	Eye disorders	
Exophthalmos	It is the protrusion of the eyeballs out of the orbital cavity as a result of the increase in retro-orbital tissue. It is generally bilateral, and presents an increase in the lid opening and with fixed gaze.	Graves-Basedow hyperthyroidism
waterfalls	Lens opacity	Hypoparathyroidism Mellitus diabetes
Hemianopia	Blindness or lack of vision that affects only half of the visual field.	Compression of the optic chiasm (pituitary tumor)
	Olfactory disturbances	
Anosmia / Hyposmia	Absence or decrease of the olfactory capacity.	Hypogonadotropic hypogonadism
Hyperosmia	Alteration where olfactory sensitivity is increased.	Pregnancy Graves-Basedow disease
	Language disorders	
Macroglossia	Increase of the tissue of the tongue for which it becomes larger than normal.	Acromegaly Congenital hypothyroidism. Down's Syndrome. Beckwith-Wiedermann

		syndrome
	Neck disorders	
Goiter	Enlargement of the thyroid gland	Congenital goiter. Hypothyroidism Hyperthyroidism Multinodular goiter. Malignant thyroid neoplasm.
Strumitis	Inflammatory processes that have been established in a goiter.	Inflammatory processes
Thyroiditis	Inflammation of the thyroid gland. It can be acute, subacute and chronic according to evolution.	Thyroid infections secondary to upper respiratory infection.
	Breast disorders	
Gynecomastia	Increase in the size of the mammary glands in males can be unilateral or bilateral. Increases breast stroma and glandular tissue.	Physiological (neonatal, pubertal, senile). Hyperprolactinemia. Feedback. Resistance to androgen action. Increased estrogen production (estrogen-secreting Leydig cell tumor, feminizing adrenocortical neoplasms). Sertoli cell tumor. Obesity. Graves-Basedown disease. Hepatic cirrhosis. Hypogonadotropic hypogonadism. Klinefelter syndrome. Congenital anorchia. Prolactinoma.
Galactorrhea	Elimination of secretions through the breast, lacteal secretions in a non-lactating woman or after 6 months postpartum in a non-breastfeeding woman.	Physiological. Craniopharyngiomas. Prolactinomas. Mixed adenomas. Sarcoidosis Dysgerminomas.

	This can be unilateral or bilateral.	Primary hypothyroidism. Nelson syndrome. Addison's disease. Primary hypothyroidism. Drugs (benzodiazepines, reserpine, tricyclic antidepressants, opiates, cimetidine, cocaine, benzodiazepines, among others). Rathke's bursa cyst.
Muscle disorders		
Muscular atrophy	Wear, loss or decrease of skeletal muscle, which can occur with or without alterations in sensitivity. It is the reduction of muscle mass.	Long-term decompensated diabetes mellitus. Cushing's disease. Adrenal cortical insufficiency. Acromegaly. Male hypogonadism due to eunucoidism or castration.
Muscle hypertrophy	Increase in muscle size due to increased number of myofibrils.	Early puberty. Marked hypothyroidism or myxedema. Early stages of acromegaly. Adrenogenital syndromes
Spasms / Tetany	It is a series of contractions of a muscle or muscle group. For its part, tetany is defined as the most prolonged or continuous contraction, which can cause altered position or be limited to a small movement.	Hypocalcemia Hypomagnesemia Dehydration Hypokalemia Pregnancy. Drugs Hypoparathyroidism
Bone alterations		
Osteoporosis	Decrease in bone mineral density that increases the risk of pathological or compression fractures.	Cushing's syndrome. Hyperthyroidism Aging.
Osteomalacia	Syndrome characterized by softening of the bones	Vitamin D deficiency. Celiac disease.

		caused by vitamin D deficiency.
Osteodystrophy	Bone atrophy with great osteoclastic activity and with replacement of bone by fibrous tissue. Radiological signs similar to primary hyperparathyroidism (subperiosteal resorption of the phalanges, bone cysts, loss of the lamina dura of the teeth, among others)	Secondary hyperparathyroidism.
Urinary volume alterations		
Polyuria	Elimination of urine greater than 3 liters in 24 hours.	Diabetes insipidus Hyperaldosteronism Hyperparathyroidism Mellitus diabetes. Primary polydipsia.
Menstrual disturbances		
Amenorrhea	Absence of menstruation for 6 consecutive months in women who have previously had menstruation or absence of menarche at 16 years of age.	Turner syndrome, Kallmann syndrome, hypothalamic anovulation, hypothyroidism, hyperthyroidism, hyperandrogenemia, anatomical defects, primary ovarian galla (gonadal dysgenesis, chromosomal mosaicisms, among others).
Oligomenorrhea	Menstrual bleeding every 35 days or more.	Polycystic ovarian syndrome. Oral contraceptives. Obesity
Neurological disorders		
Paresthesia	Abnormal sensation of tingling, shooting sensations, tingling, cold or heat, which may be experienced on the skin by subjects with nervous or	Diabetic neuropathy. Hypothyroidism Vitamin deficiency (group B). Malnutrition.

	circulatory disorders.	
Tremors	These are rhythmic movements such as involuntary jerks in one or more parts of the body. It occurs due to muscle contractions.	Hyperthyroidism Pheochromocytoma Excess catecholamine secretion. Anxiety or panic Drugs (caffeine, corticosteroids, amphetamines, others).
Osteotendinous hyperreflexia	Increase or exaltation of the tendon reflexes.	Hyperthyroidism
Slow reflexes	Slow response speed when stimulating reflexes and with a delayed recovery phase.	Hypothyroidism
Convulsions	Involuntary, violent and pathological tonic-clonic contractions.	Hypoglycemic crisis. Hypocalcemia Brain neoplasm Brain infections Phenylketonuria
Eat	Alteration of the state of consciousness characterized by a deep state of unconsciousness. It causes an inability to respond to external stimuli or internal needs.	Eat hyperosmolar. Diabetic cetoacidosis Severe hypoglycemia Kidney failure (diabetic nephropathy). Severe hyperparathyroidism Dehydration Hemoconcentration Nephrolithiasis Nephrocalcinosis. Cushing's disease complicated by renal atherosclerotic manifestations. Acute adrenal cortical insufficiency
Sexual disturbances		
Decreased libido	Reduction of interest in sex or in sexual relations both in initiative, frequency and intensity of responses to	Hypogonadism Depression Menopause Mellitus diabetes.

	erotic stimuli. It can occur in both men and women.	Drugs (beta-blockers, clonidine, diuretics, methyldopa, oral contraceptives, benzodiazepines). Prostate cancer. Chronic kidney disease
Impotence	Also called erectile sexual dysfunction. It is the failure to achieve an erection or to maintain it firmly enough to allow sexual intercourse.	Obesity. Heart disease. Mellitus diabetes. Metabolic syndrome. Multiple sclerosis Psychological factors Drugs (propanolol, ketoconazole, spironolactone, finasteride, others). Primary testicular disorders. Hyperprolactinemia. Hypopituitarism.

Bibliographic references

1. Shlomo Melmed, Richard J. Ahúchas, Alison B. Golfines, Ronald J. Konin, Lifford Rosen. Williams Text book of Endocrinology 14Th edition. ELSEVIER, 2020.
2. Argente. Alvarez. Medical semiology. Physiopathology, Semiotechnics and Propedeutics. Teaching based on the patient. 6th edition. Editorial Panamericana, 2011.
3. Raimundo Llanio Navarro, Gabriel Perdomo González. Clinical propaedeutics and Medical Semiology. Editorial Medical Sciences, 2003.
4. Yu J. (2014). Endocrine disorders and the neurologic manifestations. Annals of pediatric endocrinology & metabolism, 19 (4), 184–190.https://doi.org/10.6065/apem.2014.19.4.184

II. Role of dynamic tests in the diagnosis of endocrinopathies

To a large extent, the proper diagnosis and treatment of endocrinology depends on the use and correct interpretation of diagnostic tests. Dynamic endocrine tests provide the physician with a broad perspective of the functional status of the endocrine glands so that, together with the clinical correlation and baseline laboratories, reach the timely diagnosis and treatment for the patient.

Pituitary gland

Dynamic tests of the anterior pituitary

Proof	Indication	Contraindication	Interpretation
Insulin tolerance test	ACTH and cortisol reserve assessment Evaluation of GH reserve in children with growth retardation. Differentiation between Cushing's syndrome from depression. GH response in adults.	Epilepsy. Untreated hypothyroidism. Serum cortisol less than 100 nmol / L. Ischemic heart disease.	The adequate GH response is the increase greater than 6 mcg / L. In adults, this may indicate hypopituitarism. In children a normal response is considered in increases greater than 12 mcg / L. In Cushing syndrome, there will be an increase of less than 170 nmol / L higher in fluctuations in cortisol level. The correct response for cortisol is greater than 170 nmol to greater than 500 nmol. The test cannot be interpreted unless hypoglycemia <2.2 mmol / L is obtained.
Glucagon test	It evaluates the reserve of GH and ACTH /	Pheochromocytoma Insulinoma. Starvation for more	The appropriate cortisol response is the higher rise from 170 nmol / L to more

1895

	cortisol, mainly when induced by insulin, hypoglycemia is contraindicated.	than 48 hours. Glycogen storage diseases. Severe hypocortisolemia (level <55 nmol / L at 09:00 hours). Thyroxine deficiency (can reduce cortisol and GH response).	than 500 nmol / L. The adequate increase in GH is values greater than 6 mcg / L.
Thyrotrophin Releasing Hormone (TRH) Test	Assess the TSH pool. Differential diagnosis of pituitary and hypothalamic causes of TSH deficiency.	Patients must stop thyroxine medication for 3 weeks prior to testing. For this reason, it is rarely used in people taking thyroxine.	The normal TSH result is the higher increase of 5 mU / L with a value of 30 minutes exceeding the value of 60 minutes. When the 60-minute sample exceeds the 30-minute value, it is indicative of primary hypothalamic disease. In hyperthyroidism, TSH remains suppressed. In hypothyroidism, an exaggerated response occurs.
GnRH / LHRH Gonadotropin Releasing Hormone Test	Confirm precocious puberty. Investigate possible gonadotropin deficiencies.		Normal peaks occur within 30 to 60 minutes. The LH must exceed 10 U / L, while the FDH must be greater than 2U / L. An indication of early hypopituitarism is an inadequate response. Gonadotropin deficiency is diagnosed at baseline rather than dynamic response. In males it is based on low testosterone levels without elevated basal gonadotropins. In females, low estradiol level without elevated basal gonadotropins without response to clomiphene. Prepubertal children should have no FSH or LH response to LHRH. If sex steroids are present, the pituitary will respond to LHRH.
Combined pituitary function test	Examines all components of anterior	Epilepsy. Untreated hypothyroidism	*Currently not used* In the "Split" protocol the response of prolactin and

	pituitary function, particularly used in pituitary tumors or after treatment of neoplasms.	(impairs the cortisol and GH response). Ischemic heart disease.	GH to TRH can be observed. In the normal response, prolactin increases by 100% to its baseline level, whereas in prolactinomas there is a subnormal response. In normal people, a decrease in GH occurs with TRH, and in people with acromegaly it increases by 80%. The "split" protocol, the loss of paradoxical increase in TRH in acromegaly is a good indicator of successful treatment.
Low-dose dexamethasone suppression test	Cushing's Syndrome Screening. Differential diagnosis between PCOS, CAH and autonomous secretion of androgen neoplasms	People taking enzyme inducers. Pregnancy. Caution in DM and psychologically unstable patients.	If the cortisol value at 09:00 is less than 50 nmol / L, the patient is suppressed. Failure to achieve suppression is observed in patients with autonomous cortisol secretion. In virilization of PCOS or partial CAH, there will be complete / partial suppression of testosterone.
Exercise test	Children with growth retardation. Preferably, based on evaluation of reduced growth rate and random GH less than 15 mU / L.		A normal GH response greater than 15 mU / L, absolves any investigation of GH deficiency and precludes the need for further testing. A GH response less than 15 mU / L indicates that the child may require a formal test or a repeated exercise test.
Arginine stimulation test	Children with defined growth retardation and GH below normal in stimulation test (<15 mU / L).		A GH response greater than 15 mU / L excludes GH deficiency. A GH response between 7 to 15 mU / L indicates partial GH deficiency (should be investigated by a second formal stimulation test). A GH response less than 7 mU / L should be confirmed with a second test, although if there are compatible clinical and auxiliary findings,

			replacement therapy may be considered. Boys with delayed pubertal growth may show a lower than normal GH response if sex hormone prep is not done.
Oral glucose tolerance test for acromegaly	Clinical suspicion of acromegaly		Healthy people have a decrease in GH levels after oral glucose. At least one of the samples during the test must present undetectable GH levels (<0.6 mcg / L). Lack of suppression or a paradoxical increase in GH indicates acromegaly.

Dynamic tests of the posterior pituitary

Proof	Indications	Contraindications	Interpretation
Water deprivation test	Principle: dehydrate until ADH secretion concentrates urine. Diabetes insipidus Primary polydipsia.	Exclude other causes of polyuria (hypokalaemia, hypercalcaemia, chronic renal failure, diuretics, hyperglycemia). Deficiency of the anterior pituitary hormones.	Normal: with dehydration, a plasma concentration occurs, but less than 300 mosmol / kg. Urine is concentrated at more than 600 mosm / kg. Primary polydipsia or partial diabetes insipidus: it begins with a low osmolarity of the plasma, which is concentrated to normal during stage I. The urine is concentrated although it may be a subnormal response. Central diabetes insipidus (CID): excessive concentration (greater than 300 mosmol / kg) with inadequate hypotonic urine. After DDAVP, the patient with DIC and ADH deficiency can concentrate urine to more than 150% of the previous highest value.

Thyroid gland

Proof	Indication	Contraindication	Interpretation
Pentagastrin test for medullary thyroid carcinoma	Suspicion of medullary thyroid carcinoma. Suspicion of MEN2. Screening of families with medullary thyroid carcinoma. People with baseline TC greater than 22.1 ng / L in men or> 10.8 ng / L in women.	Allergy or anaphylaxis on repeated administration.	Stimulated CT between 30 to 100 ng / L: Recommend follow-up screening. Patients with stimulated CT between 100 to 200 ng / L: C-cell hyperplasia or probable early MTC. Stimulated CT> 200 ng / L: probable TCM.
Calcium test for medullary thyroid cancer	Suspicion of acalcitoninemia. Suspicion of medullary thyroid carcinoma. Suspicion of MEN2.	Bleeding disorders	In medullary thyroid carcinoma, there is often an increase in fasting serum calcitonin (> 90 ng / L), although it may be in the normal range. Provocative tests improve the sensitivity to the measurement of calcitonin. The normal range for the peak of calcitonin after calcium infusion ranges from 100 to 200 ng / L.
Radioactive iodine uptake test	Differentiate between types of high and low uptake hyperthyroidism. Graves disease not evident.		Normal: Average for 24 hour RAIU test are 8-25%. High RAIU: Graves disease, toxic multinodular goiter, toxic adenoma. Hashimoto toxicosis, Choriocarcinoma. Low RAIU: subacute, painless thyroiditis, acute iodine-loading Graves

	disease, iodine-induced hyperthyroidism, metastatic functioning thyroid carcinoma.

Parathyroid glands

Pathology	Proof	Result (examples)
Familial hypocalciuric hypercalcemia	Calcium in urine Creatinine in urine Plasma creatinine. Plasma calcium	1.0 mmol / L 6.3 mmol / L 130 umol / L 2.65 mmol / L
Primary hyperparathyroidism	Calcium in urine Creatinine in urine Plasma creatinine Plasma calcium	2.2 mmol / L 1.4 mmol / L 74 umol / L 3.3 mmol / L
Calcium clearance	*Formula* [Calcium in urine (mmol / l) x volume of urine (ml)] / [Calcium in plasma (mmol / l) x 1440]	
Creatinine clearance	*Formula* [Urine creatinine (mmol / l) x urine volume (ml)] / [Plasma creatinine (mmol / l) x 1440]	

Kidney glands

Proof	Indication	Contra-indicated	Interpretation
Synacthen Short Test	Hypoadrenalism due to pituitary hypofunction. Adrenal function after a prolonged course of corticosteroids or after suppression due to Cushing's Syndrome, after removal of adrenal adenoma. Diagnosis and characterization of 21-hydroxylase deficiency and other causes of adrenal hyperplasia. Diagnosis of non-	Cortisol greater than 550 nmol / L. Random cortisol greater than 450 nmol / L.	Normal response (test performed at 09:00): stimulated plasma cortisol greater than 550 nmol / L and incremental increase of at least 170 nmol / L. Altered cortisol response and ACTH greater than 200 ng / L, indicates primary adrenal insufficiency. If ACTH is less than 10 ng / L, it indicates a diagnosis of secondary adrenal insufficiency. Response of 17-OH progesterone in suspected 21-hydroxylase deficiency

Test	Indications	Contraindications	Interpretation
	classical congenital adrenal hyperplasia (hyperandrogenic woman if basal 17-hydroxyprogesterone follicular phase is greater than 6.0 nmol / L).		(non-classical): there is an increase after stimulation with ACTH greater than 30 nmol / L, which varies according to whether the patient is heterozygous or homozygous.
Synacthen Long Test	Difference between primary and secondary hypoadrenalism. Confirmation of the diagnosis of hypoadrenalism.		Normal response: basal cortisol greater than 170 nmol / L increasing to more than 900 nmol / L (peak). Samples from 09:00, 09:30 and 10:00 can be interpreted as the Synacthen short test. Little or no response occurs in primary adrenal insufficiency. In secondary adrenal insufficiency some patients show an increase in cortisol, which may be delayed. A subnormal response does not exclude this. ACTH must be measured.
Plasma aldosterone and plasma renin activity: Saline infusion test	Accelerated hypertension. Drug resistant hypertension. Hypertension with incidental arenaloma. Hypertension with hypokalemia.		Plasma aldosterone levels after infusion less than 140 pmol / L indicate an unlikely diagnosis of hyperaldosteronism. Levels above 280 pmol / L are a likely sign of hyperaldosteronism. Values between 140 to 280 pmol / L are indeterminate results.
Pentolinium suppression test	Practically obsolete Excludes diagnosis of pheochromocytoma with hypertension.	In frail patients and / or with severe coronary or carotid diseases, as well as vascular diseases, it should be done with care.	Normal: plasma epinephrine and noradrenaline initially elevated, but within the normal range with pentolinium. Autonomous secretion is not suppressed in pheochromocytoma.
Clonidine suppression test	Excludes diagnosis of pheochromocytoma.	Frail patient with a history of hypotension or severe coronary or carotid	Normal: plasma catecholamine suppression a = 50% of its initial value and a = 2.96 nmol / L. Patients with

| | disease. | | pheochromocytoma should not suppress and the diagnosis is indicated. |

Endocrine pancreas

Proof	Indication	Contra-indicated	Interpretation
Glucose tolerance test	Suspected diabetes mellitus (not required when fasting venous blood glucose is greater than 7.0 mmol / L or random blood glucose greater than 11.1 mmol / L). Acromegaly (establish diagnosis and follow-up after treatment). Suspicion of reactive hypoglycemia.		MD:> 7.0 mmol / L (fast) or> 11.1 mmol / L (2 hours after glucose loading). Glucose intolerance:> 7.8 to 11.0 mmol / L (2 hours after glucose loads). Altered fasting glucose: greater than 6.1 to 7.0 mmol / L (fast). Normal: 6.1 mmol / L (fast) and 7.8 mmol / L (2 hours after glucose load).
Autonomic functioning tests	Suspicion of diabetic autonomic neuropathy. Shy-Drager syndrome. Suspicion of autonomic failure due to other causes.	Patients with proliferative retinopathies (do not perform the Valsalva maneuver). Atrial fibrillation (non-interpretable tests).	Tests Valsalva relationship Normal = 1.21 Limit 1.11 to 1.20 Abnormal = 1.10 HR (max - min): Normal> 15 Limit 11 to 14 Abnormal <10 Ratio 30: 15 Normal> 1.04 Limit: 1.01 to 1.03 Abnormal = 1.00 Drop in BP: Normal = 10 Limit: 11 to 29 Abnormal = 30

1902

Bibliographic references

1. Lavin N, editor. Manual of endocrinology and metabolism. 4th ed. Philadelphia: Wolters Kluwer / Lippincott Williams & Wilkins Health; 2009. 837 p.
2. Andrew Hattersley Maria Barnard John Wilding Stephen Gilbey Peter Hammond, et al. Endocrine Unit. Imperial College Healthcare NHS. Trust Charing Cross, Hammersmith and St. Mary's Hospitals Endocrinology Handbook. March 2010.

III. Interaction and referral of the endocrinologist with other specialists

Mainly, the function of a multidisciplinary team consists of bringing together a group of doctors specialized in various health fields, to determine a specific treatment and follow-up plan for each patient.
The interaction between different areas of medicine includes cooperation with the aim of improving the efficiency of treatment, improving the quality of life and covering all possible alterations caused by a common pathology according to the affected devices and systems.

Receiving referrals from major medical specialties

Clinical nutritionist
Clinical nutrition consists of a discipline that allows an approach based on the nutritional status of people, correlating biological, psychological and social aspects. This branch can cover both the prevention of more frequent nutritional problems, as well as guiding the patient in the treatment of diseases associated with eating and its complications.

Reasons for the most frequent referrals from the clinical nutritionist to endocrinology
Clinical nutritionists can identify signs and symptoms associated with underlying endocrine disorders or identify a

person's risk factor for the development of certain endocrine pathologies.

The clinical nutritionist can refer his patients to the endocrinology consultation when he suspects any of the following pathologies or when he considers appropriate a screening assessment in patients at risk:

- ✓ Obesity.
- ✓ Metabolic syndrome.
- ✓ Prediabetes.
- ✓ Mellitus diabetes.
- ✓ Hypoglycemic patient.
- ✓ Child with thinness.
- ✓ Child with obesity.
- ✓ Celiac Disease.
- ✓ Acanthosis nigricans patient.
- ✓ Patient with eating pattern disorders (anorexia nervosa, bulimia).
- ✓

Nephrology

Nephrology, a subspecialty of internal medicine specialized in the treatment of kidney diseases, collaborates in the treatment of kidney problems also associated with endocrine disorders, such as the kidney complications of diabetes mellitus. However, the nephrologist may indicate referral to the endocrine physician in the following conditions:

- ✓ Central diabetes insipidus.
- ✓ Type 1 and 2 diabetes mellitus.

Cardiology

Cardiovascular diseases, together with endocrine diseases, constitute the chronic pathologies with the highest morbidity and associated with higher mortality rates in the entire world population.

In addition, cardiovascular diseases represent the main cause of morbidity and mortality among type 2 diabetic patients, this being one of the most important reasons for consultation in endocrinology consultations.

Endocrine disorders can influence the cardiovascular system in various ways. An experienced cardiologist can observe clinical features among his patients that simulate cardiovascular diseases of endocrine etiology or that this coexists with a disease of the cardiovascular system itself.

Among the most common reference pathologies are:

- ✓ Prediabetes.
- ✓ Obesity.
- ✓ Mellitus diabetes.
- ✓ Hyperthyroidism.
- ✓ Hypothyroidism
- ✓ Hypertension refractory to treatment.
- ✓ Primary aldosteronism.
- ✓ Cushing's syndrome.
- ✓ Pheochromocytoma

Gynecology and Obstetrics

Endocrinology plays a fundamental role in various gynecological and reproductive disorders, acquiring considerable practical importance in the consultations of these areas of medicine. It is estimated that around 40% of patients in gynecological clinical practice have some problem associated with endocrinological disorders, whether it be family planning problems, female virilization traits, menstrual disorders, infertility, hormone replacement therapy in menopause, among others.

Some of the indications that a gynecologist or obstetrician might consider for referral to endocrinology are:

- ✓ Hormone replacement.
- ✓ Hirsutism
- ✓ Amenorrhea
- ✓ Galactorrhea.
- ✓ Sheehan syndrome.
- ✓ Feminine infertility.
- ✓ Recurring abortions.
- ✓ Polycystic ovarian syndrome.
- ✓ Turner syndrome.
- ✓ Hypogonadotropic hypogonadism.

Pediatrics

It constitutes in the area of medicine in charge of the study and / or evaluation of patients during their first evolutionary stages of development and maturation. Chronologically, it encompasses the ages of patients from birth to adolescence, which, depending on the country, can be up to 18 or 21 years of age.

In this pediatric stage, various endocrine pathologies are evident, among which those of genetic and / or autoimmune etiology stand out, such as type 1 diabetes mellitus, although cases of type 2 diabetes mellitus are seen more frequently as well as others Endocrine disorders associated with adulthood due to environmental factors coexisting with genetic susceptibility.

Endocrinological pathologies in pediatric age are not uncommon and different types of disorders can be diagnosed from the moment of birth. Among the most frequent reasons for referral are:

- ✓ Cryptorchidism.
- ✓ Type 1 diabetes mellitus.
- ✓ Early puberty.
- ✓ Delayed puberty.
- ✓ Suprarrenal insufficiency.
- ✓ Turner syndrome.
- ✓ Klinefelter syndrome.
- ✓ Ambiguous genitalia.
- ✓ 21-hydroxylase deficiency.

Geneticists

Genetic medicine consists of the study of heredity, that is, the process by which a father transmits certain genes to his offspring, including the traits associated with their mental and developmental capacities, the probability of contracting certain diseases, among others.

Various diseases of genetic origin can alter endocrine function at various levels. For this reason, the reasons for referral to endocrinology can be diverse. Some of them are found in Table 363-1.

Main clinical situations that the endocrinologist should refer to medical specialties

Each patient can present a wide variety of clinical manifestations typical of different areas of medical specialties. It is essential for the doctor to make a timely identification of the underlying clinical situations and make a timely referral.

References to any medical specialty must consider, in addition to the underlying endocrine pathology, the risk factors associated with lifestyle, family and personal history, among other variables.

Medical speciality	Description	Reason for referral
Clinical nutritionist	The treatment of pathologies mainly of metabolic and nutritional base, should be treated in conjunction with a clinical nutritionist or dietician nutritionist, so that a more efficient treatment plan can be established for the patient. The treating physician must make referral to nutrition in the following conditions.	Diabetes type 1. Type 2 diabetes. Gestational diabetes. Nephrolithiasis. Complications of diabetes. Patients with irritable bowel. Obesity. Patients with metabolic or bariatric surgery. Lactose intolerance. Nutritional deficiencies Infertile couple. Pregnant Celiac Disease. Elderly with sarcopenia. Child with thinness or extreme thinness. Metabolic syndrome. Prediabetic patient.
Genetic medicine	Every physician should consider referring his patients to the genetic specialty when he suspects that his patient is at risk of	Patients with one or more family members with a developmental disability, mental retardation, or a common congenital defect. Premature deaths in one or more family

	having a genetic disorder, or that he is affected by it in the current consultation.	members due to known or unknown medical conditions. Onset of endocrine diseases earlier than expected for it. Parents with confirmed offspring of genetic disease. Close consanguineous couples. *Most frequent pathologies that the endocrine should refer to genetic medicine:* Diabetes mellitus: monogenic, LADA, MODY. Hashimoto's chronic thyroiditis. Congenital hypothyroidism. Graves Basedow disease. Thyroid carcinoma Di George syndrome. Paget's disease of the bone (when other causes have been excluded). ACTH resistance syndrome. Congenital adrenal hyperplasia. Multiple endocrine neoplasia 1 and 2. Craniopharyngiomas. Turner syndrome. Klinefelter syndrome. Noonan syndrome. Kallmann syndrome. Ambiguous genitalia. Recurring abortions.
Psychology / psychiatry	Although the endocrine doctor can treat the hormonal imbalance caused by these disorders, the basic treatment is aimed at the resolution of the underlying psychological factors, for which the reference to the mental health unit should not be excluded.	Anorexia nervosa. Bulimia.
Nephrology	Endocrine disorders that require assessment by the nephrology service often include an assessment, indication for joint treatment, and long-term	Uncontrolled type 2 diabetes mellitus. Diabetic nephropathy. Nephrolithiasis. Nephrogenic diabetes insipidus. Thyroid storm. Turner syndrome.

	follow-up in a coordinated manner.	
Cardiology	Cardiology referral is common in patients admitted to the hospital unit for non-cardiac causes. On the other hand, endocrine pathologies of various etiologies can cause alterations in cardiovascular functioning, while others of genetic etiology can present with underlying cardiac malformations.	Mellitus diabetes. Hyperthyroidism Hypocalcemic crisis. Thyroid storm. Turner syndrome. Klinefelter syndrome. Noonan syndrome
Oncology	The effective treatment of endocrine gland neoplasms must be established by a multidisciplinary team.	Adrenal gland metastasis. Papillary thyroid carcinoma. Follicular carcinoma of the thyroid Medullary thyroid carcinoma. Anaplastic thyroid carcinoma. Endocrine neoplasms.
Ophthalmology	Referral to the ophthalmology service is useful for diagnosing the evolution of pathologies and their complications associated with the retina, compression of the ocular nerves and others, in order to establish a therapeutic and / or reduce the risk of evolution of visual damage .	Hypothalamic, sellar, pituitary and pituitary neoplasms. Thyroid orbitopathy. Diabetic retinopathy. Turner syndrome.
Pathological anatomy	Mainly, the diagnostic referral is performed to analyze samples of tissue suspected of malignancy in order to establish the most appropriate treatment based on the behavior of the suspicious lesion.	Neuroendocrine neoplasms. Thyroid neoplasms. Adrenal neoplasms. Others.
Nuclear medicine	Useful for the study and administration of treatments with I131 and Tc99	Thyroid disorders. Parathyroid disorders. Others.

Surgery: Neurosurgery, Plastic surgery, Other	Many of the endocrine pathologies include both diagnostic and therapeutic surgical interventions.	Clitoromegaly. Ambiguous genitalia. Endocrine tumors. Congenital anatomical alterations. Acromegaly. Central hypothyroidism. Central adrenal insufficiency. Cushing's disease.

Table 363 - 1.

Bibliographic references

1. Genetic Alliance; The New York-Mid-Atlantic Consortium for Genetic and Newborn Screening Services. Understanding Genetics: A New York, Mid-Atlantic Guide for Patients and Health Professionals. Washington (DC): Genetic Alliance; 2009 Jul 8. CHAPTER 6, INDICATIONS FOR A GENETIC REFERRAL.
2. Taberna, M., Gil Moncayo, F., Jané-Salas, E., Antonio, M., Arribas, L., Vilajosana, E., Peralvez Torres, E., & Mesía, R. (2020). The Multidisciplinary Team (MDT) Approach and Quality of Care. Frontiers in oncology, 10, 85.https://doi.org/10.3389/fonc.2020.00085
3. Shlomo Melmed, Richard J. Auchus, Allison B. Goldfine, Ronald J. Kowning, Clifford Rosen. Williams Text book of Endocrinology 14Th edition. ELSEVIER, 2020.

IV. Epidemiology of endocrine diseases according to the stages of life

Metabolic endocrine diseases are currently among the most common human health problems in different populations, responsible for causing significant morbidity and mortality in different ethnic groups.

Defining the epidemiology of the most common pathologies is essential for estimating the risk and probability of incidence of endocrine pathologies in the population. Likewise, the identification of risk factors and an approach to their correction can delay or prevent the development of risky endocrine pathologies.

Pituitary disorders		
	Age group	Risk factor's
GH deficiency	*Neonate and childhood:* Prevalence 1 in 40,000 to 1 in 10,000. Reversible in about 25 to 65% of patients.	Not modifiable: Family history of hypopituitarism. History of brain tumor. 30 Gy radiation exposure at the cranial level. History of organic pituitary alteration.
	Adolescence: Between 15-20% occurs in the transition from child to adult.	
	Adult 1 in 100,000 people a year. At least 6000 diagnoses occur each year.	Not modifiable: History of cancer. Family history of GH deficiency. Cranial radiation therapy.
Pituitary tumors	*Children and adolescents* 3.5 to 8.5% are diagnosed before the age of 20. Annual incidence in children is 0.1 to 4.1 per 100,000 children.	Multiple endocrine neoplasia type 1 (MEN1). Carney complex. Familial acromegaly.
	Adults Approximate prevalence of 1 case	

	per 1000 people.	
	Pregnancy They represent 10 to 20% of intracranial tumors.	
	Elderly Its prevalence in people over 65 years of age is 0.16%.	
Thyroid disorders		
Hypothyroidism	*Neonates* Congenital hypothyroidism occurs in 1 in 3,000 live newborns. The ratio is women to men 2:1. More common in Hispanic populations.	Multiple pregnancy. Female gender. Autoimmune maternal thyroid disease. Intrauterine growth retardation. Advanced maternal age
	Children and adolescents The global prevalence of hypothyroidism in those under 21 years of age is 0.135%. In the 11 to 18 age group it is 0.113%.	Exposure to radiation. Hodgkin's disease survivors. History of LUPUS, Addison's disease, celiac disease, vitiligo, others.
	Adults Although it can occur at any age, primary hypothyroidism mainly occurs between the ages of 40 to 60. The incidence of autoimmune hypothyroidism is 80 per 100,000 men and at least 350 cases per 100,000 women.	
	Pregnant At least 30 to 60% of hypothyroid pregnant women have TPOAb or TgAb. In populations with a good iodine supply, the main cause is Hashimoto's thyroiditis.	
	Older adults The prevalence increases with age. 15% of elderly women and 17% of elderly men had not been previously diagnosed with hypothyroidism.	

		Between 7 to 12% of older adults housed in nursing homes have hypothyroidism.	
Thyroid nodule		*Children and adolescents* 5% prevalence	Not modifiable Genetic susceptibility.
		Adults It predominates in women with an incidence of 6.4% than in men with 1.5%. Palpable nodule prevalence of 2.33%. Incidence of 21.1 per 100 subjects.	Modifiable factors. Environmental factors. Demographic factors.
Hyperthyroidism		*Neonatal* More than 95% of newborns of mothers with Graves' disease have hyperthyroid symptoms in the first month of life.	History of autoimmune disease. Family history of thyroid disease. Maternal history of Graves disease.
		Children Graves' disease occurs rarely in children, although it accounts for more than 95% of hyperthyroidism in children.	
		Teenagers Low remission rate despite treatment. 15% of remission occurs in prepubertal and 30% of remission in puberty. In people over 12 years of age, the prevalence is 1.3%.	
		Adults Overall prevalence is 4.6 per 1000 women. Hispanics have lower incidence rates (1.3%).	Severe hyperthyroidism History of Graves disease. Previous treatment with radioiodine.
		Pregnant It occurs between 0.5 to 1% of women of childbearing age. 0.1 to 0.2% of pregnant women have Graves' disease.	
		Elderly It occurs in 10% of those over 80 years of age. 1.3% of those over 65 have clinical hyperthyroidism. Another group of 2.1% presents	Unmodifiable: History of autoimmune disease. History of Graves disease, History of non-toxic nodular goiter.

	subclinical hyperthyroidism.	Modifiable: Use of amiodarone.
Lymphocytic thyroiditis (postpartum)	*Postpartum women* Incidence of 11.3% during 1.4 months.	
Acute thyroiditis	*Children and adolescents* 15% incidence in children undergoing piriformis sinus fistula surgery.	Autoimmune disease. Immunosuppression status. Chemotherapy treatments.
	Adults 1% of post radiation patients.	
Subacute thyroiditis	*Children and adolescents* Rare.	Positive HLA-Bw35. History of upper respiratory disease.
	Adults More frequent in women than in men with a 4 to 1 ratio.	
Hashimoto's thyroiditis	*Children and adolescents* Non-endemic cause of goiter.	Diabetes type 1. Family history of autoimmune disease. LUPUS.
	Adults Prevalence greater than 45 to 64 years. 0.3 to 0.5 cases per year per 1000 people. Common cause of hypothyroidism in iodine-deficient regions.	
Calcium and metabolic bone disorder		
Hypercalcemia	*Children and adolescents* Prevalence from 0.4 to 1.3%. *General population* 1 to 2% prevalence	Cancer. Genetic susceptibility.
Primary hyperparathyroidism	*Children and adolescents* It rarely occurs before age 15.	History of radiation to the neck or head. Family history of primary hyperparathyroidism.
	Adults More common in women than men. Incidence of 66 cases per 100,000 women and 36 cases per 100,000 men.	
	Elderly Maximum incidence in the sixth decade of life between 65 and 74 years.	
Osteoporosis and osteopenia	*Adults* The incidence increases with	Modifiable: Weight gain.

	age.	Smoking Sedentary.
	Elderly More than 70% of adults over the age of 80 have osteoporosis. It is more common in women than in men.	Alcoholism. Not modifiable: White race. Early menopause Family history of osteoporosis
	Endocrine pancreas	
Diabetes mellitus (DM)	*Children and adolescents* It is rare for it to occur before the first year of life. The incidence of type 1 DM increases until 12 to 14 years of age. In Europe and the United States, less than 10% of non-Hispanic children have type 1 A diabetes. Monogenic diabetes accounts for 1% to 5% of all diabetes in young people. Monogenic diabetes occurs in 1 in 100,000 to 500,000 live newborns.	Genetic susceptibility
	Adults Type 2 DM represents 90% of diabetes cases. The prevalence is different for each ethnic origin: 8.5% non-Hispanic Caucasians. 10.2% non-Hispanic Asian. 13.6% Hispanic. 13.9% Afro-descendants.	Modifiable: Overweight and obesity. Sedentary. Hypercholesterolemia Hypertriglyceridaemia. Insulin resistance or prediabetes. Not modifiable: History of polycystic ovary syndrome. Hispanic, Indo-American, Afro-descendant, or Asian race or ethnicity.
	Pregnant Gestational diabetes occurs in 3-10% of pregnancies. The prevalence of gestational diabetes is 7.5%.	Modifiable: Maternal obesity or overweight. Not modifiable: History of fetal macrosomia. Poor obstetric history. Women from high-risk ethnic

		groups. Older women.
	Elderly In people older than 70 years, the prevalence of diabetes was 24.2%. The prevalence of diabetes increases with age. It is estimated that ¼ of those over 65 have diabetes.	Genetic susceptibility. Modifiable factors (smoking, overweight and obesity, alcoholism, others).
Adrenal disorders		
Pheochromocytoma	*Children and adolescents* They are unusual in this age group, although their presence could indicate an underlying inherited disorder. *General population* The global incidence is 0.8 per 100,000 people for 30 years. It occurs mainly between the 3rd and 5th decade of life.	Family history of pheochromocytoma.
Other endocrine disorders		
Polycystic ovarian disease	It occurs between 5 to 10% of women of reproductive age. It can be inherited in up to 70% of cases. About 40% of women with polycystic ovary syndrome suffer from infertility. The general prevalence is 6.6% and it is higher in Afro-descendant women by 8%, while in Caucasian women it is 5%.	Modifiable: Obesity. Metabolic syndrome. Not modifiable: Reproductive age. Family history of polycystic ovary syndrome.

Bibliographic references

1. Shlomo Melmed, Richard J. Auchus, Allison B. Goldfine, Ronald J. Kowning, Clifford Rosen. Williams

Text book of Endocrinology 14Th edition. ELSEVIER, 2020.
2. Golden, SH, Robinson, KA, Saldanha, I., Anton, B., & Ladenson, PW (2009). Clinical review: Prevalence and incidence of endocrine and metabolic disorders in the United States: a comprehensive review. The Journal of clinical endocrinology and metabolism, 94 (6), 1853–1878.https://doi.org/10.1210/jc.2008-2291
3. L. Audí, M. Bueno. R. Calzada, et al. Pombo. Treatise on pediatric endocrinology. Mc Graw Hill, 4th edition. 2009.

V. Endocrine: Specialist in nutrition, metabolism, hormones and reproduction

Endocrinology is a scientific and medical discipline that has a unique focus on hormones and presents a multidisciplinary approach to understanding the normal and pathological production and action of hormones, as well as diseases associated with abnormal hormonal signaling.

Key points of endocrinology

- ✓ The endocrine and paracrine systems differ in important ways that illustrate those evolutionary pressures on these different signaling strategies between cells.
- ✓ Hormones in the circulation are often associated with binding proteins to improve their solubility.
- ✓ The control of hormone secretion involves integrated inputs from multiple distant objects, as well as input from local paracrine and autocrine factors and from the nervous system, which lead to complex patterns of circadian secretion, pulsatile secretion, secretion driven by homeostatic stimuli. leading to secular changes in life expectancy.
- ✓ Endocrine disorders or diseases are classified according to hormonal behavior in the overproduction or underproduction of hormones, the altered tissue response to hormones or tumors that arise from the endocrine tissue.

- ✓ Both hormones and synthetic molecules, designed to interact with hormone receptors, can be administered for the diagnosis and treatment of endocrine disorders.

What does the endocrinologist do?

An endocrinologist or endocrine doctor, is a doctor who specializes in the diagnosis and treatment of hormonal, metabolic and endocrine disorders. The endocrinologist applies knowledge in biochemistry, cell biology and genetics directly to patient care.

Among the areas of competence that an endocrine doctor intervenes, is the evaluation, diagnosis and treatment of people with diabetes, thyroid diseases, osteoporosis, disorders of the pituitary glands, and adrenal glands, infertility, and also deals with disorders that affect the growth, development and metabolism of an individual.

The elements of approach that an endocrine physician uses for clinical practice consist of the clinical evaluation of the patient, the use of laboratory tests, tissue sampling, genetic analysis, as well as high-resolution medical images. Dynamic endocrine tests are also frequently performed to examine the functioning of the endocrine glands in vivo, for this they stimulate or inhibit hormonal pathways in order to interpret the results and diagnose various endocrine functional pathologies.

Likewise, the endocrine physician can perform and appropriately interpret bone mineral density tests in the evaluation of people with bone and metabolic diseases.

Likewise, among its competences are the performance of specialized imaging studies for the ultrasound evaluation of the thyroid gland, as well as the taking of samples by means of ultrasound-guided needle aspiration for biopsy, in patients who require thyroid evaluations suspicious of malignancy.

Endocrine working environment

The endocrine doctor is frequently found in outpatient settings or in an urban environment through the consultation service. However, some may also carry out consultations in hospitalized patients, although in general, in clinical practice, there are few hospital emergencies that require the presence of an endocrine doctor, although they are well prepared to solve such circumstances should they arise.

This allows the endocrine physician to have more options to work in a variety of healthcare settings, including hospitals, academic medical centers, clinics, and private practices simultaneously.

Because endocrine pathologies are often chronic disorders, patients are followed long-term, so they can maintain close and long-term relationships with their patients, unlike other medical specialties.

Most frequent inquiries:

Reasons for consultation	Observations
Diabetes	Chronic disease associated with pancreatic insufficiency of

	insulin production or resistance of peripheral tissues to insulin. The number of diabetic patients increased from 108 million in 1980 to 422 million by 2014. The global prevalence of diabetes in adults increased from 4.7% (1980) to 8.55% (2014). Diabetes is one of the leading causes of blindness, kidney failure, myocardial infarction, lower limb amputation and stroke. Diabetes can be treated, avoided or delayed through endocrinological consultations with periodic examinations, monitoring of diet, physical activity and appropriate medication.
Thyroid diseases	The thyroid is a component of the hypothalamic-pituitary-thyroid axis, which allows to maintain normal levels of hormones. Thyroid problems are estimated to be the second most common cause of consultation in the United States. For every 1000 people 8 have hypothyroidism and another 130 have subclinical hypothyroidism. For every 1000 people at least 5 have hyperthyroidism and another 4 have subclinical hyperthyroidism. For the year 2006, in the United States, 92,931 thyroidectomies were performed, 39% more than those registered for the year 1996.
Obesity	Obesity is frequently associated with various endocrine disorders, which suffer from the hypothalamic-pituitary axis. In addition to the role of storing energy, adipose tissue has important functions mediated through hormones and / or substances released by adipocytes. Obesity has tripled globally since 1975. By 2016, around 1.9 billion adults were overweight, of which at least 650 million were obese. 38 million children under the age of 5 were overweight obesity in 2019. Obesity can be prevented.
Dyslipidemias	It occurs due to the presence of abnormal amounts of lipids in the blood. This represents an important risk factor for cardiovascular disease. Dyslipidemia can be caused by genetic, environmental factors, or a combination of these.

	Dyslipidemia is associated with more than 4 million deaths a year worldwide.
Polycystic ovarian syndrome.	It is one of the most common hormonal problems among women of childbearing age. It also consists of one of the main causes of infertility and also increases the risk of type 2 diabetes mellitus and gestational diabetes. Up to 80% of women with polycystic ovary syndrome have insulin resistance. It affects 6 to 12% of American women of reproductive age. This represents around 5 million women and this figure can be increased globally.

Different origins of endocrinopathies

The endocrine system is made up of a complex and extensive set of elements that interact with each other for the proper functioning of the secretion and regulation of hormones. A large amount of these hormones, secreted by the endocrine system, are involved in many functions of the body, including growth, development, metabolism, electrolyte balance, reproduction, among others.

It is for this reason that the development of endocrinopathies can have its origin at various levels, among which stand out, genetic and nutritional origins, metabolism disorders, autoimmune behavioral pathologies, peripheral resistance in receptors to their corresponding hormones, development of neoplasms, degenerative disorders, hypersecretion of hormones, among others.

Examples of the most common and general driving behaviors

Origin	Examples	General driving behaviors
Genetics	Wilson's disease.	Prevention of short stature.

	Turner syndrome. Klinefelter syndrome.	Early approach for the prevention of intellectual deficit. Prevention and correction of aspects associated with alteration in pubertal development.
Nutritional	Child with thinness. Deficiencies Hypertriglyceridaemia. Hypercholesterolemia Hypercalcemia	Specific dietary guidance and corrections. Control and specific treatment for metabolic involvement. Start of specific therapy in case of hormonal involvement detected. Body image through lifestyle modification.
Metabolic	Obesity. Dyslipidemias. Metabolic syndrome. Hyperinsulinemia Diabetes mellitus type 2. Non-alcoholic fatty liver.	Prevention of cardiovascular risk and other complications. Lifestyle-related measures (diet, physical activity). Specific medical treatment.
Autoimmune	Type 1 diabetes mellitus. Hashimoto's thyroiditis. Celiac Disease. Autoimmune poliendocrine syndrome type 1 or 2. Addison's disease.	Stabilization of the patient through resuscitation and specific hormone replacement therapy, when required. Initiation of long-term preventive therapy. Indication of specific consultations for medical specialties. Establish long-term follow-up controls. Treatment of the consequences or complications present in the patient at the time of diagnosis.
Resistors	Insulin resistance Thyroid hormone resistance syndrome.	Lifestyle modification initiating exercise and diet therapy for the specific treatment required (weight loss or other). Indicate specific treatment according to the patient's condition.
Tumor	Thyroid carcinoma Pituitary neoplasms.	Radiotherapy. Chemotherapy.

		Surgical excision.
Hormonal excesses **Hormonal deficits**	Hyperthyroidism Hyperandrogenism. Cushing's syndrome. Hypothyroidism Hypogonadism Hypoparathyroidism	Indicate general therapies such as lifestyle changes for specific correction of the disorder. Establish preventive measures for the development of complications. Indicate hormone replacement therapy specific to the disorder. Radioiodine therapies or surgical excision as needed.
Degenerative	Sarcopenia	Evaluate underlying metabolic states that accelerate the degenerative process. Relationship with age, discomfort, potential disability
Sexual or reproductive	Feminine infertility. Polycystic ovarian syndrome. Amenorrhea Sexual dysfunctions. Gender dysphoria.	Reference to the specific medical specialty (surgery, psychologist, gynecology or other), to establish a multidisciplinary team to indicate the most appropriate treatment for the patient's peculiarities and fertility wishes or not.

Bibliographic references

1. Shlomo Melmed, Richard J. Auchus, Allison B. Goldfine, Ronald J. Kowning, Clifford Rosen. Williams Text book of Endocrinology 14Th edition. ELSEVIER, 2020.
2. Lavin N, editor. Manual of endocrinology and metabolism. 4th ed. Philadelphia: Wolters Kluwer / Lippincott Williams & Wilkins Health; 2009. 837 p.
3. Sidhu S, Parikh T, Burman KD. Endocrine Changes in Obesity. [Updated 2017 Oct 12]. In: Feingold KR, Anawalt B, Boyce A, et al., Editors. Endotext [Internet].

South Dartmouth (MA): MDText.com, Inc.; 2000-. Available from: https://www.ncbi.nlm.nih.gov/books/NBK279053/

Final thoughts

Volume III of Endocrinology 360, closes with the discussion of two key sections in the study of this medical specialty, such is the case of the Hypothalamus, the Hypophysis, and the Ovaries and testes.

In part VII of this book we have reviewed the glands that stimulate, control and regulate the secretion of other endocrine glands, in addition to fulfilling various functions in the homeostasis of the body, it is the hypothalamus and the pituitary.

Hypothalamus-pituitary is the endocrine axis that is responsible for initiating and regulating the function of other glands. The hypothalamus, a specialized region in the diencephalon, produces and secretes releasing and inhibiting peptides, which acting on the pituitary gland, induce the secretion and release of hormones intended to regulate thyroid function (TSH), body growth (GH), function adrenal (ACTH), and the ovaries and testes (FSH, LH), as well as lactation (prolactin and oxytocin).

After reviewing the anatomical, embryological and physiological aspects, the pathologies and conditions that affect the function of this gland are presented, considering congenital situations, neoplasms, or systemic conditions such as vascular disorders that can compromise the hypothalamic-pituitary function, remembering that the effects will be seen in various organs and systems of the body, such as thyroid, adrenal and gonads, whose endocrine function is regulated by this pair.

Up-to-date diagnostic methods and therapeutic alternatives are discussed, covering clinical and surgical aspects, together with recommendations for the follow-up of these cases.

We end this text with section VIII, dedicated to contemplating aspects related to sexual endocrinology, considering anatomical, physiological, pathological and therapeutic aspects of the ovaries and testes. The chapters go through topics that begin in the development and sexual differentiation, covering their function in the maturation of the human being, both physical and mental, presenting for discussion gender identity, sexual dysphoria, and current therapies for feminization and masculinization.

In addition, the last section discusses congenital genetic syndromes that affect maturation and sexual development, environmental conditions that affect the regulation of the hypothalamic-pituitary gonadal axes, and considers issues related to fertility, pregnancy and lactation.

In this way, we culminate the 360° journey around Endocrinology, reviewing its seven major areas, taking anatomical, physiological, pathological and therapeutic considerations, based on the strongest and most up-to-date evidence, with the purpose of expanding the knowledge of the health professional , whether a general practitioner or specialist, even from other areas of health action.

Dr. Mario Vega Carbó
Endocrinologist

ENDOCRINOLOGY 360

General index

Volume I. Dietetics, Nutrition, Metabolism and Diabetes mellitus

Part I. Dietetics

1. Macronutrients
2. Foods rich in vitamins
3. Mineral rich foods
4. Label reading
5. Healthy plate diet
6. Mediterranean diet
7. Vegetarian diet and variants
8. Vegan diet and variants
9. Low-calorie obesity diets
10. Diet in morbid obesity
11. Diet in bariatric surgery
12. Ketogenic diet
13. DASH diet
14. Carbohydrate counting
15. Low glycemic index diet
16. Diet in type 1 diabetes
17. Diet in type 2 diabetes
18. Diet in gestational diabetes
19. Diet in dyslipidemias
20. Diet for elevated homocysteine
21. Diet in nephrolithiasis
22. Diet in diabetic kidney disease
23. Gastric Protection Diet
24. Biliary protection diet
25. Diet for irritable bowel control

26. Diet in steatiosis and liver cirrhosis
27. Diet in thyroid diseases
28. Diet low in calcium and phosphorus
29. Diet in osteopenia and osteoporosis
30. Diet and polycystic ovary syndrome
31. Appropriate diet for the infertile couple
32. Diet to prevent and slow sarcopenia
33. Hypercaloric diets in thinness
34. Diet in celiac disease
35. Diet and lactose intolerance
36. Anti-inflammatory diet
37. Diet and phenylketonuria

Part II. Nutrition and metabolism

38. Endocrine disruptors
39. Hormones, exercises and athletes
40. Preconception nutrition
41. Child with thinness
42. Extreme thinness
43. Anorexia nervosa
44. Bulimia
45. Celiac Disease
46. Sarcopenia
47. Lipodystrophy and endocrinopathies
48. Cardiovascular risk
49. Adult obesity
50. Secondary dyslipidemias
51. Atherogenic dyslipidemia
52. Hypercholesterolemia
53. Hypertriglyceridemia
54. Low HDL cholesterol
55. Elevated transaminases
56. Nonalcoholic fatty liver
57. Adipomastia, fat flaps and rings

58.	Child with obesity
59.	Obesity and pregnancy
60.	Obesity in older adults
61.	Morbid obesity
62.	Endocrine obesity
63.	Bariatric surgery
64.	Metabolic surgery
65.	Anti-obesity medication
66.	Metabolic syndrome
67.	Insulin resistance in pediatrics
68.	Acanthosis nigricans
69.	Skin tags
70.	Fasting hypoglycemia
71.	Reactive hypoglycemia
72.	Hyperinsulinemia
73.	Congenital hyperinsulinism
74.	Peptide C
75.	Gout and hyperuricemia
76.	Wilson disease
77.	Hemochromatosis
78.	Phenylketonuria

Part III. Mellitus diabetes

79.	Endocrine pancreas
80.	Control of blood glucose
81.	Concept and classification of diabetes
82.	Diabetes pathophysiology
83.	Investigation in people without symptoms
84.	Prediabetes
85.	Type 1 diabetes mellitus
86.	Type 2 diabetes mellitus
87.	Gestational diabetes
88.	Monogenic diabetes
89.	LADA diabetes

90.	Secondary diabetes
91.	Diabetes and alcohol
92.	Diabetes and glucocorticoids
93.	Gestational prediabetes
94.	Neonatal diabetes
95.	Child of diabetic mother
96.	Hyperinsulinemia and insulin resistance
97.	Obesity and diabetes
98.	Diabetes in older adults
99.	Type 2 diabetes in pediatrics
100.	Diabetic hypoglycemia
101.	Hyperosmolar hyperglycemic state
102.	Diabetic cetoacidosis
103.	Lactic acidosis
104.	Heart and diabetes
105.	Diabetic foot
106.	Diabetic peripheral neuropathy
107.	Diabetic autonomic neuropathy
108.	Diabetic kidney disease
109.	Diabetic retinopathy
110.	Sweeteners and diabetes
111.	Control of the diabetic patient
112.	Self-monitoring of glucose
113.	Hemoglobin A1c
114.	Continuous glucose monitoring
115.	Antihyperglycemic agents
116.	Insulin treatment
117.	Insulin analogs
118.	Inhaled insulin
119.	Insulin pumps
120.	Replacement pancreas
121.	Stem cells and diabetes
122.	Surgery in the person with diabetes
123.	Remission of diabetes

Volume II. Thyroid, Parathyroid- Calcium and Adrenals

Part IV. Thyroid diseases

124.	Thyroid gland
125.	Thyroid growth and puberty
126.	Ectopic thyroid
127.	Iodine deficiency and endemic goiter
128.	Non-toxic nodular goiter
129.	Cystic or degenerative goiter
130.	Endothoracic goiter
131.	Acute thyroiditis
132.	Subacute Quervain's thyroiditis
133.	Hashimoto's chronic thyroiditis
134.	Postpartum thyroiditis
135.	Riedel's thyroiditis
136.	Post-radioactive thyroiditis
137.	Thyroiditis in childhood and adolescence
138.	Subclinical thyroid dysfunction
139.	Primary hypothyroidism
140.	Congenital hypothyroidism
141.	Pendred syndrome
142.	Hypothyroidism during pregnancy
143.	Hypothyroidism in older people
144.	Levothyroxine and liothyronine
145.	Thyrotoxicosis and hyperthyroidism
146.	Graves Basedow disease
147.	Toxic adenoma
148.	Toxic multinodular goiter
149.	Hyperthyroidism due to amiodarone
150.	Primary hyperthyroidism of the child
151.	Hyperthyroidism during pregnancy
152.	Hyperthyroidism in older people
153.	Hyperthyroidism treatment
154.	Thyroid orbitopathy
155.	Thyroid storm
156.	Thyrotoxic periodic paralysis

157.	Ultrasound and fine needle biopsy
158.	Papillary thyroid carcinoma
159.	Follicular carcinoma of the thyroid
160.	Anaplastic carcinoma of the thyroid
161.	Medullary thyroid carcinoma
162.	Thyroid Cancer in Childhood
163.	Thyroid cancer and pregnancy
164.	Thyroid cancer in the elderly
165.	Thyroid ablation with radioiodine
166.	Radioiodine teratogenicity
167.	Thyroidectomy
168.	Thyroglobulin
169.	Euthyroid disease syndrome

Part V. Parathyroids, osteology and minerals

170.	Parathyroid glands
171.	Hypercalcemia
172.	Severe hypercalcemia
173.	Parathyroid tumors
174.	Primary hyperparathyroidism
175.	Neck ultrasound
176.	Sestamibi 99 mTc scan
177.	Parathyroidectomy
178.	Hypocalcemia
179.	Neonatal hypocalcemia
180.	Hypocalcemic crisis
181.	Primary hypoparathyroidism
182.	Postsurgical hypoparathyroidism
183.	Post-ablation hypoparathyroidism
184.	Pseudohypoparathyroidism
185.	Di George syndrome
186.	Vitamin D deficiency
187.	Childhood rickets

188.	Vitamin D poisoning
189.	Osteomalacia
190.	Bone paget disease
191.	Hyperphosphatemia
192.	Hypophosphatemia
193.	Hypermagnesemia
194.	Hypomagnesemia
195.	Nephrolithiasis and nephrocalcinosis
196.	Hypercalciuria nephrolithiasis
197.	Hyperoxaluria nephrolithiasis
198.	Hyperuricosuria nephrolithiasis
199.	Cysthenuric nephrolithiasis
200.	Struvite nephrolithiasis
201.	Osseous remodeling
202.	Bone densitometry
203.	Osteopenia and osteoporosis
204.	Postmenopausal osteoporosis
205.	Secondary osteoporosis
206.	Treatment of osteoporosis
207.	Osteoporosis in childhood and adolescence
208.	Osteoporosis and pregnancy
209.	Osteoporosis in the elderly

Part VI. Adrenals, neuroendocrines and electrolytes

210.	Kidney glands
211.	Steroidogenesis
212.	Congenital adrenal hyperplasia
213.	Non-classical congenital adrenal hyperplasia
214.	Endocrine hypertension
215.	Lipothymias
216.	Suprarrenal insufficiency
217.	Glucocorticoid replacement
218.	Use of mineralocorticoids

219.	Addison's disease
220.	Addison's disease and pregnancy
221.	Acute adrenal crisis
222.	Adrenal incidentaloma
223.	Cushing's syndrome
224.	Cyclic hypercortisolism
225.	Cushing syndrome and pregnancy
226.	Pheochromocytoma
227.	Pheochromocytoma and pregnancy
228.	Primary hyperaldosteronism
229.	Hyperaldosteronism and pregnancy
230.	Adrenal gland metastasis
231.	Autoimmune polyglandular syndrome
232.	Multiple endocrine neoplasia type 1
233.	Multiple endocrine neoplasia type 2
234.	Dynamic tests
235.	Adrenal imaging
236.	Adrenalectomy
237.	APUD
238.	Neuroendocrine tumors
239.	Carcinoid syndrome
240.	Insulinoma
241.	Gastrinoma
242.	Vipoma
243.	Glucagonoma
244.	Somatostinoma
245.	Endocrine tumor surgery
246.	Dehydration
247.	Hyponatremia
248.	Hypernatremia
249.	Hypokalemia
250.	Hyperkalemia

Volume III. Hypothalamus, Pituitary, Ovaries and Testicles

Part VII. Hypothalamus and pituitary

251.	Pineal gland, hypothalamus, and pituitary
252.	Neuroendocrinology
253.	Oxytocin
254.	Melatonin, serotonin, dopamine
255.	Pineal tumors
256.	Endocrine syndromes - hypothalamic
257.	Images of the Sellar region
258.	Pituitary incidentaloma
259.	Hypothalamic pituitary dysfunction
260.	Polydipsic polyuric syndrome
261.	Central diabetes insipidus
262.	Nephrogenic diabetes insipidus
263.	Primary polydipsia
264.	Syndrome of inappropriate ADH secretion
265.	Short stature
266.	GH deficiency in the child
267.	GH deficiency in adults
268.	Secondary adrenal insufficiency
269.	Secondary hypothyroidism
270.	Secondary hypogonadism
271.	Panhypopituitarism
272.	Sheehan syndrome
273.	Craniopharyngioma
274.	Non-functioning pituitary tumor
275.	Galactorrhea
276.	Hyperprolactinemia
277.	Hyperprolactinemia and pregnancy
278.	Prolactinoma
279.	Prolactinoma and pregnancy
280.	Thyrotropinomas
281.	Gonadotropic adenomas
282.	Cushing's disease

283.	Nelson syndrome	
284.	Acromegaly	
285.	Tall statue	
286.	Pituitary metastasis	
287.	Pituitary tumor in pediatrics	
288.	Pituitary tumor and pregnancy	
289.	Rathke's pouch cysts	
290.	Pituitary granulomas	
291.	Sellar arachnoidocele	
292.	Pituitary apoplexy	
293.	Hypophysitis	
294.	Pituitary surgery	
295.	Radio and pituitary chemotherapy	

Part VIII. Gonadal conditions

296.	Endocrinological Gynecology	
297.	The ovaries	
298.	Disorder of sexual development	
299.	Normal puberty	
300.	Early thelarchy	
301.	Precocious adrenarche	
302.	Pubertal gynecomastia	
303.	Early puberty	
304.	Delayed puberty	
305.	Turner syndrome	
306.	Primary amenorrhea	
307.	Oligomenorrhea and amenorrhea	
308.	Premenstrual syndrome	
309.	Dysfunctional uterine bleeding	
310.	Polycystic ovarian syndrome	
311.	Adolescent with polycystic ovaries	
312.	Hydroxyprogesterone	
313.	Hyperandrogenism	

314. Hyperhidrosis
315. Hirsutism
316. Acne
317. Androgenic alopecia
318. Clitoromegaly
319. SHBG
320. Antiandrogens
321. Hormonal contraception
322. Feminine infertility
323. Ovarian and anti-Mullerian reserve
324. Anovulation
325. Ovulation inducers
326. Endometriosis
327. Recurrent abortions
328. Artificial insemination
329. In vitro fertilization
330. Hormonal adjustments of pregnancy
331. Female sexual dysfunction
332. Fibrocystic breast condition
333. Functional ovarian tumors
334. Climacteric syndrome
335. Premature ovarian failure
336. Female hormone replacement
337. Transgender teenager
338. Transgender woman
339. Transgender man
340. Andrology
341. The testicles
342. Anabolic steroids
343. Ambiguous genitalia
344. Prepubertal male hypogonadism
345. Micropenis
346. Cryptorchidism
347. Kallman syndrome
348. Klinefelter syndrome
349. Noonan syndrome
350. Functional testicular tumor

351.	Feminine infertility
352.	Spermatogram
353.	Oligospermia
354.	Erectile dysfunction
355.	Orchiectomy
356.	Chemical castration
357.	Adult gynecomastia
358.	Andropause
359.	Male hormone replacement

Special Section: Key Topics in Endocrinology. Abstracts

I. Suspicious clinical symptoms and signs of endocrine disease

II. Role of dynamic tests in the diagnosis of endocrinopathies

III. Interaction and referral of the endocrinologist with other specialists

IV. Epidemiology of endocrine diseases according to the stages of life

V. Endocrinologist: specialist in nutrition, metabolism, hormones and reproduction

Epilogue

Endocrinology 360
A trilogy for the study of this medical subspecialty

Endocrinology 360 It is the result of a lifetime of study, preparation, work and experience in the field of this medical subspecialty, synthesized in three volumes that cover the eight major branches of endocrinology; 360 chapters of the topics that are necessary to master for clinical practice are presented.

It is a unique collection of texts that presents, in a schematic and summarized way, the most recent and most impactful evidence on the latest studies carried out on pathophysiology and therapeutics in all areas of study of endocrine diseases.

The day begins by reviewing the knowledge about physiology and metabolism, in order to understand the bases of pathophysiology and better understand therapeutics. With the first volume, in addition to exploring metabolism, we learn about diet and nutrition, exposing therapeutic alternatives that demonstrate, with sufficient scientific evidence, how nutritional monitoring and specific dietary plans can improve the course of endocrine-metabolic diseases, as well as other apparatus and systems of the body, offering greater motivation to healthy change in eating habits and lifestyle in general.

Also, it presents the most used dietary recommendations as a nutritional complementary treatment indicated for specific diseases, eating disorders, innate errors of metabolism, among other conditions.

Next, the physiological and pathological concepts that lead to the development of diabetes mellitus are reviewed, analyzing the traditional therapeutic measures and the great advances and international consensus for its management, with the introduction of gene therapy, pancreatic surgery and the new presentations of insulin in infusion and inhaled pumps.

The second station of the journey in the study of endocrinology covers the knowledge of the hormonal system that activates the metabolism of all the cells of the body and maintains the ionic and water balance of the internal environment. It's about the function of the glands *thyroid, parathyroid and adrenal*, organs whose function maintains the homeostasis of the organism, regulating the levels of ions such as sodium, potassium, calcium, whose concentration is essential to maintain the membrane potential of the cells. In addition, these hormones regulate cellular metabolism, controlling the processes of respiration and production of ATP (thyroid), as well as the maintenance of the bone system (parathyroid), and the control of carbohydrates, fluids and electrolytes and immunological processes through secretion of adrenal hormones.

This review of topics on thyroid diseases, their causes and treatments, calcium metabolism, diseases of the adrenal glands, electrolyte and acid base disorders, synthesizes the most recent treatment and approach guidelines for practice.
We conclude the study of endocrinology by studying the processes of sexual differentiation and reproductive health, by exploring the function of the axis *hypothalamus-pituitary-gonadal (ovaries and testes)*.

New approaches to neuroendocrinology are addressed to review physiological or "normal" sexual development in both sexes, and to detect at which points of this axis different types of alterations occur that lead to disorders of sexual development, fertility problems and hormonalization, posing the influences of other health conditions and metabolism on sexual function; and even dealing with issues related to personal identity and gender "dysphoria".

Endocrinology 360 represents a synthesis of knowledge and academic, clinical and practical experience aimed at all health professionals to complement their training in an area as extensive and influential as this subspecialty.

Dr. Mario Vega Carbó
Endocrinologist

Copyright © 2021 Mario Vega Carbó
All rights reserved

About the Author

Dr. Mario Vega Carbó
Physician- Endocrinologist

- ✓ Cuban doctor graduated in 1994.
- ✓ Specialist in Endocrinology and Family Medicine.
- ✓ Master in Longevity and Ultrasonographer.
- ✓ Professor of Medical Pathophysiology.
- ✓ Lover of doing good, family and nature.

Other books

1. A bet on natural endocrinology.
2. Answering 1,500 questions about: Hormones, metabolism and nutrition.
3. Where hormone reigns... fiction based on clinical cases.
4. S.O.S Hormonal toxics.
5. Reveling myths: Metabolism, Endocrinology and Reproduction.
6. Hormones, glands and endocrine diseases. Its story.
7. Coffee, tobacco and alcohol: Metabolic and hormonal disorders.
8. Endocrine alerts.
9. Novel-coronavirus guide
10. Endocrinology 360

Social Network:

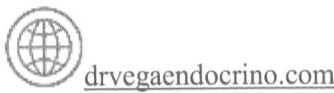 drvegaendocrino.com

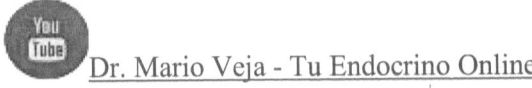 Dr. Mario Veja - Tu Endocrino Online

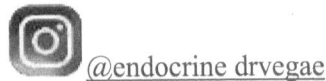 @endocrine drvegae

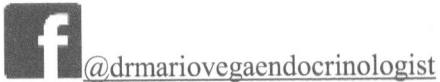 @drmariovegaendocrinologist

Endocrinology 360

A trilogy for the study of Endocrinology

A new collection of updated texts that begins with 5 introductory summaries, grouped in 8 parts, a total of 360 chapters, in turn divided into three volumes that cover all areas of study of endocrine diseases.

Dietetics, Nutrition, Metabolism and Diabetes mellitus, addressing the types of diets most used as nutritional medical treatment indicated for specific diseases, eating disorders, innate errors of metabolism, and everything about diabetes, including the most recent advances and international consensus on the matter.

Thyroid, Parathyroid and Calcium, and Adrenals, presents topics such as thyroid diseases, their causes and treatments, calcium metabolism, diseases of the adrenal glands, as well as the body's water-electrolyte and basic acid balance.

Hypothalamus-Pituitary, Ovaries and Testicles It presents the topics related to neuroendocrinology, sexual development in both sexes, fertility disorders and hormonalization in the well-known gender "dysphoria".

Available in 10 languages, it is an essential tool that aims to improve learning, clinical results and patient satisfaction who go to the endocrine doctor. This time, aimed at medical students, general practitioners, residents of medical clinics, endocrinologists and other specialists for the purpose, whose maxim is to synthesize the best diagnostic guides and the most robust evidence. Here its author, Dr. Mario Vega Carbó, graduated more than 25 years ago, invites us to take a trip with maximum depth, to safely handle the entire field of "Endocrinology 360".

www.ingramcontent.com/pod-product-compliance
Lightning Source LLC
Chambersburg PA
CBHW031602210526
45464CB00004B/1390